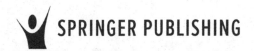

SPRINGER PUBLISHING

GET THE MOST FROM YOUR BOOK

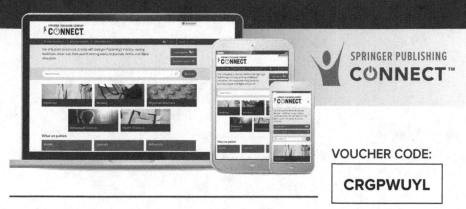

SPRINGER PUBLISHING
CONNECT™

VOUCHER CODE:

CRGPWUYL

Online Access

Your print purchase of *Quality Caring in Nursing and Health Systems, Fourth Edition*, includes **online access via Springer Publishing Connect**™ to increase accessibility, portability, and searchability.

Insert the code at http://connect.springerpub.com/content/book/978-0-8261-3696-1 today!

Having trouble? Contact our customer service department at cs@springerpub.com

Instructor Resource Access for Adopters

Let us do some of the heavy lifting to create an engaging classroom experience with a variety of instructor resources included in most textbooks SUCH AS:

INSTRUCTOR MANUAL

POWERPOINTS

TEST BANK

Visit **https://connect.springerpub.com/** and look for the **"Show Supplementary"** button on your **book homepage** to see what is available to instructors! First time using Springer Publishing Connect? Email **textbook@springerpub.com** to create an account and start unlocking valuable resources.

Quality Caring in Nursing and Health Systems

Joanne R. Duffy, PhD, RN, FAAN, is the executive vice president and senior consultant at QualiCare in Winchester, Virginia, adjunct professor at the Indiana University School of Nursing in Indianapolis, Indiana, and a member of the graduate faculty at the University of Missouri, Kansas City. Her extensive career encompasses clinical, administrative, and academic roles. Dr. Duffy has directed five graduate nursing programs in critical care nursing, care management, nursing administration, executive leadership (DNP), and a PhD program. Formerly, she was a cardiovascular clinical specialist, a university department chair, interim associate dean for research, and endowed chair for research and evidence-based practice. Dr. Duffy continues to regularly participate as a member of DNP and PhD committees.

In addition to her academic roles, Dr. Duffy has held various administrative positions in service directing medical, rehabilitation, critical care, emergency, psychiatric, and transplantation nursing services at both community and academic medical centers. She also directed a center for outcomes analysis, a nurse-led department for improving the quality of cardiovascular services. She has published extensively across the nursing literature, but is best known for her work in maximizing patient outcomes. Dr. Duffy was the first to link nurse caring to patient outcomes, designed and tested multiple versions of the Caring Assessment Tool© and developed the Quality-Caring Model© (QCM) a middle-range theory.

Dr. Duffy was the principal investigator on the national demonstration project, "Relationship-Centered Caring in Acute Care," where the QCM was evaluated at two sites. She was the principal investigator for the "Telehomecare and Heart Failure Outcomes" pilot study, which tested a caring-based intervention on the readmission rates and quality of life of heart failure patients; and the principal investigator for the "Improving Safety and Quality in Vulnerable Acute Care Patients Through Interprofessional Collaborative Practice" project. She evaluated the feasibility of using the e-CAT on hospitalized older adults, completed a study on nurses' research capacity and use of evidence, assessed the impact of a joint academic–service journal club, studied factors associated with missed nursing care, longitudinally compared hospital nurses' values, knowledge, and implementation of evidence-based practice and recently finalized a self-caring study of nurses. Dr. Duffy regularly leads research councils and journal clubs, assists staff nurses and nurse leaders in research and performance improvement projects, provides consultation on professional practice model integration, leadership development, courses and curriculum revision, faculty development, and evaluation methods.

Dr. Duffy was a consultant to the American Nurses Association in the development and implementation of the National Database of Nursing Quality Indicators (NDNQI) and was the former chair of the National League for Nursing's Nursing Educational Research Advisory Council. She is a Commonwealth Fund Executive Nurse Fellow, a Fellow in the American Academy of Nursing, a frequent guest speaker, a former Magnet® appraiser, and a recipient of several awards, including the American Heart Association's Nursing Advisory Council Clinical Article of the Year Award, Virginia's Outstanding Nurse Award, and the National Institute of Healthcare Management's Annual Healthcare Research Award.

The first and third editions of this book, *Quality Caring in Nursing: Applying Theory to Clinical Practice, Education, and Leadership,* received the AJN Book of the Year award in 2009 and 2018 respectively. The QCM has been embraced by over 60 healthcare organizations, several of which have attained Magnet status, and three professional nursing organizations.

Quality Caring in Nursing and Health Systems

Implications for Clinicians, Educators, and Leaders

Fourth Edition

Joanne R. Duffy, PhD, RN, FAAN

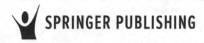
SPRINGER PUBLISHING

Springer Publishing Company, LLC
11 West 42nd Street, New York, NY 10036
www.springerpub.com
connect.springerpub.com/

Acquisitions Editor: Joseph Morita
Compositor: Transforma

ISBN: 978-0-8261-3686-2
ebook ISBN: 978-0-8261-3696-1
DOI: 10.1891/9780826136961

SUPPLEMENTS:

A robust set of instructor resources designed to supplement this text is located at http://connect.springerpub.com/content/book/978-0-8261-3696-1. Qualifying instructors may request access by emailing textbook@springerpub.com.

Instructor Manual ISBN: 978-0-8261-3712-8
Instructor PowerPoints ISBN: 978-0-8261-3707-4

Printed by BnT

The author and the publisher of this Work have made every effort to use sources believed to be reliable to provide information that is accurate and compatible with the standards generally accepted at the time of publication. The author and publisher shall not be liable for any special, consequential, or exemplary damages resulting, in whole or in part, from the readers' use of, or reliance on, the information contained in this book. The publisher has no responsibility for the persistence or accuracy of URLs for external or third-party Internet websites referred to in this publication and does not guarantee that any content on such websites is, or will remain, accurate or appropriate.

Library of Congress Control Number: 2022041848

Contact sales@springerpub.com to receive discount rates on bulk purchases.

Publisher's Note: **New and used products purchased from third-party sellers are not guaranteed for quality, authenticity, or access to any included digital components.**

Printed in the United States of America.

Contents

Practice Exemplar Contributors

Genesis R. Bojorquez, PhD, RN, NE-BC, PCCN, Advance Practice Specialist, UC San Diego Health

Dawn Carroll, DNP, NE-BC, WHNP, Nurse Manager, UC San Diego Health

Judy E. Davidson, DNP, RN, MCCM, FAAN, Nurse Scientist, UC San Diego Health Sciences; Health Scientist, UC San Diego School of Medicine, Department of Psychiatry, La Jolla, California

Heather Davis, MSN, RN, PCCN, SCRN, Advance Practice Specialist, East/West Inpatient Medicine Services Line, UC San Diego Health

Abigail Edilloran, RN, DNP, Assistant Nurse Manager, 3F and 5H Neuro ICU/PCU, UC San Diego Health

Lindsay Holt, PhD, RN, CPAN, Nurse Educator, UC San Diego Health

Jacqueline Imus, BSN, RN, Clinical Nurse II, UC San Diego Health

Kristina James, MSN, RN, CNL, PCCN, Assistant Nurse Manager, Thornton 2 West, UC San Diego Health

Joan Meunier-Sham, RN, MS, Director, MA SANE Program, Co-Director National TeleNursing Center, Massachusetts Department of Public Health

Tamara Norton, BSN, RN, CCRN, Clinical Nurse IV, Sulpizio 3A Cardiovascular ICU, TH Cardiovascular IUC 2, UC San Diego Health

Randi Petricone, MSN, CNP, RN, WHNP-BC, SANE Associate Director, National TeleNursing Center, TeleSANE Services, Massachusetts Department of Health

Stacy Street, BSN, RN, CCRN, Clinical Nurse II, UCSD Jacobs 3GH ICU, UC San Diego Health

Preface

Despite the 20-plus years since the Institute of Medicine's *Crossing the Quality Chasm* (2001) was published, the U.S. health system continues to deliver inconsistent and sometimes inadequate person-centered care, inflicts unnecessary harms, omits or fails to provide best and up-to-date evidence-based services, and struggles to authentically connect to its customers, including its employees. The relationships that patients and healthcare professionals hold with each other, the cornerstone of healthcare, remain variable depending on the context. More importantly, in spite of the fundamental caring relationships that undergird healthcare delivery, they are not routinely evaluated in real time, emphasized as significant performance improvement indicators, or analyzed robustly for improvement.

In many contemporary U.S. health systems, dedicated time spent with patients and families is limited, sometimes detached, and often rushed and impersonal. Nameless and often distracted clinicians unknowingly exacerbate unnecessary patient uncertainty, stress, limited opportunities for participation in decisions, and incomplete care. Many people, at some of the most vulnerable times of life, reluctantly adapt to expectations of the system, and are frequently left to wonder whether they and their families are safe and whether anyone would be there for them when they need it most. Interestingly, these exact words described hospitalized patient experiences in earlier editions of this book, prior to the SARS-CoV-2 pandemic!

In spite of the pandemic that devastated many individuals, families, and communities, swarms of dedicated health professionals brought lifesaving interventions, connection, and hope to many. Although suffering victims were dependent and isolated from family members, the enthusiastic, courageous, and moral choices that dedicated health professionals made to purposely work together in the delivery of expert care brought some healing to those suffering. In other words, they cared enough for others, even with scant resources and unhealthy work environments, to work together, to try novel approaches, and to accomplish "what really mattered." And this was witnessed over and over again by countless individuals the world over.

Professional nurses, in particular, have expertly responded on the frontlines of patient care throughout the SARS-CoV-2 pandemic. They upheld the delivery of 24/7 healthcare, despite experiencing fear, stress, moral distress, and exhaustion. Notwithstanding the risk for their own personal safety, professional nurses performed in the manner they always do: responsibly, voluntarily, ethically, proudly, patriotically, and with a sense of duty to their communities.

Regardless of the suffering of their patients, their own social isolation from family members, guilt over not being able to deliver optimum care, physical and mental exhaustion, and constant reminders of their own personal risk, nurses and other health professionals activated their best selves to deliver healthcare during a time of great international need. It is indeed inspiring and reminds us of the reason why so many of us became nurses (or other health professionals) in the first place!

Nonetheless, the rapid international spread of the virus coupled with unprepared health systems, in many cases, further marginalized relationships as the central organizing aspect of healthcare. Evidence of this can be found in numerous professional publications, anecdotal evidence from patients, families, and healthcare professionals as well as the empirical literature. For example, in the context of hospitals, nursing homes, schools, and some clinics, healthcare professionals' direct contact with patients and families was reduced, limiting personal touch, nonverbal communication techniques, the experience of making eye contact and actively listening to another, problem-solving together, providing in-person health education and teach-back methods, and routinely engaging with family members. In most instances, advancing healthcare quality and safety as well as transitioning healthcare delivery to a more relationship-centric practice took a back seat during the pandemic. Although most of this was necessary owing to the nature of the illness, the restrictions and mandates imposed, limited human and material resources, the isolation, access, and equity issues created uncertainty and angst about health, healthcare, and health professionals, negatively impacting people's mental and physical health.

On a positive note, almost immediately after the pandemic started, emphasis shifted to rapid vaccine development, virtual health services, securing equipment, vaccinations, qualified personnel, remote teaching, learning and working, advancing prevention, curing, and learning. Unfortunately, all of this occurred in a more globalized, politically charged, and technologically connected society, influencing the virus' dispersion and society's resulting response, perhaps overshadowing nursing's most publicly observed contribution. These forms of rapid innovation, while necessary, are not usual occurrences in health systems, demanding the question, "Why wait for disasters (or pandemics) to learn from our work, use our expertise, and the power of relationships to adapt our practices?"

As we are approaching the autumn of 2022, the virus continues to mutate, but hospitalizations are reduced, masks are off, and the world is tentatively watching as a war continues in Eastern Europe. Some have stated that the pandemic is over while others are mobilizing resources for the upcoming winter. Healthcare, as we know it, will be changed forever, and nurses at all levels are struggling with how to move forward when there seems to be no history on which to draw from. Perhaps, taking note of the lessons learned during the pandemic may help.

For example, those living in the community during the pandemic began to engage virtually with their providers. As society quickly became receptive to virtual care, increased use of telehealth visits, patient portals, direct collaborations between primary and tertiary care, and the communities they served were observed. Some of these services have been reported to positively influence health outcomes, and many patients are now clamoring for more of this. In addition, technological approaches such as smart wearable devices, artificial intelligence (AI) various learning platforms, and others are here to stay, shaping how the delivery of care is changing. Lessons were learned in health systems related to employee well-being, the importance of teamwork, and the need for advocacy, particularly in terms of support for health equity, adequate nurse staffing, and patient safety. Many individual health professionals have shared important lessons learned as they cared for vulnerable populations, such as specific new skills acquired or a sense of gratitude or renewed commitment to nursing (personal conversations). Their work has inspired increased numbers of college applicants to nursing and medical programs throughout the country! However, lurking on the horizon is a remodeled healthcare system that is forming but not yet known. As caring relationships form the foundation of nursing, and dare I say, healthcare professionals' delivery of services to patients and families; the question arises, how will future professional nurses and other health professionals, battered by the pandemic, respond to the fundamental human need to "feel cared for?"

This relational core of health services is significant and may be linked to important health outcomes. Not only has limited time spent "in relationship" challenged patients and families, but health professionals themselves, leading to work dissatisfaction, burnout, diminished personal health, and lack of engagement in the work. Today's newly emerging, but resource constrained health system, renders caring relationships, including teamwork, self-caring, and community engagement, obscure. Despite our best intentions, patients and families continue to suffer not only from their illnesses but also from the healthcare system itself. Although most health professionals strive to deliver excellent care, many lack the competencies required to regularly incorporate best evidence or timely practice improvement into their workflows. Relationships among health professional students, faculty, and clinical preceptors are, in some cases, considered uncivil; and healthcare leadership practices at all levels are not routinely attuned to the fundamental relational nature of health systems work.

This is particularly difficult for new health professionals who have been educated "to care" and suddenly find themselves working in health systems that do not advance relationships, have little supportive infrastructure, are focused on maximizing reimbursement, and offer few incentives for professional development. Nurses, who are the largest group of healthcare professionals and spend the longest time with patients and families, are in a unique position to advance more relationship-centric approaches to healthcare.

The SARS-CoV-2 pandemic has jumpstarted a major remodeling in how healthcare is learned and delivered, how healthcare innovation is sparked and nurtured, and how the quantity, expertise and overall well-being of healthcare professionals, particularly nurses, contribute to health outcomes. The long-term ability of health professionals to continue their professional roles in society, along with the access, utilization, inclusivity, quality, and funding of health services presents a radical experiment in how society will receive care in the future.

For some 20-plus years, the healthcare system has been focused on what needs to be done to improve the quality of healthcare. We are past due on the commitment to improve healthcare quality! The time to act on what needs to be done is now. The healthcare system has never been more poised and adaptable to remodeling! Workforce competencies have been developed to support knowledge and skill requirements, robust technology is available, and sufficient opportunity exists. Furthermore, due to the pandemic, the public continues to view nurses and other health professionals in a favorable light, increasing the chances of success.

This book provides an overview and updates the continuing quality crisis in healthcare, emphasizes its foundational relational core through an evolving middle-range theory, and offers opportunities for application at several levels. In this edition, background literature is updated; objectives are included for each chapter; components of the Quality-Caring Model© (QCM) are mapped to current and relevant standards and competencies; an update on self-caring has been added; examples of caring behaviors in action are used; practice analyses appear; and additional instructor resources have been added.

The intent of the book is to continue the focus on the significance of caring relationships in improving the safety and quality of health systems. It is also a call to health professionals, particularly nurses, to act. Safe and quality healthcare, meaningful work, and overall well-being are at stake. Through exploration of several theoretical concepts drawn from multiple sources, the QCM is clarified. The important relationships with self, the community served, patients and families, and the healthcare team are illuminated and updated for current and future practice. Applying the model in clinical, educational, and leadership practice offers possibilities for advancing the value of the nation's health systems while providing the context for meaningful work. Finally, using the QCM as a foundation for research may point to new evidence regarding the contribution of caring relationships to quality health outcomes.

Part I focuses on the continuing problems inherent in complex health systems, including the continuing, disturbing facts about safety and quality and the state of professional practice, particularly in hospitals. The text continues by describing the QCM, a middle-range theory that emphasizes the value of caring relationships to quality health outcomes. It is a hope-filled approach that is repeatedly emphasized throughout the text with specific exemplars. Part II concentrates on those relationships necessary for quality caring, namely, relationships with self, patients and families, members of the healthcare team, and the community. Concepts in the model are described in depth with several exemplars. The system characteristics of professionalism, relational capacity and practice improvement are addressed. Finally, self-advancing systems—those that naturally evolve with focused attention to caring relationships—end the section. Part III centers on leading and learning in quality-caring health systems, with emphasis on those relational processes that support professional clinical practice. To conclude, the future of self-advancing systems—those that add individual and system value—is tied to the caring relationships that nurses have always known to be the enduring foundation for professional practice.

HOW TO USE THIS BOOK

This revised edition is intended for use by nursing students, and nursing scholars as well as clinical nurses, nurse educators, nurse researchers, and those in nursing leadership positions. Health professionals in other disciplines may also find it helpful. Each chapter contains objectives, an introductory section followed by specific narratives holding new information or applications. Areas of special emphasis are boxed to highlight their importance, and specific "Calls to Action" are included at the end of each chapter. The text offers multiple case examples and includes reflective questions and practice analyses for use in formal education programs, continuing education, workshops and conferences, and general clinical practice. Although these additions are organized for nurses in clinical practice, educators, and nurse leaders, they are not mutually exclusive and may be used by health professionals in many different roles. The Appendices provide additional resources for those interested in caring relationships or improvement in health systems.

During this salient remodeling phase in healthcare history, where rapid, real-time approaches are drastically needed to meet our social mandate, health professionals at all levels are called to choose caring relationships as the cornerstone of their practice. In particular, professional nurses, the largest group of health professionals, who are educated "to care" and spend the majority of their time with patients and families, are called to prioritize a more person-centered health system by practicing from a quality-caring base, educating and leading health professionals and health systems to positively impact all human persons.

Acknowledgments

Foremost, I wish to thank Steve, who, for 49 years, has always placed priority on caring for me as I continue to advance quality caring scholarship. His support, humor, and tolerance has afforded me the opportunity to pursue this work; to him, I owe my deepest gratitude.

Secondly, I sadly wish to recognize all those who have lost their lives due to SARS-COVID-19 or are living with "long COVID," as well as those with other illnesses who experienced delays in their care during the last three years. These individuals, their families, and others who are ill remind me often of the reason I continue to be passionate about nursing and healthcare, its worth, and its enduring commitment to society.

And, with admiration, I wish to acknowledge all the caring clinical nurses, other health professionals, and first responders who continue to "give it their all," even as the pandemic continues. These warriors exemplify conviction, bravery, courage, grace, and sacrifice. Most used their relational expertise to connect, comfort, and support ill persons and their families during the last three years. They continue to inspire me and society at large when others do not. To them, I give my deepest appreciation, continued respect, and all the encouragement necessary to lead a remodeled healthcare system.

SPECIAL ACKNOWLEDGMENTS

My sincerest recognition and gratitude goes to the following exceptional nurses who have provided exemplars of caring professional practice that appear throughout this text. Their work provides selected evidence of the ongoing theory-practice translation that is taking place in many contemporary health systems:

Genesis R. Bojorquez, PhD, RN, NE-BC, PCCN
Dawn Carroll, DNP, NE-BC, WHNP
Judy E. Davidson, DNP RN MCCM FAAN
Heather Davis, MSN, RN, PCCN, SCRN
Abigail Edilloran, RN, DNP
Lindsay Holt, PhD, RN, CPAN
Jacqueline Imus, BSN, RN
Kristina James, MSN, RN, CNL, PCCN
Joan Meunier-Sham, RN, MS
Tamara Norton, BSN, RN, CCRN
Randi Petricone, MSN, CNP, RN, WHNP-BC
Stacy Street, BSN, RN, CCRN

Instructor Resources

 A robust set of instructor resources designed to supplement this text is located at http://connect.springerpub.com/content/book/ 978-0-8261-3696-1. Qualifying instructors may request access by emailing textbook@springerpub.com.

Available resources include:

- Instructor's Manual, including a crosswalk of Quality Caring Model concepts, core competencies, and performance standards, along with student assignments, reflections, and value exercises.
- Chapter-Based PowerPoint Presentations
- Mapping to AACN Essentials: Core Competencies for Professional Nursing Education

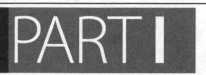

PART I

Nursing and Health Systems

CHAPTER 1

Quality, Caring, and Health Systems

"America's healthcare system is neither healthy, caring, or a system."

—Walter Cronkite

CHAPTER OBJECTIVES:

1. Describe the crisis of quality in health systems
2. Analyze the association between the recent pandemic and the crisis of quality in health systems
3. State three challenges pertinent to the quality of nursing care

PERSISTENT CRISIS OF QUALITY IN HEALTH SYSTEMS

The U.S. healthcare system was slowly progressing in its pursuit of safe, high-quality care, while simultaneously dealing with rising patient age and acuity, emerging global infections, societal and political pressures, reimbursement challenges, and workforce issues before the arrival of the novel SARS-CoV-2 virus (COVID-19). In fact, since the early Institute of Medicine (IOM) safety and quality reports (IOM, 2001a, 2001b; Kohn et al., 2000), major efforts and the consumption of massive resources have been expended to measure and improve healthcare, particularly in hospitals. Despite these actions, adverse events, as well as decreased patient functional performance related to hospitalization (including nursing homes, home care, clinics, schools, and outpatient centers), remained a major source of harm, death, and disability for Americans. It is widely recognized that patients were at risk for errors from healthcare itself (Makary & Daniel, 2016) and also suffered from preventable failures or omissions of care, leading to unintended harm (Panagioti et al., 2019). For example, in 2020, it was reported that 27% of Medicare beneficiaries were harmed during their stay in acute care hospitals, 29% in rehabilitation hospitals, 39% in skilled nursing facilities (SNF), and 46% in long-term-care institutions (U.S. Department of Health and Human Services, Office of Inspector General, 2020). Furthermore, chronic understaffing and burnout of hospital-based nurses *prior* to COVID-19 already presented risks to the public's health (Lasater et al., 2021; Weston, 2022).

Thus, hospitalization in and of itself was and continues to be linked to unintentional harms. Moreover, during hospitalization, many patients experience disruption of sleep cycles, prolonged bedrest, disruption in routine hygiene practices, and separation from families, often leading to unnecessary suffering. Despite some reports of improved performance in hospitals immediately prior to COVID-19, serious concerns were raised at many hospitals, causing unnecessary burden to patients and families as well as increased expenditures to the U.S. health system.

In nursing homes, quality and safety harms have been longstanding issues, extending beyond national boundaries. Older adults frequently bounce between nursing homes and hospitals for healthcare, creating continuity and transition issues. Despite public reporting systems, nursing home residents continue to experience adverse events such as pressure ulcers, falls, and injuries from falls that are not always the result of illness but rather consequences of the residence itself; and many require unanticipated interventions, generating a significant financial burden (Quach et al., 2021).

Since early 2020, however, the healthcare system has been overwhelmed by the COVID-19 pandemic, an unexpected deviant whose sudden onset instigated new ways of delivering care, while also exposing some fundamental flaws that those of us in healthcare have known about for some time. For example, in a recent U.S. Health and Human Services (HHS) Inspector General's report, the presence of COVID-19 has actually "created new and different problems ... and exacerbated longstanding challenges in health care delivery, access, and health outcomes" (HHS, 2021, p. 1). First, hospitals quickly became overrun with very sick, unanticipated patients, and the already existing staffing shortages exacerbated by these demands necessitated adjusted work hours, re-training and re-assigning personnel, surges in overtime, and changes to staffing ratios. The physical and emotional trauma associated with these sudden workflow changes, coupled with limited material resources, high acuity, and death, dampened employee morale and overall health, inducing increased burnout and resulting turnover (Associated Press, 2021). During this time, many "mature" RNs pursued early retirement while others engaged in temporary or travel work. The exit of so many experienced RNs presented quite a loss in terms of mentorship, onboarding, and leadership to many healthcare systems.

Second, problems with vaccine distribution and vaccine hesitancy among employees and the community have added to the prevalence of patients with COVID-19. Third, existing racial disparities and inequities were exposed. Black, Hispanic, and Asian populations were reported to have substantially higher rates of infection, hospitalization, and deaths due to COVID-19 (Lopez et al., 2021). Some health systems reported financial instability because of the forced reduction in surgical and other procedures and difficulties in discharging COVID-19 patients, affecting bed space for other patients. Many providers also lost revenue due to decreased demand for services, and the long neglected public health system struggled to respond adequately. The report also highlighted some erosion of trust in hospital safety due to patients contracting COVID-19 while hospitalized for other illnesses.

During this time, maintaining patient safety and quality in hospitals was reported as challenging, and with projected increases in the nursing shortage, was expected to worsen (Esposito, 2021). The pandemic disproportionately affected nursing home residents, particularly in communities with a higher concentration of racial and ethnic minorities (Cai et al., 2021). To further add to the burden, the education of future health professionals during the pandemic was suddenly forced to operate virtually, decreasing direct clinical time with patients and in some cases, relaxed graduation requirements. It is not yet known how these quickly crafted educational strategies will affect health professionals' future practice, the care of patients, or their long-term careers. In fact, the pandemic has left a lasting impact on the nursing workforce (Weston, 2022), making planning for the future in terms of hiring, procuring products and equipment, rightsizing of beds, and delivering care even more complicated.

The newly exposed quality and safety concerns, layered on top of those already known, presents many new and sometimes frightening worries. For example, although some progress had been made in hospital-acquired infections prior to COVID-19 (Centers for Disease Control and Prevention [CDC], 2019), "significant increases in 2020 were observed for hospital associated infections, compared to 2019" (Weiner-Lastinger et al., 2022, p. 1), indicating the need to vigorously and immediately improve infection prevention and control practices to be able withstand future pandemics. In fact, a special issue from the CDC reported a significant increase in antimicrobial use and hospitals with higher rates for four out of six types of healthcare-associated infections (HAIs; CDC, 2022). The health disparities and other vulnerabilities in the U.S. healthcare system exposed during COVID-19 has heightened Americans' awareness of and attention to health equity, social determinants of health, and social needs (National Academies of Sciences, Engineering, and Medicine. 2021). For example, overall U.S. life expectancy rates declined by 1.5 years from 2019 to 2020, but declined two to three times further for Black and Latino populations compared to White populations, primarily due to COVID-19 (Andrasfay & Goldman, 2021; Centers for Disease Control and Prevention National Center for Health Statistics, 2021). Despite two decades of concerted efforts to improve person-centeredness, the pandemic's burdens on hospitals may have impacted how they performed on selected quality indicators. A Beryl Institute report documented that Hospital Consumer Assessment of Healthcare Providers and Systems (HCAHPS) scores were reduced slightly from 2019 to 2020 with the greatest change related to "responsiveness of staff" (Silvera et al., 2021). Press Ganey's recent survey of 1,000 plus U.S. adults showed that during the pandemic, a third of those questioned reported that they trusted the healthcare industry less than they once did (Kelly, 2022). Finally, across facilities that report findings to The Leapfrog Group, a recent analysis suggested that: (1) fewer parents felt comfortable raising concerns about errors related to their child's care; (2) on average, only half of the patients who responded indicated that they clearly understood their transition to home; and (3) adult inpatients were less likely to report higher ratings related to communication about medications (The Leapfrog Group, 2021). Although outpatients reported better experiences in this report, acute-care patient experience data continues to show challenges that health systems must better understand.

Even worse, the proliferation of electronic health records (EHRs), whose intent was to benefit healthcare, has been linked to sustained documentation burden, work-arounds, and even some medical errors (Moy et al., 2021; Bell et al., 2020). Continuing cybersecurity issues challenge health systems to protect sensitive patient data. Although reduced from the last analysis, a recent report estimated 161,250 preventable deaths occur each year in U.S. hospitals (The Leapfrog Group, 2021). This needless harm has persisted despite the large investment in safety and quality programs over the last two decades, with the pandemic exacerbating these concerns. A radical disruption of healthcare is occurring, and it is re-setting how healthcare, as we know it, will be delivered in the next 10 or 20 years. Many believe that care delivery models will be completely transformed much sooner.

Quality reporting requirements were relaxed during the pandemic but will remain a high priority focus through this drastic period of change. Of concern, however, is the archaic way healthcare quality reporting is currently being performed. Longstanding issues such as quality reporting *after* care is delivered rather than in real-time, long time lags for improvement actions, little standardization of results allowing comparisons, and resource intensive requirements that may be interfering with timely learning and improvement need to be addressed. In fact, health systems, insurers, and the general public may have to wait a long time to understand the impact of COVID-19 on healthcare quality. Nevertheless, patient safety and quality will remain a high priority focus area throughout this drastic remodeling period. In particular, preventable adverse health outcomes, health disparities, true person-centeredness, and nursing-sensitive indicators (NSIs) will continue to be reported and acted upon (Boissy, 2020; Geyman, 2021; Stifter et al., 2021). The methods for measurement, analysis, and findings of reportable healthcare processes and outcomes may be revised, but will continue to consume limited resources, in the ever-increasing pursuit of high quality and patient safety.

Although the value of the American health system remains stagnant, and some would say shifting downward, others argue that the radical upheaval generated by the COVID-19 pandemic will create the conditions for health systems to rise to the opportunities presented. However, payment mechanisms in place *before* COVID-19 may need to be re-examined in light of new learnings from the pandemic.

Since the first edition of this book, the complex Patient Protection and Affordable Care Act [ACA] (2010), with its emphasis on shared accountability for high-quality care among all providers, disciplines, and associated healthcare organizations, has been implemented. Pay-for-performance programs and value-based purchasing were provisions in the law expected to reimburse and reward health systems that attained certain quality scores and provided better care for five of the most prevalent conditions. Most hospitals now have initiatives for improving these scores, although the pandemic has negated some of this work. After 10 years, implementation has evolved considerably. According to several studies, the ACA has reduced uninsurance and improved affordability of coverage for Americans (Gruber & Sommers, 2019; LaFontaine et al., 2019). However, some would argue that Emergency Department (ED) visits have increased (Garthwaite et al., 2019), and the affordability of coverage is still too high for many individuals and families (LaFontaine et al., 2019). Although the law continues to be a subject of intense discussions and controversy, it is clear that expanding coverage and quality while containing costs will continue to be top priorities for legislators.

In the context of a continuing pandemic, the U.S. healthcare system that was already strained is suffering. Uncertainty about future variants amidst financial and workforce constraints suggests tough decisions in the immediate years ahead. Yet, this crisis offers an opportunity to reshape healthcare in ways that may not have seemed possible just a few months ago. Advancing patient safety and quality *despite* the crisis, consistently prioritizing human persons, including the healthcare workforce, and drastically reducing disparities requires remembering and *using* our core values. Embracing a more relational approach, where person-centered priorities are embedded in the clinical workflow, and patients have the power to drive them is fast becoming the preferred approach in the neverending battle of pursuing value. The valuable role of the professional nurse in such a remodeled system is radically evolving.

QUALITY AND PROFESSIONAL NURSING CARE

Nursing as we know it is in the midst of several challenges. For example, *prior* to COVID-19, reports surfaced regarding nursing employers having increasing expectations for RNs to be prepared for the growing scope of professional nursing practice, including safe, high-quality, and value-based healthcare. These concerns, together with the body of evidence linking education to quality outcomes, coalesced into nurses' needs to be adequately prepared to help repair and renew the fragmented care delivery system. The American Association of Colleges of Nursing (AACN) conducted an environmental scan that summarized the social and institutional trends affecting nursing work. Their findings, along with data about the continuing academic–practice gap and concerns about nursing clinical judgement (Huston et al., 2018; Jessee, 2021) resulted in new and competency-based educational criteria. With the goal of meeting the needs of a dynamic and global society, this AACN vision for nursing suggested that the competency levels of new graduate RNs were inadequate for current practice, slightly exacerbated by the impact of the COVID-19 pandemic as many traditional in-person clinical and classroom experiences were adapted or abbreviated (Kavanagh & Sharpnack, 2021). As a result, new AACN core competencies were developed (AACN, 2021). Known as *The Essentials: Core Competencies for Professional Nursing Education,* they provide a framework for preparing potential professional nurses, including expectations across the trajectory of nursing education and applied experiences. They intend to bridge the gap between education and practice and were disseminated in the spring of 2021. In universities across America, faculty members are currently adapting their various curricula and evaluation strategies to meet the new requirements. Of importance is the focus on competency-based education where students are held accountable for the mastery of competencies deemed critical for an area of study. The outcomes of the educational experience and performance expectations are clearly delineated to ensure that stakeholders' expectations for nursing competencies are met. It is hoped that enactment of the new guidelines will increase nursing graduates' preparation for modern-day healthcare employment.

A second challenge to nursing is the continuing quality problem in care delivery. For example, in hospitals and nursing homes, patient falls (some with injury), pressure injuries, catheter-associated urinary tract infections (CAUTIs), problems related to transitions in care, alarm fatigue, struggles with early mobility, inadequate medication teaching, hand hygiene, infections, workplace violence, and medication errors continue to plague the system. In many cases the presence of COVID-19 exacerbated these problems (Grimley et al., 2021). A common theme in these nursing quality of care issues is the lack of, limited, or missed basic nursing care.

Missed nursing care is defined as any aspect of required patient care that is omitted (either in part or in whole) or delayed (Kalisch et al., 2009). Missed nursing care is considered an error of omission that potentially leads to negative outcomes, varies across hospitals, and is impacted by several variables (Kalisch et al., 2011). Missed nursing care is considered a process indicator, and it appears to be occurring on a regular basis in hospitals worldwide, impacting important and reimbursable health outcomes. For example, Recio-Saucedo et al. (2018) in a review of studies linking missed nursing care to patient outcomes, concluded that poorer experiences of care, increased risks of infection, 30-day readmissions, and complications due to critical incidents from undetected physiological deterioration were realized. Nurse characteristics (i.e., gender, age, experience and education) have not consistently been linked to missed nursing care occurrences (Chaboyer et al., 2021). In an integrative review, missed nursing care was reported to be not only a patient safety issue but one connected to decreased job dissatisfaction and increased intention to leave, which may be reflective of inadequate staffing levels (Alsubhi et al., 2021). According to Kalisch et al. (2011), the health system has allowed a "culture of missing care" to evolve over time, and nurses who have practiced more than 20 years point to a major decline in completeness of nursing care over the last several decades. The COVID-19 pandemic may have exacerbated these findings. For example, in one acute care hospital, critical care nurses were overheard saying, "We are only attending to oxygenation and medications these days" (personal conversation). Personal hygiene, including mouth care, regular peripheral IV maintenance care, ambulation, psychosociospiritual care, and other basic aspects of basic nursing care that impact patient outcomes may have been compromised during this time.

Interestingly, the unmet care needs associated with missed nursing care fall in the categories of patient teaching, discharge planning, comfort, inadequate patient–nurse interactions, ambulation, oral hygiene and skin care, adequate documentation, and updating care plans—all basic responsibilities of nursing (Duffy, 2018). Taken together, the complexity of forces impacting professional nursing and other health professionals today has never been greater; this is true not only in hospitals but also in nursing homes and all community-based health systems where nursing is delivered. Undoubtedly, the slow creep of unmet nurse staffing levels *prior* to COVID-19 has contributed to this greatly.

However, the severest staffing crisis in recent years is currently emerging in the nation's health system, which is being tested again and again by the pandemic. Although nurses performed bravely and with dedication during a time of national need and more than 1,200 of them died from the virus (Hunter, 2022), many have been faced with ethical challenges never encountered before. Numerous nurses have suffered post-traumatic stress disorder (PTSD) and moral injury, while others were asked to assume a professional identity immediately after graduation without the benefit of sufficient hands-on clinical experience (DeGagne et al., 2021). Many nurses today say they are worn out, frustrated, and angry. Across the country, the shortages are complicating efforts to treat hospitalized patients, leading to longer emergency room waiting times and rushed or inadequate care as health professionals struggle to treat patients who often require round-the-clock attention. The staffing shortages have a hospital-wide domino effect, affecting, for example, efficient diagnostic testing, discharges, and procedures for all patients. In September 2021, the American Nurses Association (ANA) asked the U.S. Health and Human Services Administration to declare a national nurse staffing crisis and immediately identify and implement solutions. The ANA suggested a whole government approach to finding and implementing solutions for the nurse staffing crisis involving all stakeholders and offered some suggestions. Additionally, others requested immediate policy reforms from the Centers for Medicare and Medicaid in terms of help for staffing long-term care facilities (Kolanowski et al., 2021).

Within this challenging context, RNs continuously show up, monitor and assess patients' illness trajectories, deliver independent and collaborative interventions to a wide variety of patients, delegate and supervise assistive personnel, participate in research, shared governance, and departmental committees, complete continuing education requirements, lead interprofessional teams, and provide services 24 hours/day, 7 days/week, creating an intense and unpredictable work environment that may or may not meet patient or their own needs. But, while awaiting a response from federal agencies to the shortage, new nurse turnover and vacancy rates are rising, and still others are leaving the profession altogether. According to Buerhaus, "a third of the nation's nurses were born during the baby boom years, with 640,000 nearing retirement; the demographic bulge of aging boomers needing intensive medical care will only increase the demand for hospital nurses. A sudden withdrawal of so many experienced nurses would be disastrous for hospitals" (New York Times, 2021). It would also be disastrous for communities, nursing homes, schools of nursing, and others! Losing the tacit knowledge of many experienced nurses so suddenly has never occurred before in this country and will likely leave a huge gap in the healthcare workforce.

A new system of elevating clinical practice, providing ongoing support, and responding to the well-being of nurses, the backbone of the healthcare system, is needed. The current value-based reimbursement model, point-of-care, and other knowledge-based systems, person-centered care delivered over multiple platforms requires collaborative, flexible, data-literate, professionally accountable, and gritty nurses who are experts in social determinants of health, evidence-based practice, and human relationships. With the pandemic, more nurses will be in demand in the community where most patients will be cared for. All this is occurring as the state of nursing quality remains problematic. Such concerns have repercussions for schools of nursing in terms of curricula and faculty competencies.

Despite this ongoing workforce crisis, the basics of professional nursing endures—advocating for patients and families, ensuring a holistic perspective, and most importantly, preserving human-to-human caring connections.

Because their continuous interactions and intimate relationships with patients and families uniquely position nurses to positively influence experiences of care and other significant health outcomes, nurses are now, more than ever, in a position to harness and leverage that power to their full advantage. In particular, the most fundamental role of all nursing processes—caring relationships with self, patients, families, other health professionals, and communities—provides the context for all healthcare actions and is tied to important patient and system outcomes (Duffy, 2018). Yet, such relationships may be in jeopardy as the world responds to the COVID-19 pandemic. How is it that the largest of all the health professions is teetering on the brink of a huge national crisis, putting many health systems and patients at risk? Is it simply a response to the pandemic or is it much more? Did schools of nursing prepare new nurses with the right blend of knowledge and skills to adapt to uncertainty and change? Do health systems really support those in direct care roles when the going gets tough? Do they even understand and value the connections between what nurses do and health outcomes? Or was the incessant focus on "getting things done" so pervasive that the nurses themselves failed to see the duty they have to self? Where does the patient's voice get heard in all this mayhem?

Improving Quality in Nursing and Health Systems

Nursing-sensitive indicators (NSI) have been used widely by many organizations, accrediting agencies, and insurers for some years now as measures of nursing care quality. This set of acute care performance indicators, first developed by the American Nurses Association (ANA, 1995), provides internal and benchmarking information related to nursing care. Described in detail in the first edition of *Quality Caring in Nursing* (Duffy, 2009), many organizations have used these indicators to improve their performance. Additional indicators have been added, for example, pediatric and behavioral health metrics. However, during COVID-19, one survey of hospital chief nursing officers (Grimley et al., 2021) documented that routine monitoring of NSIs was limited without an alternative solution, and routine standards of practice were interrupted, increasing opportunities for missed or disrupted care. More solutions during times of intense crisis must be found to adequately respond to the data and quality needs of patients and families.

Another gold standard of nursing excellence and patient quality has been the attainment of Magnet® designation. Some research has demonstrated that Magnet-designated hospitals provide positive work environments and may improve nurse satisfaction levels. However, little is known about other nurse performance indicators. A recent secondary data analysis showed no differences between Magnet-designated and non-Magnet-designated nurses in evidence-based practice (EBP) competency scores, and average scores for the 24 EBP competency items were less than competent in both groups (Melnyk et al., 2020). Research on *patient* outcomes in Magnet hospitals is unclear. For example, in one observational comparative study, Magnet hospitals had lower patient falls with injury rates than the non-Magnet hospitals, lower CAUTI rates, and lower central line associated blood-stream infections (CLABSI) rates; however, no statistically significant differences were noted in the hospital-acquired pressure ulcer (HAPU) rates between the Magnet and non-Magnet hospitals (Fischer & Nichols, 2019). In a post-hoc analysis of data from an existing administrative national database, no differences in mortality between the two groups were found, despite stratifying for patient characteristics and acuity (Rettiganti et al., 2018).

Nonetheless, a systematic review of 21 studies that met all eligibility criteria documented favorable outcomes for nurses and patients in Magnet-designated hospitals (Rodríguez-García, 2020). For example, Magnet hospitals were associated with lower levels of job dissatisfaction, burnout, nurse turnover, and better work environments. Additionally, the rates of patient mortality, falls, hospital-acquired infections, and pressure ulcers were also lower. Within this review, one study found greater retention and satisfaction rates among nurses in Magnet hospitals, with less intent to leave while another found that Magnet status was associated with significantly fewer instances of forgotten, omitted, or unfinished nursing care during shifts. Magnet hospital culture was shown to have a preventive effect on bullying and other hostile behaviors between professionals.

In terms of patient outcomes, this systematic review found that, compared with non-Magnet hospitals, Magnet hospitals were associated with 5% fewer falls, 21% fewer pressure ulcers, and a 14% reduction in mortality. Significantly lower central line–associated bloodstream infection rates in Magnet hospitals compared with non-Magnet hospitals were identified, and Magnet status was associated with lower rates of methicillin-resistant *Staphylococcus aureus* bloodstream infections, but higher-than-expected rates of Clostridium difficile infections. Moreover, the patients in Magnet and Magnet-aspiring hospitals reported higher levels of satisfaction with care and services received, better nurse communication, better pain management, and better health-related information, and they would "definitely recommend" such hospitals to others.

Not all data in the review, however, showed positive outcomes in Magnet hospitals. For example, no significant differences in pressure ulcers and failure-to-rescue rates between Magnet and non-Magnet hospitals was shown in one study, while another documented better outcomes in non-Magnet hospitals, including lower rates of infections associated with medical care, postoperative sepsis, or postoperative metabolic derangements. Although this review is interesting, *it is important to note* that the designs of the reviewed studies were mostly retrospective or descriptive, and their sample sizes and characteristics differed; thus, causality or generalizability could not be established. It is also not known how long these results were sustained.

Therefore, although striving for excellence through the attainment of external designations or certifications and routinely examining internal performance is laudable and often required, the use of external evidence—such as that found in the professional literature in the form of practice guidelines and research—provides the basis from which to *activate* practice changes; however, the implementation of evidence-based nursing is variable.

Professional nurses have been educated to apply evidence-based practice, which remains a standard for Magnet designation, and nursing leaders have touted its benefits. Yet, its use remains inconsistent across health systems in the United States. In fact, deficits in RN competence and practice have been reported (Melnyk et al., 2018), and nursing leadership support has been lacking (Melnyk et al., 2016). It may have only worsened during COVID-19.

To significantly improve safety and quality while effectively meeting patient needs (and ultimately patient outcomes) in a timely fashion, imagining new approaches to nursing practice and its improvement are needed. Of importance is the recognition that quality and safety (based on evidence) are continuously embedded in the daily work of healthcare rather than activities pursued occasionally or as projects. Some examples of approaches to better ingrain quality and safety activities in daily work are active learning communities at the unit/department level, improvement activities included in staffing plans, mentoring activities, multisite improvement collaboratives, academic–service partnerships, authentic simulations, real-time data collection and analysis (learning from the work), nurse leader focus on person-centeredness, and an emphasis on positive (versus adverse) indicators. Such approaches may provide the performance data and actionable practice changes necessary to accelerate improvements in practice.

Assessing the quality of and continuously improving patient–provider relationships remain crucial concerns for health systems today as new and improved platforms are emerging for delivering care (e.g., telehealth), health professionals are in short supply, and national priorities for high quality and equitable care are growing. A recent study cited the important role nurses and physicians play in patient experience and intent to return, with most actions related to communication and trust. These aspects of patient experience were also the largest contributors to the overall ratings of a provider or facility (Quigley, 2021).

RNs, who represent the most continuous and stabilizing force that engages with patients, monitors and validates their progress, provides encouragement, ensures dignity and confidentiality, guarantees safety, coordinates care among multiple healthcare providers, and performs specialized interventions are vital to this relationship. Thus, "the patient–nurse relationship provides the context for care as vulnerable patients and families depend on RNs for safe and high-quality services" (Duffy & Brewer, 2011, p. 79). However, little data are routinely collected informing RNs of the quality of the patient–nurse relationship.

BOX 1.1: Attending to the regular evaluation and improvement of the patient–RN relationship can demonstrate the significance of the RN's role in the provision of person-centered care (and the patient experience) and facilitate the attainment of high-reliability health systems, where consistently safe and high-quality services thrive.

Sustaining a Valuable Health System

Because the U.S. health system today is at a crossroads between older approaches and recent novel methods of delivering healthcare, while simultaneously trying to control enormous costs during a pandemic, the problem of sustaining a high-value system is demanding. Americans still must wait long time periods for important diagnostic test results and procedures; read about or experience adverse outcomes such as hospital-acquired infections, pressure ulcers, or wrong-site procedures; endure multiple providers who do not adequately talk to one another; receive outrageous charges for services; experience sleeplessness, unnecessary pain, and anxiety during hospitalization; and worst of all, be made to feel as if they don't matter, are unimportant, or are not invited to participate in the decision making about their own health.

A sustainable high-value health system will not be realized with continued use of EHRs created for billing data, overuse of travel nurses, or new payment mechanisms alone. All of these will relieve some immediate stress or contribute in some way; however, at its core, delivering high-value healthcare depends on faithfully *caring* for ourselves, patients and families, health professionals, and communities. Cultivating caring relationships with patients and families, other health professionals, and the self requires responsiveness, acknowledgement of shared vulnerabilities among us all, and empathy skills. Caring for others, while rewarding, can also be harmful if our own needs for caring and wellness are not adequately met. It is no longer okay to avoid caring for self—our patients depend on us. Acknowledging the tensions between adequate staffing, evidence-based practice, and caring relationships is a first step. There is an urgency not to get complacent about the significance of caring relationships in healthcare. Actively placing patients and families at the center of practice by accepting that healthcare is a collaborative service, addressing systematic problems associated with staff and patient dissatisfaction, enhancing teamwork (caring relationships with other health professionals), ensuring safety and using evidence will advance the health of communities. Nurses, the largest group of health professionals who interact 24/7 with patients and their families, are key. The increasing evidence that caring patient–nurse relationships are worthy contributors to valuable health systems provides a unique, but brief, opportunity to showcase their potential.

Yet, most nurses are not aware of the value they provide or the resources they consume. The cost and benefits of clinical care directly related to nursing services must be better understood to leverage the power of nursing that continues to be invisible and underused. Strengthening the nursing workforce through expertise gained in educational programs and advanced in the workforce is paramount. Caring relationships, the most often described value associated with nursing, must remain a major thrust of healthcare systems with appropriate attention to resources, learning opportunities and recognition to better understand, cultivate, and appreciate its significance in safe and quality health systems.

BOX 1.2: We must hold each other accountable for caring professional practice, including recognizing, listening, observing, and confronting unacceptable caring behaviors and attitudes. Although many nurse educators are working on curricular change as this text is being written, careful attention to the need for "relational capacity" (described in Chapter 6) is necessary to effectively prepare the next generation of nurses. More comprehensive and efficient program evaluation with explicit learning competencies are needed by nurse educators to assess whether the curricula they design is meeting the needs of a *valuable* health system. Attending to the evidence related to valuable health systems, how best to help students learn, and one's own teaching abilities will ensure responsible curricular changes and, hopefully, engaged, caring nurse graduates.

Nursing leaders at all levels must consistently model caring relationships, being clear and direct in terms of what defines and is acceptable nursing professional practice, and how caring professional practice will be recognized and rewarded. Increasing time that professional nurses spend in direct patient care, facilitating high-quality patient–nurse relationships as the basis for professional practice, enhancing the work environment, stimulating career development, and demanding that those who assist professional nurses effectively contribute to the team are some approaches that nursing leaders may find advantageous. Of course, using evidence to showcase nursing contributions is paramount.

Capitalizing on the unique, intimate human connections between patients and those delivering services to them is the key to valuable health systems. To meet this demand, clinical nurses, nurse leaders, and nurse educators must appreciate, display, educate, and reward the human caring relationships that are central to professional practice and effectively translate those theoretical frameworks that support them. With unique, relating, human persons at its core, nursing's unique caring professional base will advance the value of the nation's health system.

SUMMARY

In this chapter, the persistent crisis of health system quality has been reviewed. Of particular concern is the downward trend in quality performance indicators as a result of the COVID-19 pandemic at a time when continuing slow progress toward its improvement was evolving. The value of the U.S. health system still lags behind many other countries, and it is not known how COVID has impacted this. Professional nursing, the largest health system discipline, continues to have quality problems as perceived by patients, families, and nurses themselves. In fact, a "culture of missing care" has evolved over time and now seems rather usual in acute-care hospitals. Although routine evaluation of nurse-sensitive indicators and attainment of certifications has stimulated some improvement, speedier translation of external evidence to the bedside will advance the value of nursing care even further. Attending to the routine evaluation, continuous improvement, and scientific investigation of patient–RN relationships may demonstrate the significance of the RN's role in the provision of patient-centered care and facilitate the attainment of high-reliability health systems. Leveraging the caring power of professional nursing that continues to be invisible and underused may prove to positively benefit the post-pandemic health system.

CALL TO ACTION

The value of the nation's health system is, in part, dependent on the accountability of its professional nurses for delivering caring patient–nurse relationships. Accept the responsibility for high-quality patient–nurse relationships.

REFLECTIVE QUESTIONS/APPLICATIONS

For Professional Nurses in Clinical Practice:

- Discuss the persistent quality problems in your healthcare institution.
- Is there an accepted "culture of missing care"? If so, who is responsible for its evolution?
- How should missed nursing care be handled (if at all)?
- How have collecting and reporting on nursing-sensitive quality indicators improved nursing care in your institution?
- What new evidence-based nursing interventions or care guidelines have recently been introduced in your unit? Was the evidence from which they were based explicit? How have they been evaluated?
- How do you hold yourself and fellow nurses accountable for caring relationships?

For Professional Nurses in Educational Practice:

- Has curricular revision taken hold in your institution? If yes, what evidence did you use to shape it? How did you attend to the relational capacity of your graduates?
- Reflect on the COVID-19 pandemic. How has your educational program changed as a result? What new knowledge and skills will be expected of nursing graduates?
- How have the learning outcomes specified in your evaluation plan improved over the past 3 years? How does/did this inform curriculum revision?
- How do you assess caring competence? Is it even necessary?

For Professional Nurses in Leadership Practice:

- How has the value of nursing care improved over the past 3 years at your institution? Should it have? Why or why not?
- What professional nurse role competencies have you revised in the last 3 years at your institution?
- Reflect on the career development activities in place at your institution. Are they working? How do you know?
- Describe the evidence base that is routinely used to make leadership decisions at your institution.
- How do you ensure accountability for caring patient–nurse relationships?

PRACTICE ANALYSIS

A large Magnet-accredited academic medical center recently completed a study aimed at determining the type and extent of self-caring practices among RNs. The findings indicated that the RNs in this sample rarely rated the frequency of their own self-caring practices at the highest levels, and the lowest scores were noted on physical and spiritual aspects of self-caring. The findings were reported in aggregate, but the principal investigator relayed that individual department results were available and could be obtained in confidence through request by the directors and department managers. Of particular interest was that the lower scores were spread throughout the system.

Upon discussion at the practice council, RNs admitted that they were not sure how they could fit in self-caring practices with the amount of clinical care they were providing. In fact, the nurses stated they often did not have enough time during their shifts to assess their patients' status adequately, so finding time to attend to themselves seemed irresponsible. Six months after the initial results were reported, no requests from clinical managers for specific data on their units had been received and the nursing department, as a whole, has not taken any action on the results.

- Is there any urgency associated with these results for this organization?
- How did the nurses' reaction to the results advance their needs for self-caring?
- Describe some approaches that nursing leadership could take to improve RNs' self-caring actions at this organization.

REFERENCES

Alsubhi, H., Meskell, P., Shea, D. O., & Doody, O. (2020). Missed nursing care and nurses' intention to leave: An integrative review. *Journal of Nursing Management*, 28(8), 1830–1840. https://doi.org/10.1111/jonm.13069

American Association of Colleges of Nursing. (2021). The essentials: Core competencies for professional nursing education. https://www.aacnnursing.org/AACN-Essentials

American Nurses Association. (1995). *Nursing report card for acute care*. Washington, DC: American Nurses Publishing.

Andrasfay, T., & Goldman, N. (2021). Association of the COVID-19 pandemic with estimated life expectancy by race/ethnicity in the United States, 2020. *JAMA Network Open*, 4(6), e2114520. https://doi.org/10.1001/jamanetworkopen.2021.14520

Associated Press. (2021). U.S. hospitals hit with nurse staffing crisis as pandemic rages. https://www.nbcnews.com/health/health-news/u-s-hospitals-hit-nurse-staffing-crisis-pandemic-rages-n1278465

Bell, S. K., Delbanco, T., Elmore, J. G., et al. (2020). Frequency and types of patient-reported errors in electronic health record ambulatory care notes. *JAMA Network Open*, 3(6), e205867. https://doi.org/10.1001/jamanetworkopen.2020.5867

Boissy, A. (2020). Getting to patient-centered care in a post-covid-19 digital world: A proposal for novel surveys, methodology, and patient experience maturity assessment. *NEJM Catalyst*, July 14, 1–26. https://catalyst.nejm.org/doi/full/10.1056/CAT.19.1106

Cai, S., Yan, D., & Intrator, O. (2021). COVID-19 Cases and death in nursing homes: The role of racial and ethnic composition of facilities and their communities. *Journal of* the *Amercan Medical Directors Association, 22*(7), 1345–1351. https://doi.org/10.1016/j.jamda.2021.05.002

Centers for Disease Control and Prevention. (2019). 2019 National and state healthcare-associated infections progress report. https://www.cdc.gov/hai/data/archive/2019-HAI-progress-report.html

Centers for Disease Control and Prevention. (2022). COVID-19: U.S. impact on antimicrobial resistance. special report 2022. https://dx.doi.org/10.15620/cdc:117915

Centers for Disease Control and Prevention National Center for Health Statistics. (2021). Life expectancy in the U.S. declined a year and half in 2020. https://www.cdc.gov/nchs/pressroom/nchs_press_releases/2021/202107.htm

Chaboyer, W., Harbeck, E., Lee, B. O., & Grealish, L. (2021). Missed nursing care: An overview of reviews. *Kaohsiung Journal of Medical Sciences, 37*(2), 82–91. https://doi.org/10.1002/kjm2.12308

DeGagne, J. C., Cho, E., Park, H. K., Nam, J. D., & Jung, D. (2021). A qualitative analysis of nursing 288 students' tweets during the COVID-19 pandemic. *Nursing and Health Sciences, 23*(1), 273–289.

Duffy, J. R. (2009). *Quality caring in nursing: Applying theory to clinical practice, education, and leadership.* Springer Publishing Company.

Duffy, J. R. (2018). *Quality caring in nursing and health systems: Implications for clinicians, educators, and leaders* (2nd ed.). Springer Publishing Company.

Duffy, J. R., & Brewer, B. B. (2011). Feasibility of a multi-institution collaborative to improve patient–nurse relationship quality. *Journal of Nursing Administration, 41*(2), 78–83. https://doi.org/10.1097/NNA.0b013e3182059463

Esposito, L. (2021). Pandemic's impact on the nursing profession nurses continue to experience effects on their health, morale and careers. US News. https://health.usnews.com/health-care/patient-advice/articles/pandemics-impact-on-the-nursing-profession

Fischer, J. P., & Nichols, C. (2019). Leadership practices and patient outcomes in Magnet® vs. non-Magnet hospitals. *Nursing Management, 50*(5), 26–31. https://doi.org/10.1097/01.NUMA.0000553496.63026.95

Garthwaite, C., Graves, J., & Gross, T. (2019). All Medicaid expansions are not created equal: The geography and targeting of the Affordable Care Act. *Brookings Papers on Economic Activity.* https://www.brookings.edu/wp-content/uploads/2019/09/Garthwaite-et-al_conference-draft.pdf

Geyman, J. (2021). COVID-19 has revealed America's broken health care system: What can we learn? *International Journal of Health Services, 51*(2), 188–194. https://doi.org/10.1177/0020731420985640

Grimley, K. A., Gruebling, K., Kurani, A., & Marshall, D. (2021). Nurse sensitive indicators and how COVID-19 influenced practice change, *Nurse Leader, 19*(4), 371–377.

Gruber J., & Sommers, B. D. (2019). The affordable care act's effects on patients, providers, and the economy: What we've learned so far. *Journal of Policy Analysis and Management, 38*(4), 1028–1052. http://dx.doi.org/10.1002/pam.22158

Hunter, L. A. (2022). Nurses in the trenches: Honoring our fallen heroes. *The Journal of Perinatal & Neonatal Nursing, 36*(1), 15–17.

Huston, C. L., Phillips, B., Jeffries, P., Todero, C., Rich, J., Knecht, P., Sommer, S., & Lewis, M. P. (2018). The academic-practice gap: Strategies for an enduring problem. *Nursing Forum, 53*(1), 27–34.

Institute of Medicine. (2001a). *Crossing the quality chasm: A new health system for the 21st century.* Washington, DC: National Academies Press.

Institute of Medicine. (2001b). *New health care system for the 21st century: Health care organizations as complex adaptive systems.* Washington, DC: National Academies Press.

Jessee, M. A. (2021). An update on clinical judgment in nursing and implications for education, practice, and regulation. *Journal of Nursing Regulation, 12*(3), 50–60.

Kalisch, B. J., Landstrom, G., & Hinshaw, A. S. (2009). Missed nursing care: A concept analysis. *Journal of Advanced Nursing, 65*(7), 1509–1517. https://doi.org/10.1111/j.1365-2648.2009.05027.x

Kalisch, B. J., Tschannen, D., & Lee, H. (2011). Does missed nursing care predict job satisfaction? *Journal of Healthcare Management, 56*(2), 117–131. https://doi.org/10.1097/00115514-201103000-00007

Kavanagh, J. M., & Sharpnack, P. A., (2021). Crisis in competency: A defining moment in nursing education. *OJIN: The Online Journal of Issues in Nursing, 26*, 1.

Kelly, J. (2022). Surviving the "Great Patient Migration": 4 ways to upgrade PX in 2022. https://info.pressganey.com/featured-resources/surviving-the-great-patient-migration-4-ways-to-upgrade-px-in-2022

Kohn, L. T., Corrigan, J. M., & Donaldson, M. S. (2000). *To err is human: Building a safer health system.* Washington, DC: National Academies Press.

Kolanowski, A., Cortes, T. A., Mueller, C., et al. (2021). A call to the CMS: Mandate adequate professional nurse staffing in nursing homes. *American Journal of Nursing, 121*(3), 24–27. https://doi.org/10.1097/01.NAJ.0000737292.96068.18

LaFontaine, P. R., Vogenberg, F. R., & Pizzi, L. T. (2019). From then until now: A top-down view of the affordable care act. *P & T, 44*(8), 467–493.

Lasater, K. B., Aiken, L. H., Sloane, D. M., et al (2021). Chronic hospital nurse understaffing meets COVID-19: An observational study. *BMJ Quality & Safety, 30*, 639–647.

The Leapfrog Group. (2021). What patients think about their hospitals and ambulatory surgery centers an analysis of patient experience surveys. https://www.leapfroggroup.org/patient-experience-report

Lopez, L., Hart, L. H., & Katz, M. H. (2021). Racial and ethnic health disparities related to COVID-19. *JAMA, 325*(8), 719–720. https://doi.org/10.1001/jama.2020.26443

Makary, M. A., & Daniel, M. (2016). Medical error—The third leading cause of death in the US. *British Medical Journal, 353*, i2139. https://doi.org/10.1136/bmj.i2139

Melnyk, B. M., Gallagher-Ford, L., Thomas, B. K., et al. (2016). A study of chief nurse executives indicates low prioritization of evidence-based practice and shortcomings in hospital performance metrics across the United States. *Worldviews Evidence Based Nursing, 13*(1), 6–14. https://doi.org/10.1111/wvn.12133

Melnyk, B. M., Gallagher-Ford, L., Zellefrow, C., Tucker, S., Thomas, B., Sinnott, L. T., & Tan, A. (2018). The first U.S. study on nurses' evidence-based practice competencies indicates major deficits that threaten healthcare quality, safety, and patient outcomes. *Worldviews on Evidence Based Nursing, 15*(1), 16–25. https://doi.org/10.1111/wvn.12269

Melnyk, B. M., Zellefrow, C., Tan, A., & Hsieh, A. P. (2020). Differences between Magnet and non-Magnet-designated hospitals in nurses' evidence-based practice knowledge, competencies, mentoring, and culture. *Worldviews on Evidence-Based Nursing, 17*(5), 337–347. https://doi.org/10.1111/wvn.12467

Moy, A. J., Schwartz, J. M., Chen, R. J., et al. (2021). Measurement of clinical documentation burden among physicians and nurses using electronic health records: A scoping review. *Journal of the American Medical Informatics Association, 28*(5), 998–1008. https://doi.org/10.1093/jamia/ocaa325

National Academies of Sciences, Engineering, and Medicine. (2021). The future of nursing 2020–2030: Charting a path to achieve health equity. Washington, D.C: The National Academies Press. https://doi.org/10.17226/25982

New York Times. (2021). Nursing in crisis: Staff shortages put patients at risk. https://www.nytimes.com/2021/08/21/health/covid-nursing-shortage-delta.html

Panagioti, M., Khan, K., Keers, R. N., et al. (2019). Prevalence, severity, and nature of preventable patient harm across medical care settings: Systematic review and meta-analysis. *British Medical Journal, 366*, l4185. https://doi.org/10.1136/bmj.l4185

Patient Protection and Affordable Care Act. (2010). Public Law No. 111-148, 124 Stat. 119. http://www.gpo.gov/fdsys/pkg/PLAW-111publ148/pdf/PLAW-111publ148.pdf

Quach, E. D., Kazis, L. E., Zhao, S., et al. (2021). Safety climate associated with adverse events in nursing homes: A national VA study. *Journal of the American Medical Directors Association, 22*(2), 388–392. https://doi.org/10.1016/j.jamda.2020.05.028

Quigley, D., Reynolds, K., Dellva, S., et al. (2021). Examining the business case for patient experience: A systematic review, *Journal of Healthcare Management, 66*(3), 200–224. https://doi.org/10.1097/JHM-D-20-00207

Recio-Saucedo, A., Dall'Ora, C., Maruotti, A., et al. (2018). What impact does nursing care left undone have on patient outcomes? Review of the literature. *Journal of Clinical Nursing, 27*(11–12), 2248–2259. https://doi.org/10.1111/jocn.14058

Rettiganti, M., Shah, K. M., Gossett, J. M., et al. (2018). Is Magnet® recognition associated with improved outcomes among critically ill children treated at freestanding children's hospitals? *Journal of Critical Care, 43*, 207–213.

Rodríguez-García, M., Márquez-Hernández, V., Belmonte-García, T., et al. (2020). How magnet hospital status affects nurses, patients, and organizations: A systematic review. *American Journal of Nursing, 120*(7), 28–38. https://doi.org/10.1097/01.NAJ.0000681648.48249

Silvera, G. A., Wolf, J. A., Stanowski, A., et al. (2021). The influence of COVID-19 visitation restrictions on patient experience and safety outcomes: A critical role for subjective advocates. *Patient Experience Journal, 8*(1), 30–39. https://doi.org/10.35680/2372-0247.1596

Stifter, J., Sermersheim, E., Ellsworth, M., et al. (2021). COVID-19 and nurse-sensitive indicators: Using performance improvement teams to address quality indicators during a pandemic. *Journal of Nursing Care Quality, 36*(1), 1–6. https://doi.org/10.1097/NCQ.0000000000000523

U.S. Department of Health and Human Services, Office of Inspector General. (2021). Hospitals reported that the COVID-19 pandemic has significantly strained health care delivery: Results of a national pulse survey. https://oig.hhs.gov/oei/reports/OEI-09-21-00140.pdf

Weiner-Lastinger, L. M., Pattabiraman, V., Konnor, R. Y., Patel, P. R., Wong, E., Xu, S. Y., Smith, B., Edwards, J. R., & Dudeck, M. A. (2022). The impact of coronavirus disease 2019 (COVID-19) on healthcare-associated infections in 2020: A summary of data reported to the National Healthcare Safety Network–ADDENDUM. *Infection Control and Hospital Epidemiology, 43*(1):137. https://doi.org/10.1017/ice.2022.10.

Weston, M. J. (2022). Strategic planning for a very different nursing workforce. *Nurse Leader, 20*(2), 152–160. https://doi.org/10.1016/j.mnl.2021.12.021

CHAPTER 2

Professionalism in Health Systems

"Professionalism is about having the integrity, honesty, and sincere regard for the personhood of the customer, in the context of always doing what is best for the business. Those two things do not need to be in conflict."

—Eric Lippert

CHAPTER OBJECTIVES:

1. State three characteristics of a profession.
2. Describe the word *professionalism* as it relates to nursing.
3. Evaluate the relationship between professional identity and conduct.
4. Explain the link between professional accountability and patient advocacy.

THE *PROFESSION* OF NURSING

Professionalism is a multifaceted concept that is not easy to articulate. In addition, it is a concept that continues to expand and evolve, requiring continuous learning, the developing of competence, and certain behavioral attributes. A *profession*, on the other hand, has been described as work that comprises a specific body of knowledge, a formalized educational program, a beneficial commitment to society, a certain autonomy with associated responsibility and accountability, regulations and standards, and ongoing knowledge development (Finkelman, 2019, p. 18).

Most nursing organizations and regulatory agencies view nursing as a profession and state this in their official documents. Nursing holds a unique set of concepts that are grounded in theory and embedded throughout most formal educational programs. The specialized education of RNs and their subsequent entry into practice are regulated via the professional licensure process. Once nurses are employed in a practice setting, the American Nurses Association's (ANA) *Code of Ethics with Interpretative Statements* (2015) drives ethical standards of practice, whereas state regulations and organization policies provide overarching rules to guide and evaluate professional nursing behavior. *The ANA Guide to Nursing's Social Policy Statement: Understanding the Profession from*

Social Contract to Social Covenant (2015) and the *Scope and Standards of Practice* 4th Edition (ANA, 2021) describe the essence of the profession through its covenant with society, the definition of nursing, the description of its knowledge base, the societal authority for practice, and the scope of the practice, including those criteria that represent professional performance. Finally, nursing enjoys a body of ongoing research that shapes its growing knowledge base for practice.

Along with the required knowledge, regulations, and ethical conduct, several societal advantages are associated with the profession of nursing. Foremost among them is the trust and respect of most Americans as evidenced by the 2021 Gallup poll that revealed that 81% of Americans rated nurses' honesty and ethical standards as "high" or "very high" (Saad, 2021). Nurses have maintained this honor since the inception of the list in 1999 (except in 2001 when firefighters were ranked higher). Such a professional perspective conveys a high level of positive regard in society. Nurses also work autonomously within the scope of their practice by designing and evaluating plans of care, making judgments and clinical decisions, coordinating services among multiple providers, and employing specific nursing interventions. In the context of clinical practice, some would argue that nursing holds special authority over patients and families. However, as most nurses are employees of health systems, full autonomy is somewhat limited. Finally, nurses engage in unique stories, language, symbols, and rights of practice, although in recent years, some of these have been modified.

While the traits and privileges associated with a profession are characteristic of professional nursing today, contrary to other professions (e.g., law, medicine), nursing is learned primarily at the undergraduate level, even as debates continue over what that entry-level education should be. Furthermore, nursing theory, although learned in some educational programs, is not typically used as the foundation for clinical practice (Zieber & Wojtowicz, 2020), and many nurses are not empowered to base their practice on evidence (Gorsuch et al., 2020). On a more practical level, most nurses are still compensated based on a shift or time worked approach, routinely clock in and out, and perform repetitive tasks. Thus, some debate about whether nursing is a true profession persists.

The rapidly shifting context of healthcare, and consequently the practice of nursing (Chapter 1), however, is demanding increasingly sophisticated nursing behaviors.

BOX 2.1: The pivotal role that nurses play in society has been revealed most recently during the COVID-19 pandemic. Their unique combination of knowledge, skills, and commitment to advancing health enables nurses to improve health and well-being, reduce suffering, significantly impact communities, and contribute to healthcare teams. The importance of aligning values with clinical practice has never been more relevant. For example, advancing a professional identity, maintaining trust, ensuring safety and quality, engaging in lifelong learning, and maintaining one's own well-being are paramount. Guidance is needed, however, on effective professional attitudes and behaviors to help nurses manage issues that arise at the societal, organizational, and clinical levels of practice. Questions, such as the following, are paramount: How do nurses protect patients and families as they navigate the complex health system during times when resources are limited? Or, How do nurses hold each other accountable in unhealthy work environments? Or even, What attitudes and behaviors need to change to effectively address health equity in healthcare organizations?

PROFESSIONALISM

Professionalism is a core competency of all health professionals and generally refers to the overall knowledge, values, and behaviors applied in the workplace. There are numerous definitions and few cohesive interpretations of the word *professionalism*. Thus, professionalism remains somewhat nebulous in terms of its development and evaluation. Although the term, professionalism, is often used to describe a broad set of behaviors, dress, language, affect, and appropriate hierarchies (Alexis et al., 2020), more specific activities have also been offered. The health professional literature has described professionalism as striving for excellence, integrity, adherence to ethical principles and codes of conduct, practicing within the legal limits of the professional, exercising responsibilities and ensuring accountability; using self-reflection and demonstrating respect; communicating effectively, being collaborative; behaving in a socially responsible fashion, and demonstrating clinical and cultural competence (Grus et al., 2018). In recent years, these attributes have been incorporated in developing measures and metrics to evaluate professionalism, describe specific strategies for learning professionalism, examining the effectiveness of curriculum changes in promoting professionalism, and changing associated institutional culture. In fact, the revised American Association of Colleges of Nursing (AACN) *Essentials: Core Competencies for Professional Nursing Education* has listed professionalism as an important competency of professional nursing education (AACN, 2021).

Interprofessional professionalism is a newer concept based on the work of the Interprofessional Professionalism Collaborative (IPC); they have envisioned that, "when practiced by all professions in all care settings, [it] will improve patient outcomes, promote a culture that values and fosters individual and team competence, and enhance practice and academic environments" (Frost et al., 2019). This concept has matured into observable behaviors that can be measured, resulting in the 26-item instrument Interprofessional Professionalism Assessment (IPA). Four factors (communication, respect, excellence, altruism, and caring) explained 85.6% of the variance in the set of variables and internal consistency reliability coefficients for the entire instrument, and its four subscales remained high (Frost et al., 2019). This assessment tool has the ability to evaluate interprofessional professionalism across multiple health professions and within different practice settings, providing an opportunity to advance collaborative team-based care.

Finally, the term *professional culture* has been used to describe health systems where professionalism is consistently displayed and embedded in workplace behaviors. More recently, cultures of professionalism in which clinicians think and act more broadly in their practices to include teamwork, population and community health, and citizenship have been advanced (Chu, 2021). Professional/organizational citizenship includes stepping up to engage in organizational shared governance, nursing organizations and their respective committee work, contributing to local, state, and national healthcare policy, and generating innovative ideas that lead to impactful changes (Fulton, 2019).

In nursing, Miller's (1988) model provides a framework for considering professionalism that remains of importance today. In essence, this model includes behaviors such as adherence to the code of ethics, participation in theory development and use, performing community service, engaging in ongoing continuing education, development, evaluation and use of research, being self-regulating, participation in professional organizations, and public dissemination and communication. These behaviors form the basis for nursing autonomy, competence, maintaining public trust, decision making, and nursing's evolving knowledge base.

BOX 2.2: At its core, professionalism is about relationships—those we have with ourselves, with patients and their families, with other healthcare providers, and with the wider community in which we serve. A professional nurse, grounded by a set of ethical values, exhibits professionalism in all of these relationships, but upholds patient–nurse relationships at the center of the practice.

In patient-nurse relationships, nurses recognize the uniqueness of human persons who are suffering and use specialized knowledge and skills to attend to their human experience of health and illness. Thus, it is within mutually reciprocal relationships that professional nurses demonstrate their commitment to, and contract with, individuals and society. Theoretically, patients and families who interact with healthcare providers who exhibit professionalism are more apt to disclose, engage, and follow recommended treatment guidelines (Duffy & Hoskins, 2003), leading to improved healthcare outcomes.

Unprofessional conduct, on the other hand, refers to behaviors that do not conform to the ethical or performance standards set by the profession and that may impede safe and quality patient care. Unfortunately, unprofessional behavior among healthcare providers is visible and of concern to regulatory bodies. For instance, improper use of social media sites, lateral violence in hospitals, inappropriate public conversations about patients, organized cheating among students enrolled in health professional programs, workplace bullying, scientific integrity among health researchers, elder abuse, and even irresponsible use of resources among healthcare leaders have dominated the literature in the last few years. The ethical challenges to professionalism associated with the use of mobile devices, adapting to remote working, or applying population health data are evolving as technology advances. Issues such as privacy/confidentiality and resultant Health Insurance Portability and Accountability Act (HIPAA) violations, microbial transmission from contact with mobile devices, maintenance of personal/professional boundaries, appropriate communication between colleagues, and inappropriate prioritization of personal affairs over patient care are serious and increasing (DeWane et al., 2019). Unprofessional conduct in health systems is linked to an organization's ability to maintain a culture of safety (Agency for Healthcare Research & Quality [AHRQ], 2019). For example, one study indicated that 91% of the variance in patient safety competency was explained by nursing professionalism (Kakemam et al., 2022). Although this study was a cross-sectional, descriptive survey, it was conducted in 10 teaching hospitals with a sample size of 358 nurses and warrants follow-up. Unprofessional patient–clinician encounters may also negatively impact reimbursement, regulatory requirements, and generate legal conflicts.

In nursing, for example, the integration of electronic health records (EHRs), use of "smart" systems, shortened lengths of stay, and the complexity of the work in the face of limited resources may trigger stress. Under these conditions, unprofessional behaviors versus the obligations to society derived from the ethical codes of conduct may flare up. Those in healthcare leadership and educational practice face similar pressures and may also act unprofessionally at times. When displayed to patients and families, such behavior may lead to anxiety and/or feelings of insecurity, potentially impacting the patient experience and other outcomes of care.

Although violations from the *Code for Nursing with Interpretative Statements* (ANA, 2015) are most often thought of when considering unprofessional behavior in nursing, nonadherence or violations of state practice acts are also considered unprofessional conduct. This is especially important today as the complex practice environment sometimes blurs health workers' roles and responsibilities. Professional nurses themselves and their leaders are responsible and accountable for adhering to state practice acts, including reporting misconduct, advocating for patients and families, and owning those responsibilities delegated to unlicensed assistive personnel.

BOX 2.3: The commitment of health professionals to put the needs of patients and families ahead of personal gain, whether that gain is monetary or just being able to complete the tasks of a particular shift, represents the duty to society that undergirds professional practice.

Contrast the professional behavior of nurses in the following scenarios:

One of the senior charge nurses on a medical surgical unit of a 450-bed community hospital, who has been considered an invaluable preceptor to countless new graduates, has recently been acting weird. For example, she has been rather oblivious to recent violent acts by patients, has shown up to work without combing her hair three times in the last week, and delayed medicating two patients with important antibiotics for over 10 hours. When confronted by the physician about the medication lapses, she just shrugged it off and said he was being unreasonable. When asked if anything was going on, she replied, "I am so tired lately; I just need a vacation." You let it go, but the odd behaviors continue and several weeks later, she misses an obvious change in a post-op patient's BP that results in a "failure to rescue." The patient developed a post-op retroperitoneal bleed that required stabilization in the operation room. You are embarrassed and troubled that you did not call attention to this nurse prior to the safety episode that endangered the patient. You are left wondering how many other patients were at risk...

The second nurse is working in a 517-plus-bed community hospital in a major northeastern suburban city. This hospital has a strong heritage and partners with a research-oriented university in a neighboring city where some of the physicians conduct ongoing studies. In one such study, you notice that a research assistant goes into the patient room and begins asking survey questions of the patient and stores the responses on his personal laptop. When you ask him about whether the study has been approved, he says, "No, this is just a survey, and we didn't want to go through that lengthy process." You realize that his practices might create risk to the patient and the organization, and so you call the Internal Review Board (IRB) and speak to the manager. As a result, the principal investigator, a physician, is notified and reports you to the Chief Nursing Executive (CNE) for interfering with his "study." During the follow-up meeting with the CNE, you explain that you observed the research assistant collecting identifiable patient data on his personal laptop, without affording the patient informed consent, which violates the health system's Human Subjects policy. The CNE supports your concerns and after discussions with the IRB chair,, the study is paused while appropriate approvals can be obtained. The physician involved has now stopped communicating with you.

How would you contrast the nursing professionalism in the two nurses? Which nurse displayed the most professional behavior? Why? In which health system would you want your family members admitted?

Unprofessional conduct by health professionals may be first observed during the educational process as academic dishonesty, incivility, and poor reporting of errors; and disruptive behaviors in the classroom, online, or during clinical courses may also be observed. It is precisely during this time of formation that the health profession's educators must prepare students for professional conduct, including the behavioral and dynamic nature of professionalism. In fact, forming a *professional identity* is a key factor in future professional practice, including providing safe and high-quality care. Professional identity has been described as "thinking, feeling, and acting like a nurse" (Godfrey & Young, 2020) and includes the integration of both personal and professional values. A concept analysis of professional identity revealed common themes and characteristics such as knowledge and skills, actions and behaviors, values beliefs and ethics, context and socialization, and group and personal identity (Fitzgerald, 2020). Successful acquisition of knowledge as evidenced by diploma/certification, the ability to perform the functions of the profession, connecting with a community of practice, exhibiting the values and ethics of the profession, and personal identification as a professional within an identified professional group are examples of the components of professional identity.

Recent studies provide some evidence that professional identity formation in health professional education programs may be thwarted by the "hidden curriculum," aka unknown influential factors at work within learning environments, including clinical courses (Hafferty & Franks, 1994). For example, in one qualitative study using focus groups of medical students in Brazil, speeding up—repetition without reflection,—negative role modeling, including educators who did not cultivate the values of professionals and did not find joy in it, created conflict among students in terms of finding meaning in the profession (Silveira et al., 2019). Other studies in nursing education have corroborated these negative aspects of the hidden curriculum (Raso et al., 2019).

The newly revised *Essentials: The Core Competencies for Professional Nursing Education* includes competencies reflecting professionalism and professional behaviors among other aspects of professional nursing (AACN, 2021). The formation and cultivation of a sustainable professional identity is a component of this domain in nursing education and includes several areas of competency. Highlights of the professionalism domain competencies include the following:

- Demonstrating an ethical comportment in one's practice reflective of nursing's mission to society.
- Employing a participatory approach to nursing care.
- Demonstrating accountability to the individual, society, and the profession.
- Complying with relevant laws, policies, and regulations.
- Demonstrating the professional identity of nursing.
- Integrating diversity, equity, and inclusion as the core of one's professional identity.
- Describing nursing's professional identity and contributions to the healthcare team.
- Demonstrating the core values of professional nursing identity.
- Demonstrating sensitivity to the values of others.
- Demonstrating ethical comportment and moral courage in decision making and actions.
- Demonstrating emotional intelligence.

(AACN, 2021, pp. 49–51)

To prepare nurses for the complexities of professional practice in a newer health system, new ways of learning and evaluating the attainment of these revised competencies are needed. Experiential and role modeling activities that help professional nursing students appreciate the meaning of good practice are warranted. Some examples may include: understanding the patient as a human person worthy of dignity and self-determination, using moral courage to report unethical or substandard behaviors, engaging in authentic caring relationships, safeguarding privacy, confidentiality, and participating in advocacy for social justice and health equity, protecting vulnerable populations, taking responsibility for actions and adhering to the RN standards of practice and organizational policies, engaging in professional activities and peer review, and promoting cultures of civility.

These central but everyday concerns of professional nursing must be addressed during the educational process in order to guide students in the formation of professional identity, a component of professionalism. As Wolf (2012) so aptly stated some years ago, "Nursing programs are the first filters of character for the profession, and modeling good nursing care begins in schools of nursing" (p. 16). Likewise, employers of nurses and nursing leaders have an obligation to influence professional identity in the workplace. Lindell et al. (2021) recently reported on the results of the International Society for Professional Identity in Nursing (ISPIN), a think tank of nurse leaders, who participated in several discussions about professional identity in nursing. As a result of their efforts, the group elaborated on the role that nursing leadership plays as a primary conduit for professional identity development in the workplace. In particular, role modeling, improving practice environments, and fostering lifelong learning were seen as influencers in the growth and sustainability professional identity in nurses, as well as in the next generation of leaders. Regular assessment and routine linkage of professional behaviors to patient outcomes may also help nurses appreciate their commitment to the values of professionalism, despite the inevitable challenges of the workplace.

Leaders and educators can expedite professionalism by creating an open, safe culture for discussion and reporting of unethical behavior, clarifying behavioral expectations, organizing ongoing education, consistently implementing policy, recognizing how their own actions guide the practice of employees or students (living the organization's values), creating peer support groups for themselves and employees/students to help stay grounded on important values and to safely reflect on their conduct, and creating an ongoing professional development program. Measuring the ethical climate in the organization and matching results of procedural audits with established ethical values may provide baseline information from which professional practice can be reframed and improved. Regular review and discussion of revised ethical codes, standards, and state nurse practice acts draws attention to professional behaviors in the context of safe, high-quality services.

Historically, healthcare professionals have been educated with a strong emphasis on individual performance, acknowledged to be a contributing factor to professionalism. However, expanding such education to include systems thinking, where health professional students are expected to advocate for patients and families beyond their own department may narrow the education-practice gap in the rapidly changing health system.

Advocacy is an action-oriented word that describes individual, interprofessional, organizational, and community activity. In 2021, the ANA added the demonstration of advocacy to the revised *Scope and Standards of Practice* (ANA, 2021). Fifteen competencies were developed for professional nurses, with additional competencies included for advance practice nurses. These competencies include the following:

- Championing the voice of the healthcare consumer
- Recommending appropriate levels of care, timely and appropriate transitions, and allocation of resources to optimize outcomes
- Promoting safe care of healthcare consumers, safe work environments, and sufficient resources

- Participating in healthcare initiatives on behalf of the healthcare consumer and the systems where nursing happens
- Demonstrating a willingness to address persistent, pervasive systemic issues
- Informing the political arena about the role of nurses and the vital components necessary for nurses and nursing to provide optimal care delivery
- Empowering all members of the healthcare team to include the healthcare consumer in care decisions, including limitation of treatment and end of life.
- Embracing diversity, equity, inclusivity, health promotion, and healthcare for individuals of diverse geographic, cultural, ethnic, racial, gender, and spiritual backgrounds across the lifespan
- Developing policies that improve care delivery and access for underserved and vulnerable populations
- Promoting policies, regulations, and legislation at the local, state, and national level to improve healthcare access and delivery of healthcare
- Considering societal, political, economic, and cultural factors to address social determinants of health
- Adopting a role-model advocacy behavior
- Addressing the urgent need for a diverse and inclusive workforce as a strategy to improve outcomes related to the social determinants of health and inequities in healthcare systems
- Advancing policies, programs, and practices within the healthcare environment that maintain, sustain, and restore the environment and natural world
- Contributing to professional organizations

(ANA, 2021, pp. 91–92)

Patient advocacy requires active support and protection for patients and families. Advocating for patients and families *proactively* is even harder and takes quite a bit of courage. Oftentimes, nurses find themselves in clinical situations that conflict with their personal or professional beliefs but are afraid to speak up for fear of repercussions that may follow. However, championing the patient is a duty (ANA, 2015) that must be honored. Doing so requires moral courage, especially in highly charged situations or when the patient's rights are being violated. Moral courage is the willingness to stand up for and act according to one's ethical beliefs when moral principles are threatened, regardless of the perceived or actual risks (such as stress, anxiety, isolation from colleagues, or threats to employment) (Smith, 2017). Taking a stand in such situations is difficult, but made easier in environments where leadership support, including adhering to clear policies that reinforce openness, multilevel communication, and staff empowerment is present.

ACCOUNTABILITY

Accountability in professional practice is a crucial component of the newly emerging health system. Accountability, an important aspect of professional practice, including maintaining competency, ethical conduct, lifelong learning, upholding professional standards, assuring quality patient care outcomes, promoting equity, and enabling caring relationships may help nurses to leverage the power that they hold, but oftentimes remains invisible and underused. In essence, accountability is about commitment—assuring the delivery of a quality product or service in a timely fashion, but also accepting the consequences if this is not accomplished. Accountability signifies intent, ownership, commitment, obligation, and willingness (Rachel, 2012), or to use a baseball metaphor, stepping up to the plate. It is no longer okay to languish in a job, to *not* engage in lifelong learning, to *not* consider caring relationships essential to professional practice, to *not* partner with professional colleagues, to *not* use data for decision making, to *not* practice caring for self, or to *not* use evidence in practice. These behaviors are pertinent to the entire practice of nursing—clinical, educational, and leadership.

To ensure health professionals are practicing at the highest levels of professionalism, all health professionals must constantly safeguard professional behavior by observing, identifying, and reporting conduct that does not conform to ethical standards. One way to facilitate professional accountability is to perform organizational nursing values clarification exercises every 3 to 5 years to clearly articulate the values that guide professional practice and then embed them in pertinent documents such as philosophy and mission statements, professional practice models, and even job descriptions and policies. Some organizations frame and post these core values on clinical units, letterheads, or even web pages as constant reminders of the foundational beliefs of the profession. Using such values for decision making (all decisions), performance evaluations, recognition programs, and continuing education provides clarity and promotes activism. Similarly, using individual performance data to increase ownership and accountability of nurses' practice or peer review principles provides specific and actionable information (Cline, 2016; Semper et al., 2016). On a personal level, individual health professionals who routinely reflect on their practice, both individually and in groups, and who maintain a level of awareness about ethical behavior may be able to recognize tendencies toward unethical behaviours early enough to impede their full development.

While institutional culture and systems influence the actions and behaviors of health professionals, professional accountability is an internally driven mindset (Sherman & Cohn, 2019) that requires owning one's actions and holding oneself answerable for the quality of care delivered (including any care that is missed or that deviates from the current evidence-based recommendations).

PROFESSIONAL NURSING IN CONTEMPORARY HEALTH SYSTEMS

COVID-19 has put a spotlight on several ongoing challenges related to professionalism in the healthcare system. A large, but often difficult-to-acknowledge problem exposed during COVID-19 was the level of disparity in health systems. In a large cohort study ($N = 9,722$) in New York City, Black and Hispanic patients were more likely, and Asian patients less likely, than White patients to test positive for COVID-19. After adjustment for comorbidity and neighborhood characteristics, however, Black patients were less likely than White patients to have a critical illness or die in the hospital, suggesting that existing factors pervasive in Black and Hispanic communities may explain the disproportionately higher out-of-hospital COVID-19 mortality (Ogedegbe et al., 2020). Likewise, a cross-sectional analysis of national nursing home COVID-19 reports (12,576 nursing homes nationally) revealed that nursing homes who cared for disproportionately higher racial/ethnic minority residents in the early period of the pandemic, reported more weekly new COVID-19 confirmed cases and/ or deaths (Li et al., 2020). These disparities across nursing homes persisted even after adjustment for nursing home and local infection rates. Although limited by the study design and unknown confounding variables, this study exposed the structural inequalities associated with nursing home care, a disturbing national phenomenon.

Consistent with these findings, a later study (N = 13,312) showed that in nursing homes with more than 40% non-White residents, COVID-19 death counts were 3.3-fold higher than those in nursing homes with lower proportions of non-White residents (Konetzka & Gorges, 2021). The differences were associated with larger nursing home size and higher infection burden in counties in which nursing homes with high proportions of non-White residents were located. This study was also limited by its observational nature and lack of individual patient data required to better understand whether within-facility risk factors are associated with worse COVID-19 outcomes in disproportionally impacted populations. Nevertheless, the documented disparities in health outcomes among non-White populations with COVID-19 were profound and alarming.

Despite past and ongoing efforts to achieve health equity in the United States, individuals from racial and ethnic minority groups were disproportionately affected by COVID-19, including experiencing increased risk for infection (Webb Hooper et al., 2020), hospitalization (Garg et al., 2020; Karaca-Mandic et al., 2021), and death (Gold et al., 2020; Rossen et al., 2020). Furthermore, within each U.S. census region, the proportion of hospitalized patients with COVID-19 was the highest for Hispanic or Latino patients (Romano et al., 2021). These data and others suggest that racial and ethnic disparities persist in the U.S. health system in spite of health professionals' best intentions. Nurses and other health professionals must recognize and help address the ways in which societal inequities perpetuate contrasting health outcomes. The importance of educating current and future nurses to engage in population health, with attention to culturally relevant care and social determinants of health has recently been called to action.

The National Academies of Sciences, Engineering, and Medicine's *The Future of Nursing 2020 to 2030 report* (2021) specifically called on nurses to acknowledge the critical importance of the relationship among social determinants of health (SDOH), health equity, and health outcomes. This consensus report has changed since its original version, whose intention was to shape nursing's role in a transformed health system. The current recommendations were informed by evidence developed during the COVID-19 pandemic and are meant to highlight social determinants of health and health equity. For example, the report documents the need for advanced preparation of nurses to "meet challenges associated with an aging population, access to primary care, mental and behavioral health problems, structural racism, high maternal mortality and morbidity, and elimination of the disproportionate disease burden carried by specific segments of the U.S. population" (p. 2). In addition, strengthening nursing's capacity to take action on these priorities was recommended. Specific recommendations include the following:

- In 2021, all national nursing organizations should initiate work to develop a shared agenda for addressing social determinants of health and achieving health equity.

- By 2023, state and federal government agencies, healthcare and public health organizations, payers, and foundations should initiate substantive actions to enable the nursing workforce to address social determinants of health and health equity more comprehensively, regardless of practice setting.

- By 2021, nursing education programs, employers, nursing leaders, licensing boards, and nursing organizations should initiate the implementation of structures, systems, and evidence-based interventions to promote nurses' health and well-being, especially as they take on new roles to advance health equity.

- All organizations, including state and federal entities and employing organizations, should enable nurses to practice to the full extent of their education and training by removing barriers that prevent them from more fully addressing social needs and social determinants of health and by improving healthcare access, quality, and value.

- Federal, tribal, state, local, and private payers and public health agencies should establish sustainable and flexible payment mechanisms to support nurses in both healthcare and public health, including school nurses, in addressing social needs, social determinants of health, and health equity.

- All public and private healthcare systems should incorporate nursing expertise in designing, generating, analyzing, and applying data to support initiatives focused on social determinants of health and health equity using diverse digital platforms, artificial intelligence, and other innovative technologies.

- Nursing education programs, including continuing education, and accreditors and the National Council of State Boards of Nursing should ensure that nurses are prepared to address social determinants of health and achieve health equity.

- To enable nurses to address inequities within communities, federal agencies and other key stakeholders within and outside the nursing profession should strengthen and protect the nursing workforce during the response to such public health emergencies as the COVID-19 pandemic and natural disasters, including those related to climate change.

■ The National Institutes of Health, the Centers for Medicare & Medicaid Services, the Centers for Disease Control and Prevention, the Health Resources and Services Administration, the Agency for Healthcare Research and Quality, the Administration for Children and Families, the Administration for Community Living, and private associations and foundations should convene representatives from nursing, public health, and healthcare to develop and support a research agenda and evidence base describing the impact of nursing interventions, including multisector collaboration, on social determinants of health, environmental health, health equity, and nurses' health and well-being.

(National Academies of Sciences, Engineering, & Medicine, 2021, pp. 13–14)

This report along with the aforementioned *Core Competencies for Professional Nursing Education* (AACN, 2021) provide compelling content for ongoing education, workforce performance goals and policies, leadership, and research action. Competencies such as advocating for social justice, using data-based, culturally relevant decisions in care, and promoting high-quality outcomes for diverse populations are desperately needed by nurses. Removing the negative reputation associated with practicing outside the hospital, and demonstrating the significant impact that nurses can bring to diverse, outpatient settings, such as those in schools, homes, community centers, so forth may help improve public health priorities, address the social determinants of health, and prepare adequately for future acute and chronic population health crises.

Another problem facing nursing professionalism that has been talked about but not really acknowledged during COVID-19 is the ongoing quality problem in nursing. Although discussed in Chapter 1, these quality problems refer to potential *declines* in nursing-sensitive quality indicators that may be occurring as a result of the abrupt systems issues associated with COVID-19. Delays in standard reporting of crucial safety measures were granted during the pandemic to allow hospitals to focus on patient care. However, as the pandemic progressed, a steady increase in the rates of hospital-acquired conditions per 10,000 adult discharges continued to be recorded (Grimley et al., 2021). Grimley and colleagues reported that 21 chief nursing officers (CNOs), consistently responded that they were concerned that declining performance in four nursing sensitive indicators could impact their ability to achieve or maintain ANCC Magnet® designation or redesignation. These responses prompted a 49-question electronic survey regarding performance on four key indicators of hospital nursing quality—catheter-associated urinary tract infections (CAUTI), central line-associated blood stream infections (CLABSI), hospital-acquired pressure infections (HAPI), and patient falls. Although not particularly systematic in the collection of data, the authors' findings indicated that most organizations reported a worsening in each of these four indicators, significantly more so in both CLABSI and HAPI. The importance of evidence-based practice and ensuring consistent delivery of current standards of care was a theme throughout.

Although more data is needed on additional nursing-sensitive performance indicators, including those obtained outside acute care settings, the need to prioritize patient safety and quality will continue to plague the profession. Owning how nurses contribute to and/or mitigate adverse patient outcomes, underscores professional accountability.

The rise of telehealth, digital solutions, accelerated pace of clinical trials and federal approvals, increased use of simulation, online learning with limited clinical time, use of virtual meetings, and remote care for patients with chronic disease states has expedited changes in healthcare delivery. All of these novel approaches, provided in the midst of the ongoing pandemic, sparked revisions in professional education (AACN Essentials, 2021), standards of performance (ANA Standards of Performance, 2021), and The Future of Nursing 2020 to 2030 report recommendations. Together with significant societal change, these important revisions will drastically impact the role of nursing, including how it is learned, licensed, researched, and lead. It is beyond time to get serious about evidence-based practice (EBP)!

Multiple studies have concluded that EBP is not well understood, championed or resourced, or routinely used in the care of patients (Melnyk et al., 2016, 2018, 2021a). Despite years of learning and continuing education, many nurses still are not confident in their EBP skills and find it difficult to use, and it is given little budgetary priority in health systems. In fact, a quick survey of the nursing literature on EBP continues to show titles about the barriers to EBP rather than any actual evidence generated or used in practice! A recent cross-sectional survey of 99 nurses in eight acute care hospitals reported nurses' willingness to engage in research-related tasks, but having low or moderate knowledge of and ability to perform them (Nowlin et al., 2021). In this survey, knowledge, attitudes, and practices of research increased with the level of education, although gaps between willingness to engage versus knowledge and ability persisted, even among doctorally-prepared nurses! Master's degree–prepared nurses ($N = 8$) reported lack of time, institutional support, and knowledge about processes for engaging in research as barriers to participation. Although this study was limited by the targeted convenience sample, it lends additional insight into the continuing problem of inadequate implementation of evidence by practicing professional nurses. The challenge facing clinical nurses and healthcare organizations regarding EBP is that the skill sets required to engage in it are lacking, and little infrastructure is provided to support nurses with their willingness to engage. The survey findings showed that nurses rated themselves low on formulating research questions, identifying data collection tools, setting up study procedures, getting administrative and IRB approval, and analyzing data. These results underscore the need for large investments in mentorships, partnerships, recognition, and dedicated protected time for clinical nurses to integrate EBP in their practice (Heitschmidt et al., 2021; Melnyk et al., 2021a). Although many studies of EBP in nurses have been conducted in acute care, as nursing roles extend outside hospital walls, the development and use of evidence in community settings is equally relevant. Without evidence of the value of nursing care and its link to important patient outcomes, it will be difficult to convince other stakeholders that increased funding is needed.

Regular and expert use of the recommended ANA standards and AACN competencies, together with adequate support from health systems may gradually extend EBP use. Educational efforts to ensure EBP competencies across all levels of education and leadership support in the form of amplified resources has never been more important! Documenting improved outcomes based on nursing interventions will build the business case for additional resources to drive innovations in patient care, enhancing the professional status of nursing. Building capacity for EBP will require individual and organizational infrastructures that eliminate barriers, facilitate the use of evidence in practice, and focus on collaboration and partnership, while simultaneously attending to employee wellness.

The failure of professional nurses and health systems to attend to employee wellness has been exposed during the COVID-19 pandemic. Although it was already documented as a problem *before* COVID-19 (National Academy of Medicine, 2016), a recent study exposed its extent. A random sample of 771 critical care nurses was used to assess overall wellness via online surveys. A majority (91.4%) of the nurses worked more than 8 hours per day, and more than two-thirds reported that their typical workday or shift was longer than 12 hours. The majority of nurses sampled reported suboptimal health, both physical and mental. A substantial proportion of nurses reported some degree of depressive symptoms (39.5%), anxiety (53.2%), and stress (42.2%). Only about a third of the nurses reported high professional quality of life. Many (60.9%) of the nurses reported having made medical errors in the past 5 years. For all of the health measures (physical and mental), the occurrence of medical errors was significantly higher among nurses in poor health than those in the better health categories (Melnyk et al., 2021b).

The declining workplace well-being of professional nurses, physicians, and other health professionals has also been emphasized in television and newspaper articles during the pandemic. Levels of stress, anxiety, and depression were reported to be particularly high among those with the greatest amount of patient contact and interaction (Shecter et al., 2020). The *Code of Ethics for Nurses with Interpretive Statements* (ANA, 2015) is unique in that it states explicitly that nurses must adopt self-caring as a duty to self in addition to their duty to provide care to patients. It is well recognized that nurses' physical and emotional health is necessary for high quality professional practice. Yet, the majority of nurses continue to work longer than 12-hour shifts with many working additional overtime shifts, without adopting healthy lifestyle behaviors and addressing workplace stressors. Health systems, on the other hand, pressure nurses to work overtime, continue to enable poor clinical workflows (such as duplicative work), and do not prioritize cultures of well-being. As research has shown, health systems with unwell employees may unknowingly be jeopardizing the quality and safety of care that clinicians provide the patients (Trockel et al., 2020).

Self-caring (see Chapter 4) is a professional responsibility that is tied to patient outcomes. Shared responsibility for nurses' and other health professional's self-caring rests on individual clinicians and health systems (see Figure 2.1). Using the caring behaviors as the basis for interactions provides the relational

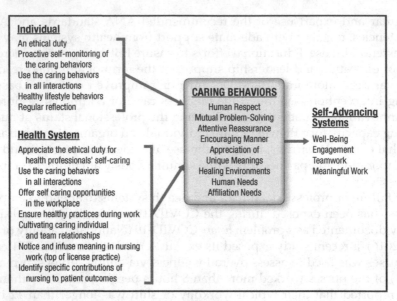

FIGURE 2.1 Shared responsibility for nurse self-caring.

space or opportunities for self-caring. For example, through interacting with self, individual nurses proactively monitor self for judgmental or mean actions, respect the self sufficiently to accept oneself as worthy of self-caring, establish boundaries, unplug (from electronic devices and other forms of passive entertainment), encourage the self through languaging, attend to human and affiliation needs, engage in healthy lifestyle behaviors both at work and at home, and practice regular reflective activities to promote greater self-awareness. Combined with system level attention to relationships, including employee and team interactions, need for relational space and wellness, and attention to what contextual forces are shaping health professional's behaviors may help to promote self-caring.

Nursing educators and leaders can lead this imperative by addressing it directly during undergraduate and graduate nursing programs (educators), giving permission for self-caring in the workplace (nursing leaders), ensuring healthy practices during work (serving healthy food, enabling outside lighting, time-out rooms, regular breaks, access to debriefing, etc.) (leaders), cultivating caring individual and team relationships (educators and leaders), calling out and infusing meaning in nursing work (leaders), and identifying the contributions of nursing to patient outcomes (educators and leaders).

The Code for Nursing with Interpretative Statements (The Code) (2015) is the nursing profession's ethical standard of practice and nursing's contract with society. Its nine provisions address the nursing's values, accountability and duties to self and others, as well as obligations at professional and societal levels. For example, "advancing the profession though research and scholarly inquiry, professional standards…and generation of health policy" (p. 14), obligates clinical nurses to know and disseminate recent research findings to support best practices, protect patient rights in research, develop and adhere to practice standards, contribute to nursing's body of knowledge, and participate in a variety of local, state, national, or global initiatives.

Thus, nurses are accountable and responsible for their decisions and actions and the quality of the care they provide, have a duty to self in terms of maintaining health and safety, preserving integrity, and ensuring professional competence through continued personal and professional development. In the evolving new healthcare system, nurses must be ready to address health inequities, document their contributions to quality health outcomes, develop and use evidence in care delivery, and practice self-caring. All of these obligations of professionalism translate into beneficial outcomes for patients and better teamwork, engagement, well-being, and meaningful work for nurses. As a final point, the sufficient translation of nursing theory into professional nursing practice may help ensure that the discipline of nursing continues to advance as a profession.

THE GROUNDING BENEFITS OF THEORY-GUIDED PROFESSIONAL PRACTICE

Theory-guided practice directs nurses in thinking about, being, and doing nursing (Smith, 2020). Based on deeply held values and beliefs about the discipline, it provides a frame of reference for clinical assessments and interventions, including ongoing professional development and evaluation, specifies curricular content for nursing faculty, assists leaders in translating nursing to other disciplines, helps researchers describe and analyze how nursing uniquely contributes to patient outcomes, and advances nursing's autonomy and accountability as a profession. Nurses use theories much of the time in practice, but often do not think of it in those terms. For example, the physiological gate control theory of pain (Melzack & Wall, 1965) is often used by nurses in the care of postoperative patients, and Lazarus & Folkman's (1984) theory of stress and coping is often used when dealing with occupational stressors (Garcia et al., 2021).

Nursing theory, on the other hand, is unique to the discipline in that it focuses on specific values and beliefs, concepts (and their definitions), and interrelated statements that frame its practice. In so doing, nursing theory provides an overall structure of the discipline to inform its members how "to be and do nursing" while simultaneously advancing the profession. Although there has been an expansion of theory development in nursing (especially middle range theory in recent years), to remain relevant, the theory must continually evolve as the context for healthcare changes, and new evidence regarding its benefits emerges. However, little recent literature was found focusing on the evolution of nursing theory in terms of how it has been revised, updated, or improved over time. This may be a reflection of the consistent struggle in the practical application of theory in health systems, the lack of integration of theory-based professional practice models, limited theory-testing research, or all three. One has to ask, is nursing practice not based on disciplinary theory best practice? Is it even nursing?

In today's world, many undergraduate nursing programs do not address theoretical components of the discipline and numerous graduate programs focus on theory in a conceptual manner with little practical application. For those Magnet®-designated hospitals who state their professional practice models are based on theory, how well that theory has actually been translated into day-to-day practice in the form of role expectations, policy-development, career advancement, or evaluation methods is questionable (personal observations).

In reality, most busy health systems (in the interest of time and resources) find it challenging and costly to embrace new processes and responsibilities, resulting in the inadequate translation of knowledge into action. This persistent phenomenon, known as the theory (knowledge)-practice gap, is a systems issue that contributes to wasted resources and disappointed users (Greenway et al., 2018). More importantly, in reference to theory-based professional practice models, their impact on nursing practice and improvement of patient outcomes relies on how well they are embedded within the culture and practices of nurses (Mensik et al., 2017).

Another example of limited theory use in nursing practice relates to performance improvement activities. In some cases, applying specific new changes to practice are implemented without a link to any foundational theory. Without theory, any contextual considerations that might impact the improvement activity or how the change will be evaluated is often left unaddressed. In fact, this last point is often quite costly to organizations and is an explanation for why many nursing contributions are left unknown (Duffy, 2016). Without a good grasp of an underlying theory and its critical components (concepts, assumptions, and propositions), it is difficult to articulate the components of a nursing intervention or demonstrate a particular intervention's impact. Thus, little is known about what differences these theories make to patient outcomes; and although conceptual underpinnings are a part of the research process, the precise link between nursing theory and research may not always be obvious.

In a recent essay on the technological contributions of nursing exposed during the pandemic and the needs of long-COVID-19 patients, Maxwell & Radford (2021) commented, "Interest in nursing theory has waned over the last 20 years, and practice is largely atheoretical at present. A refocus on the theoretical underpinnings of nursing and a wider discourse on the nature of nursing would challenge the prevailing narratives beyond the technical" (p. 364). In a more practical but compelling way, Nickitas & Frederickson (2015) have asked what is the impact of nursing knowledge and theory on improving quality? They even suggested (*in 2015*) that theoretically driven and consistent nursing knowledge and behaviors must be fully realized for nursing care to be valuable in today's value-based environment.

Using nursing theory to guide research is crucial in knowledge development and advancing nursing as a profession. For example, the Quality-Caring Model© (QCM) has been used in the evaluation of Caring Assessment Tools© (Duffy et al., 2010; Wolverton et al., 2018) and in the development and pilot testing of a caring-based intervention for older adults with heart failure (Duffy et al., 2005). In two national demonstration projects, the model was embedded into nursing practice and used to improve patient and nurse outcomes. However, the expansion of nursing's disciplinary knowledge is dependent upon more robust research that clearly demonstrates nursing's contribution to patient outcomes.

This translates to good designs, relevant sample types and sizes, suitable metrics and analyses, and clear conclusions that provide directions for practice and future research.

To meet the challenge of professionalism in the post-pandemic health system, the nursing disciplinary domains must be explicitly tied to significant patient and employee outcomes. Middle range theory tends to be less abstract than grand theory and helps nurses focus on more specific phenomena in different care settings. Middle range theory in particular adds meaning to practice as it is applied in daily care, used in research studies, and in performance improvement. Of note, many middle range theories are amenable to empirical testing, making evaluation of outcomes easier and actionable practice changes faster. However, selecting theories for application are decisions that require evaluation, including analysis of a theory's value, worth, and significance (Smith, 2020) and its alignment with nurses' values and beliefs, the organization's mission, and its feasibility for implementation and evaluation. It is critical that nurses step up to the plate with leadership, research, and service delivery. If not now, then when?

BOX 2.4: QCM is a middle range theory that is congruent with nursing's disciplinary beliefs and values, the ANA Standards of Performance (2021; Appendix B, p. 135), and offers language and concepts consistent with professional nursing practice. It has literature support, empirical measures for evaluation, and has been implemented in numerous sites, several of which have successfully attained Magnet designation. This model can be used as a basis for nursing assessment, to guide job descriptions and advancement programs, as a basis for nursing interventions, and as a foundation for research and improvement. And, most importantly, as the model is integrated into practice and used to routinely evaluate and improve quality, professionalism is advanced.

Theory unique to nursing (aka nursing theory) focuses nurses on the important aspects of their role and its importance (value) to health outcomes; helps label what it is that nurses actually do, clarifying its uniqueness; grounds nursing work within enduring values and traditions; provides meaning to nursing work, adding purpose and connection; and advances the discipline, an attribute of a profession. There is increasing evidence of caring and relationship-centered processes as central to healthcare practice in the current literature, the revised definition of nursing (ANA standards of practice and AACN Essentials), the growing use of instruments in the measurement of caring, the adoption of caring theories as the basis of professional practice models, and lately as the basis for self-caring.

It is especially crucial in this global and emerging remodeled health system that healthcare professionals maintain their focus on the human experience of individuals in need of and serving in health systems. To meet this professional obligation, however, health systems must recognize and mitigate contextual forces that may impede the human experience. The holistic and contextual nature of humans and health systems demands grounded, healthy, and accountable health professionals who know how their work impacts health outcomes and are valued for it, can quickly adjust to changing societal needs, advocate for diverse populations, and who generate and use evidence in their work. The need for grounding frameworks has never been greater.

SUMMARY

Characteristics of professionalism are described and examined in relation to nursing and healthcare. Relationships form the basis of professionalism, guided by ethical codes of conduct, standards, and regulatory mechanisms. Unprofessional behaviors in nursing and healthcare are discussed and linked to poorer patient outcomes. The accountability of health professionals, educators, and leadership for professional conduct is highlighted in light of the transitioning health system. Selected topics pertinent to the emerging post-pandemic health system are presented with recommendations. Finally, the value of grounding frameworks for professional practice is presented.

CALL TO ACTION

Professionalism is a social mandate based on strong ethical foundations. Professional nursing validates the nature of humans as they exist in union with larger contexts. **Consider** how nursing serves society. **Assume** accountability for placing the needs of patients and families first.

REFLECTIVE QUESTIONS/APPLICATIONS

For Professional Nurses in Clinical Practice:

- Discuss professionalism in your healthcare institution. How is it displayed?
- Is there an accepted code of behavior? If so, who is responsible for its application and evaluation?
- Should unprofessional nursing care be corrected? If so, then how?
- How are health outcomes reported in your institution? Are nurses held accountable for nursing-sensitive health outcomes? How do you know?
- Are you active in EBP? Provide some examples.
- What nursing theory is used on your unit? How was it chosen? How has it been evaluated? Provide some examples.
- How do you hold yourself and fellow nurses accountable for professional conduct?
- How have you integrated diversity, equity, and inclusion into your professional identity?

For Professional Nurses in Educational Practice:

- What specific curricular revisions have you developed that address ethical comportment among nursing students? What evidence did you use to shape them? What teaching strategies will you use to help undergraduate and graduate students develop competency in ethical comportment?

- Reflect on today's nursing practice environment. How do you think your educational program helps graduates stay focused on disciplinary domains of nursing as the central components of practice? What new knowledge and skills will be required to meet the societal obligations associated with professionalism?

- Have the learning outcomes specified in your evaluation plan informed curricular revision regarding professionalism over the last 3 years?

- How do you assess professionalism competencies in students?

- What evidence do you use to support the teaching strategies used in your curriculum?

For Professional Nurses in Leadership Practice:

- How has professionalism in nursing improved/worsened over the last 3 years at your institution?

- How have you articulated the specific professional conduct required of professional nurses at your institution?

- Reflect on the developmental activities in place at your institution. Do they include aspects of professionalism? Are they working? How do you know?

- How are data on patient outcomes used to advance professionalism at your institution?

- How do you ensure accountability for professional behavior?

- What resources and infrastructure have you personally put in place to facilitate EBP at your health system? List two examples of evidence used in nursing leadership practice in the least year.

PRACTICE ANALYSIS

A day-shift nursing director in a large tertiary hospital was reporting off to the night nursing director when an RN called in sick. The RN was scheduled to work on a busy medical–surgical unit. Since there were no other RNs available, the day-shift nursing director communicated this via telephone to the unit charge nurse suggesting that she rearrange assignments to accommodate for the absent RN (the unit was originally intended to be staffed with five RNs [two with <6 months of experience] and two NAs for 36 patients, leaving them with four RNs and two NAs. Furthermore, there were four empty beds and several admitted patients in the emergency department). Specifically, the nursing director asked the charge nurse to assign some extra duties to the two NAs to lighten the remaining RNs' workloads and assign herself to a couple of patients. About 15 minutes later, the charge nurse called the day-shift director to express that one of her scheduled night RNs was distraught about having to work short. She threatened to leave if another RN was not assigned to care for the 36 patients on the unit. Furthermore, the charge nurse communicated that the nurse stated, "I will not continue to put up with this constant shortage of help. It is the number 1 reason everyone quits around here. We are overworked and underpaid, and the hospital management does nothing about it. The patients deserve better. This place needs to be investigated." A senior baccalaureate student who was completing a clinical assignment on the unit and overheard the charge nurse, asked her instructor, "Does this happen often? Doesn't the nursing director have some responsibility for providing the unit with more RNs?" The day-shift director, who had just worked for the last 12 hours, asked the charge nurse to do the best she can to calm down the employee and suggested that the night nursing director would come to check on them as soon as she was able.

- What behaviors did the day nursing director and the distraught staff RN display that were professional and/or unprofessional?
- What about the nursing student?
- Was moral courage displayed in this situation? If so, by whom?
- Were any ethical codes, practice acts, or professional responsibilities violated? If so, what were they?
- How did the relational aspects of the situation demonstrate and/or not demonstrate professionalism?
- If you were the nursing instructor, what would you have communicated to the student?
- What advice do you have for the nurses in this situation?

REFERENCES

Agency for Healthcare Research & Quality. (2019). *Disruptive and unprofessional behavior.* Patient Safety Network. Available at: https://psnet.ahrq.gov/primer/disruptive-and-unprofessional-behavior

Alexis, D. A., Kearney, M. D., Williams, J. C., et al. (2020). Assessment of perceptions of professionalism among faculty, trainees, staff, and students in a large university-based health system. *JAMA Network Open, 3*(11), e2021452. https://doi.org/10.1001/jamanetworkopen.2020.21452

American Association of Colleges of Nursing. (2021). *The essentials: Core competencies for professional nursing education.* Washington, DC: Author. Available at: https://www.aacnnursing.org/Portals/42/AcademicNursing/pdf/Essentials-2021.pdf

American Nurses Association. (2015). *Code of ethics for nurses with interpretive statements.* Washington, DC: Author.

American Nurses Association. (2021). *Nursing: Scope and standards of practice* (4th ed.). Washington, DC: Author.

Chu, L. C. (2021). The influence of compassion fatigue on job performance and organizational citizenship behaviors: The moderating effect of person–job fit. *Journal of Nursing Scholarship, 53,* 500–510. https://doi.org/10.1111/jnu.12644

Cline, M. (2016). Increasing RN accountability in professional practice. *JONA: The Journal of Nursing Administration, 46*(3), 128–131. https://doi.org/10.1097/NNA.0000000000000311

DeWane, M., Waldman, R., & Waldman, S. (2019). Cell phone etiquette in the clinical arena: A professionalism imperative for healthcare. *Current Problems in Pediatric Adolescent Health Care, 49*(4), 79–83. https://doi.org/10.1016/j.cppeds.2019.03.005

Duffy, J. (2016). *Professional practice models in nursing: Successful health system integration.* Springer Publishing Company.

Duffy, J., & Hoskins, L. (2003). The quality-caring model©: Blending dual paradigms. *Advances in Nursing Science, 26*(1), 77–88. https://doi.org/10.1097/00012272-200301000-00010

Duffy, J., Brewer, B., & Weaver, M. (2010). Revision and psychometric properties of the caring assessment tool. *Clinical Nursing Research.* https://doi.org/10.1177/1054773810369827

Duffy, J., Hoskins, L., & Dudley-Brown, S. (2005). Development and testing of a caring-based intervention for older adults with heart failure. *The Journal of Cardiovascular Nursing, 20*(5), 325–333.

Finkelman, A. (2019). *Professional nursing concepts: Competencies for quality leadership* (4th ed.). Jones and Bartlett Learning.

Fitzgerald, A. (2020). Professional identity: A concept analysis. *Nursing Forum, 25*(3), 447–472. https://doi.org/10.1111/nuf.12450

Frost, J. S., Hammer, D. P., Nunez, L. M., et al. (2019). The intersection of professionalism and interprofessional care: Development and initial testing of the interprofessional professionalism assessment (IPA). *Journal of Interprofessional Care, 33*(1), 102–115. https://doi.org/10.1080/13561820.2018.1515733

Fulton, J. (2019). Professional citizenship. *Clinical Nurse Specialist, 33*(4), 153–154. https://doi.org/10.1097/NUR.0000000000000463

Garcia, A. S., Carotta, C. L., Brown, R., et al. (2021). Parenting stress, self-efficacy and COVID-19 health risks as predictors of general stress among nurses. *International Journal of Nursing Practice*, e13009. https://doi.org/10.1111/ijn.13009

Garg, S., Kim, L., Whitaker, M., et al. (2020). Hospitalization rates and characteristics of patients hospitalized with laboratory-confirmed coronavirus disease 2019—COVID-NET, 14 states, March 1–30, 2020. *MMWR Morbidity & Mortality Weekly Report, 69*, 458–464. https://doi.org/10.15585/mmwr.mm6915e3

Godfrey, N., & Young, E. (2020). Professional identity. In J. F. Giddens (Ed.), *Concepts of nursing practice* (3rd ed.). Elsevier Publishing.

Gold, J. A., Rossen, L. M., Ahmad, F. B., et al. (2020). Race, ethnicity, and age trends in persons who died from COVID-19—United States, May–August 2020. *MMWR Mortality & Morbidity Weekly Report 2020, 69*, 1517–1521. http://dx.doi.org/10.15585/mmwr.mm6942e1 external icon.

Gorsuch, C., Gallagher Ford, L., Koshy Thomas, B., et al. (2020). Impact of a formal educational skill-building program based on the ARCC model to enhance evidence-based practice competency in nurse teams. *Worldviews on Evidence-Based Nursing, 17*(4), 258–268. https://doi.org/10.1111/wvn.12463

Greenway, K., Butt, G., & Walthall, H. (2018). What is a theory-practice gap? An exploration of the concept. *Nurse Education in Practice, 34*, 1–6.

Grimley, K. A., Gruebling, N. M., Kurani, A., & Marshall, D. (2021). Nurse sensitive indicators and how COVID-19 influenced practice change. *Nurse Leader, 19*(4), 371–377. https://doi.org/10.1016/j.mnl.2021.05.003

Grus, C. L., Shen-Miller, D., Lease, S. H., et al. (2018). Professionalism: A competency cluster whose time has come. *Ethics & Behavior, 28*(6), 450–464. https://doi.org/10.1080/10508422.2017.1419133

Hafferty, F. W., & Franks, R. (1994). The hidden curriculum, ethics teaching, and the structure of medical education. *Academic Medicine, 69*(11), 861–871.

Heitschmidt, M., Staffileno, B. A., & Kleinpell, R. (2021). Implementing a faculty mentoring process to improve academic-clinical partnerships for nurse led evidence-based practice and research projects. *Journal of Professional Nursing, 37*(2), 399–403. https://doi.org/10.1016/j.profnurs.2020.04.015

Kakemam, E., Ghafari, M., Rouzbahani, M., Zahedi, H., & Roh, Y. S. (2022). The association of professionalism and systems thinking with patient safety competency: A structural equation mode. *Journal of Nursing Management.* https://doi.org/10.1111/jonm.13536

Karaca-Mandic, P., Georgiou, A., & Sen, S. (2021). Assessment of COVID-19 hospitalizations by race/ethnicity in 12 states. *JAMA Internal Medicine, 181*(1), 131–134. https://doi.org/10.1001/jamainternmed.2020.3857

Konetzka, R. T., & Gorges, R. J. (2021). Nothing much has changed: COVID-19 nursing home cases and deaths follow fall surges. *Journal of the American Geriatric Society, 69*(1), 46–47. https://doi.org/10.1111/jgs.16951

Lazarus, R. S., & Folkman, S. (1984). *Stress, appraisal, and coping.* Springer.

Li, Y., Cen, X., Cai, X., & Temkin-Greener, H. (2020). Racial and ethnic disparities in COVID-19 infections and deaths across U.S. nursing homes. *Journal of the American Geriatrics Society, 68*(11), 2454–2461. https://doi.org/10.1111/jgs.16847

Lindell, M. J., Cusatis, B., Edmonson, C., et al. (2021). The nurse leader's role: A conduit for professional identity formation and sustainability. *Nurse Leader, 19*(1), 27–32. https://doi.org/10.1016/j.mnl.2020.10.001

Maxwell, E., & Radford, M. (2021). Long COVID and the ghost of nursing theory. *Journal of Research in Nursing, 26*(5), 362–366. https://doi.org/10.1177/17449871211037473

Melnyk, B. M., Gallagher-Ford, L., Zellefrow, C., et al. (2018). The first U.S. study on nurses' evidence-based practice competencies indicates major deficits that threaten healthcare quality, safety, and patient outcomes. *Worldviews on Evidence-Based Nursing, 15*(1), 16–25. https://doi.org/10.1111/wvn.12269

Melnyk, B. M., Tan, A., Hsieh, A. P., & Gallagher-Ford, L. (2021a). Evidence-based practice culture and mentorship predict EBP implementation, nurse job satisfaction, and intent to stay: Support for the ARCC© model. *Worldviews on Evidence Based Nursing, 18*(4), 272–281. https://doi.org/10.1111/wvn.12524

Melnyk, B. M., Tan, A., Hsieh, A. P., et al. (2021b). Critical care nurses' physical and mental health, worksite wellness support, and medical errors. *American Journal of Critical Care, 30*(3), 176–184. https://doi.org/10.4037/ajcc2021301

Melnyk, B. M., Gallagher-Ford, L., Thomas, B. K., et al. (2016). A study of chief nurse executives indicates low prioritization of evidence-based practice and shortcomings in hospital performance metrics across the United States. *Worldviews on Evidence-Based Nursing, 13*(1), 6–14. https://doi.org/10.1111/wvn.12133

Melzack, R., & Wall, P. D. (1965). Pain mechanisms: A new theory. *Science, 150*(3699), 971–979.

Mensik, J. S., Martin, D. M., Johnson, K. L., et al. (2017). Embedding a professional practice model across a system. *Journal of Nursing Administration, 47*(9), 421–425. https://doi.org/10.1097/NNA.0000000000000508

Miller, B. K. (1988). A model for professionalism in nursing. *Today's or Nurse, 10*(9), 18–23.

National Academies of Sciences, Engineering, and Medicine. (2021). *The future of nursing 2020–2030: Charting a path to achieve health equity.* Washington, DC: The National Academies Press. https://doi.org/10.17226/25982

National Academy of Medicine. (2016). Action collaborative for clinician well-being and resilience. Available at: https://nam.edu/action-collaborative-on-clinician-well-being-and-resilience-network-organizations/

Nickitas, D. M., & Frederickson, K. (2015). Nursing knowledge and theory: Where is the economic value. *Nursing Economics, 33*(4), 190.

Nowlin, S., Rampertaap, K., Lulgjuraj, D., et al. (2021). Willing but not quite ready: Nurses' knowledge, attitudes, and practices of research in an academic healthcare system. *JONA Journal of Nursing Administration, 51*(10), 495–499.

Ogedegbe, G., Ravenell, J., Adhikari, S., et al. (2020). Assessment of racial/ethnic disparities in hospitalization and mortality in patients with COVID-19 in New York City. *JAMA Network Open. 3*(12), e2026881. https://doi.org/10.1001/jamanetworkopen.2020.26881. Available at: https://jamanetwork.com/journals/jamanetworkopen/article-abstract/2773538

Rachel, M. M. (2012). Accountability: A concept worth revisiting. *American Nurse Today, 7*(3), 36–40.

Raso, A., Marchetti, A., D'Angelo, D., et al. (2019). The hidden curriculum in nursing education: A scoping study. *Medical Education, 53*(10), 989–1002. https://doi.org/10.1111/medu.13911

Romano, S. D., Blackstock, A. J., Taylor, E. V., et al. (2021). Trends in racial and ethnic disparities in COVID-19 hospitalizations, by region—United States, March–December 2020. *MMWR. Morbidity and Mortality Weekly Report, 70*(15), 560–565. https://doi.org/10.15585/mmwr.mm7015e2

Rossen, L. M., Branum, A. M., Ahmad, F. B., et al. (2020). Excess deaths associated with COVID-19, by age and race and ethnicity—United States, January 26–October 3, 2020. *MMWR Morbidity & Mortalality Weekly Report, 69*(42), 1522–1527. https://doi.org/10.15585/mmwr.mm6942e2

Saad, L. (2021). Military brass, judges among professions at new image lows. Gallup News. Available at: https://news.gallup.com/poll/388649/military-brass-judges-among-professions-new-image-lows.aspx

Semper, J., Halvorson, B., Hersh, M., Torres, C., & Lillington, L. (2016). Clinical nurse specialists guide staff nurses to promote practice accountability through peer review. *Clinical Nurse Specialist, 30*(1), 19–27. https://doi.org/10.1097/NUR.0000000000000157

Shechter, A., Diaz, F., Moise, N., Anstey, D. E., Ye, S., Agarwal, S., … , & Abdalla, M. (2020). Psychological distress, coping behaviors, and preferences for support among New York healthcare workers during the COVID-19 pandemic. *General Hospital Psychiatry, 66*, 1–8. https://doi.org/10.1016/j.genhosppsych.2020.06.007

Sherman, R., & Cohn, T. (2019). Promoting professional accountability and ownership. *American Nurse Today, 14*(2), 24–26.

Silveira, G. L., Campos, L. K. S., Schweller, M., et al. (2019). "Speed up"! The influences of the hidden curriculum on the professional identity development of medical students. *Health Professions Education, 5*(3), 198–209. https://doi.org/10.1016/j.hpe.2018.07.003

Smith, M. A. (2017). The ethics/advocacy connection. *Nursing Management, 48*(8), 18–23. https://doi.org/10.1097/01.NUMA.0000521571.43055.38

Smith, M. A. (2020). *Nursing theories and nursing practice* (5th ed.). F.A. Davis.

Trockel, M. T., Menon, N. K., Rowe, S. G., et al. (2020). Assessment of physician sleep and wellness, burnout, and clinically significant medical errors. *JAMA Network Open, 3*(12), e2028111. https://doi.org/10.1001/jamanetworkopen.2020.28111

Webb Hooper, M., Nápoles, A. M., & Pérez-Stable, E. J. (2020). COVID-19 and racial/ethnic disparities. *Journal of the American Medical Association, 323*, 2466–2467. https://doi.org/10.1001/jama.2020.8598

Wolf, Z. R. (2012). Nursing practice breakdown: Good and bad nursing. *MedSurg Nursing, 21*(1), 16–36.

Wolverton, C. L., Lasiter, S., Duffy, J. R., Weaver, M. T., & McDaniel, A. M. (2018). Psychometric testing of the caring assessment tool: Administration (CAT-Adm©). *SAGE Open Medicine.* https://doi.org/10.1177/2050312118760739

Zieber, M., & Wojtowicz, B. (2020). To dwell within: Bridging the theory–practice gap. *Nursing Philosophy, 21*(2), 1–4. https://doi.org/10.1111/nup.12296

CHAPTER 3

Evolution of the Quality-Caring Model©

"Caring can be learned by all human beings, can be worked into the design of every life, meeting an individual's need as well as a pervasive need in society."

—Mary Catherine Bateson

CHAPTER OBJECTIVES:

1. Evaluate the relationship between complex adaptive systems and health systems
2. Describe the evolution of the Quality-Caring Model
3. Define the four major concepts in the Quality-Caring Model
4. Analyze the role of the nurse reflected in the Quality-Caring Model

COMPLEX HEALTH SYSTEMS

A complex system comprises a large number of parts, often called agents, that continuously interact, adapt, and learn (Holland, 2006, p. 24), much like health systems. Complexity in this sense refers to the valuable and dynamic interconnectivity among the many parts of a system that often transforms them in unexpected and irreversible ways (Uhl-Bien & Arena, 2017). Health systems, in particular, are composed of multiple systems—individuals, groups, departments (or units), organizations, the larger community and societal systems. Furthermore, health systems are open systems allowing for contextual information and feedback to interact with the system's many agents. It follows, then, that the delivery of healthcare is not a linear process, but rather a complex and dynamic process that allows for continual interaction, contextual influences, relationship forming and remodeling, feedback among the many parts and the larger society, pattern development, and adaptation. Thus, healthcare systems are unpredictable; processes and practices emerge in unexpected ways, unit-based rules arise and adapt over time, and the system is sometimes beset by random events that occasionally generate turmoil.

Complexity science is the study of complex systems, especially adaptations to the constantly changing context or environment. Complex adaptive systems

(CAS) refer to the application of complexity science to living, dynamic systems (e.g., health and health systems). As such, emerging patterns can be grasped as the many agents (or individual parts) use "simple rules" from the "bottom up" without external control (Martin, 2018). The emerging patterns in a CAS are often unobservable until their effects are made manifest as "self-organizing" systems. Emerging patterns inform behaviors and over time, these accumulated experiences and their resultant performance enable adaptations that shape the evolution of the system. Often during this process, unexpected behaviors surface in ways that can neither be predicted nor controlled. This dynamic allows for the process of self-organization as new patterns of behavior, labeled *emergence or co-emergence* form (Institute of Medicine, 2001; Mahajan et al., 2017).

In essence, emergence refers to the collective ability of individual agents who work and relate together to spontaneously generate dramatically different actions that are greater than the sum of their individual parts (Pines, 2014). In this way, emergent behavior is a property of a system that is at a different scale than the parts of the system (Carmichael & Hadžikadić, 2019). Finally, emergence transpires in concert with the environment and without a specified leader.

Thus, CASs are flexible and often ambiguous systems with feedback loops open to energy and information from the environment enabling adaptation, learning, and growth (Begun & Jiang, 2020). As human experiences in health systems are often unpredictable or nonlinear, health professionals who work in them are constantly co-emerging. For example, during the COVID-19 pandemic, a seemingly small, unexpected event in one part of the world spread at a rapid pace, generating a substantial influence on the daily operations of health systems internationally. Individual agents adapted to this by reaching out to others and sharing and networking with health professionals globally (interaction and connection). Gradually, new relationships and interdependencies formed. Over time, through continuous interaction, new patterns of behavior formed (emergence) and manifested in new treatment modalities and innovative adjustments to supply chains, staffing, and capacity. In some cases, new leaders emerged, and more tightly knit groups of health professionals were formed. Interestingly, these diverse agents interacted in a manner that allowed for creative adaptations and did so in an unpredictable manner that did not require centralized control. The nursing profession has long emphasized and valued connections and interactions within a systems paradigm and has a long, rich tradition of appreciating patterns. Healthcare in general is now recognized as a CAS because of the dynamic network of interactions needed to execute complex plans of care, both for individuals and groups (i.e., patient populations; Ratnapalan & Lang, 2020).

In fact, in the larger health system context, connections and relationships continuously occur in a complex, dynamically changing environment. Over time, the interaction of multiple individuals fosters collective learning from that context and re-influences the context to better prepare for future advancement. However, as a health system is embedded within its context, when one part of the health system changes, so does the context in a constant interplay of coexisting correction or revision. This intricacy of interdependent related parts, together with the constant flux of the external environment, creates a natural cycle of coevolution such that the system and the agents within it evolve (or coevolve) together over time (Lindberg et al., 2008; Marshall & Broome, 2016). For example, in a health system where a new service is introduced, operationalization of the new service (including the involved patients and employees) will coevolve over time as each interacts with the other and learns to adapt.

In the social systems of healthcare, interactions among various team members affect the processes and outcomes of work. Sociologists have labeled this phenomenon the social network theory and use this as a framework for analysis (Freeman, 2004; Knoke & Yang, 2020; Scott, 2000; Valente & Pitts, 2017; Wasserman & Faust, 1994). In social networks, individuals (nodes) and their relationships/connections (ties) influence how information is relayed, the performance of professionals, and ultimately quality and safety outcomes (Cunningham et al., 2012). In fact, in this systematic review, evidence for cohesive and collaborative health professional networks facilitating the coordination of care and contributing to improved quality and safety of care was apparent (Cunningham et al., 2012).

Individual health professionals are often influenced by their social networks to adopt new practices that affect their work life, some positive and others negative. Change of shift reporting between hospital nurses in a department, for example, can be influenced by the social relationships among the nurses, ultimately affecting the accuracy and efficiency of the patient information that is transmitted. In this case, the shift report can take on a life of its own, explaining how a report on one hospital unit differs from the shift report on other units, undermining quality. Increasingly, the many complexities of modern health systems and society, in general, warrant attending to the complexity, communication and collaboration, groups, interactions, processes, and distributed control, aka *relationships*!

Accordingly, because of the many connections among nursing (and other health professions), patients, organizations, and communities, including interactions among their respective social groups, the Quality-Caring Model© (QCM) has evolved from its initiation in 2003. Once depicted in a linear format between patients and care providers, it is now situated within several relationships, social structures, and the environment (context). These relationships form a complex web of connections common to healthcare with open boundaries among them. The many relationships that characterize health systems and their environments (see Figure 3.1) influence the application of the QCM, enabling adaptations that shape the evolution of healthcare professionals, the performance of departments and the system, the community, and the model itself.

Healthcare providers and patients, however, serve as individual systems (or agents) who cocreate social systems during healthcare encounters. For example, healthcare encounters typically occur between agents within hospital departments or units, medical offices, or homes/schools (microsystems) that coexist in larger healthcare organizations that are connected yet again to local communities, and ultimately, to the larger global society. These multiple social systems continually interact, form relationships, interact with the changing context, and generate feedback that informs the development of new ways of being. Interestingly, the ongoing interaction, relationship-building, and continuous learning that occurs among the many connections in health systems (interdependencies) organizes from the bottom up, shaping them and their environment. Thus, relationships between and among healthcare subsystems emerge on their own, with varying

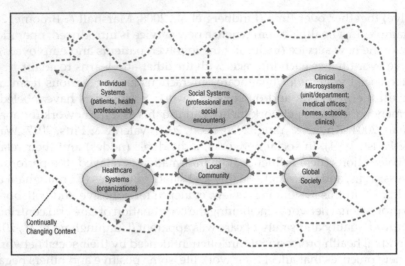

FIGURE 3.1 Complex web of social connections in health systems.

features that influence their performance. This is not complicated, but rather a straightforward tenet that affirms the significant influence that relationships and connections play in the progress of health systems. It also demonstrates the lack of outside control that is necessary to evolve or advance. This is a particularly difficult concept for health professionals and their leaders, who are used to continually anticipating and controlling. The continual interaction, reshaping, feedback, and adaptation common to relationships in complex systems actually creates the energy (or flow) required to sustain the system and expedite its advancement.

As an example, seemingly small improvements in a unit (such as improved responses to patients' pain), if attended to and nurtured, may take hold, multiply, and shift to other departments. For this to happen in an efficient manner, however, reactions to this new behavior must be quick, direct, and show benefit. Thus, for those in leadership positions, feedback mechanisms that are delayed or generated through a third party will not be as effective as those that are disseminated directly to clinicians who are providing the care. In this example, the leadership effort is best concentrated at the local level (vs. upper organizational levels), supporting health professionals in their efforts to improve response times to patients' reports of pain. Another example of the power of relationships is that observed among nurses in a particular unit consistently and genuinely collaborating with physicians during rounds. Over time, the physicians will actively seek out nurses and their opinions, and the nurses will integrate it into their routines (personal observation).

At all points in the larger health system, application of the QCM can be observed and evaluated for effects on overall system progress or advancement. Developed as an approach to the professional practice of nursing, the QCM has also been used at the organizational level with many health professionals attuned to its concepts. For example, in one large organization that uses the model to guide overall professional practice, board members who greatly believed in the QCM model, devoted an entire annual meeting to its integration in the system!

THE EVOLVING QUALITY-CARING MODEL

The philosophical and theoretical underpinnings of the QCM remain rooted in models of healthcare quality (Donabedian, 1966; Institute of Medicine [IOM], 2001; Lachman et al., 2020); the relational aspects of nursing (Irvine et al., 1998; King, 1981; Peplau, 1988; Swanson, 1993; Watson, 1979); but more recently are influenced by the complexity theory (Plsek & Greenhalgh, 2001), often associated with the continuously evolving health system. The model also reflects and is consistent with the newly developed professional nursing model (American Nurses Association [ANA], 2021, p. 10), which espouses the continuously evolving and transforming nature of nursing.

Human experiences of health and illness are not simple, linear, or predictable. The interaction of physiological, psychological, sociocultural, and spiritual systems, together with environmental situations, force us to recognize the complexity of not only healthcare itself, but also of our place in it, including the meaning of our work to the larger world. In essence, the relationships and interactions among the agents in the healthcare system are viewed as fundamental and central to its operations and require different approaches to clinical practice, leadership, education, change, and ongoing professional development. Although the term *quality* was originally defined as excellence or worthiness of a service (Duffy, 2009), it is now seen as a broader construct that incorporates the concepts of safety, value, adaptive capacity, and centers on patients and their families. In this perspective, quality is not an endpoint per se, but a relational *process* of connecting, continuously interacting, collaborating, appreciating and learning, translating, adjusting practice (adaptation), emerging and co-emerging, and self-organizing or self-advancing. Such a broad view connotes a dynamic system that mutually interacts with patients as full partners, in which teams of health professionals collaborate with patients/families to coproduce health and healing, where health professionals attend to their own health and well-being, and where transparent service, founded on enduring values, serves the larger community (Lachman et al., 2020).

Through continuous improvement processes, individual patients and healthcare providers attend to revising their behaviors using internal and external evidence as guides, generating practice changes that are ongoing and innovative, allowing for natural self-advancement. Collectively, these individual agents facilitate continuous learning, contributing to ongoing progress or quality.

Healthcare learning organizations are characterized as systematic, data driven, knowledge-based, using best evidence, innovative, focused on value, engaged, and active. They are powered by a culture that focuses on shared learning that is integrated into everyday work activities/routines. Additionally, healthcare learning organizations align science, informatics, patient-clinician partnerships, incentives, and culture to enable continuous, *real-time* improvement in both effectiveness and efficiency (Institute of Medicine, 2013, p. 17). As such, healthcare learning organizations are able to leverage organizational knowledge to innovate, compete, co-create, and build capacity (behavioral, social, and informational) for rapid improvements that generate value for patients and families as well as employees. From an individual healthcare professional perspective, continuous learning and the resultant change in practice not only meets a professional responsibility, but also adds meaning to the work, influencing quality—see Chapter 8 for more information on learning health systems.

Today's technological advances enable patients, individual health professionals, departments, and whole health systems to regularly gather, analyze, and disseminate internal data. Furthermore, regular external benchmarking and access to current research are customary features of health systems that are available to guide practice improvement. From the individual health professional's perspective, this implies that all are actively involved in improving their practice, including those parts that interact with other health professionals. Using knowledge to advance practice helps one learn about themself and ensures that patients and families are provided the highest value. An open and safe environment for inquiry and regular reflection facilitates such a practice.

An environment of inquiry engages health professionals in discussions, allows for education and development of new ideas, regular reflection on practice, and encourages pilot studies that test feasibility of new approaches. Of course, leadership is key to *promoting* an environment of inquiry through supportive infrastructure, but uses the natural properties of complex systems to work together with direct care clinicians. Thus, healthcare learning organizations focus their efforts on supporting continuous inquiry, the use of internal and external data, regular reflection, and relationships to forge learning among its agents. Such learning facilitates safety, improvements in efficiency and effectiveness, and most importantly adds value, all features of *valuable* health systems that serve larger communities. A key feature of this process is the *quality* of relationships among its agents.

BOX 3.1: Caring is often used to characterize healthcare relationships as it is implicitly tied to the relational nature of human beings, who are multidimensional beings worthy of our ongoing consideration. Caring relationships, when attended to and sustained, facilitate advancement of individual, social, micro, organizational, community, and societal systems.

In healthcare, caring relationships are fundamental to service. In fact, caring relationships have been described as therapeutic, and when not applied, are often reported to increase psychological distress, anxiety, feelings of dehumanization, and even some physical symptoms (Dieppe et al., 2020). Many individuals equate caring with adjectives such as kindness, concern, and empathy—considered an intangible concept or "soft" science by some. However, real caring is hard work and is nursing's primary work, as explicitly stated in the newly revised definition of nursing (ANA, 2021, p. 1). Other health professionals also establish caring relationships with patients and must be recognized for this; however, nursing, in many healthcare environments, is the only health profession that maintains a 24/7 presence, has the most direct contact with patients and families, is a stabilizing force in a fragmented health system, and remains very influential in the prevention of adverse outcomes (Carthon et al., 2021; Lasater et al., 2020; Rosenkoetter, 2016). Caring is the foundation of nurses' work and remains a crucial phenomenon that is expressed daily in the attitudes, behaviors, and skills of professional nurses.

Caring is a process that involves the human person of the nurse connecting to the human person of the patient. This reciprocal relationship forms the foundation for all nursing practice and generates "feeling cared for," a positive emotion experienced by both the patient and the nurse. It is this feeling of being "cared for" that gives rise to patients' sentiments that they *matter* in the complex health system and is an important performance indicator of high-quality nursing care. This mattering concept is also fundamental to nurses themselves in terms of lower levels of burnout (Haizlip et al., 2020).

For such a fundamental component of practice, caring relationships are not often measured as an indicator of professional performance (Duffy et al., 2012). However, patients and families know when it is lacking (Baird et al., 2016). It is most often associated with "basic nursing care" or those seemingly inconsequential routine activities that professional nurses often delegate to unlicensed assistive personnel. Yet, caring relationships honor the dignity of human persons and provide the energy for future interactions (required for person-centered care), create a spirit of transparency (necessary ingredient for safety cultures), and enable the conditions for advancement (may help patients better participate in care and attain health goals while engaging employees in meaningful practice). These are beneficial and progressive consequences that contribute to the value of a health system. However, since the health system is still so focused on disease, cures, technology, and finances, we often fail to notice the advantages associated with its more routine (or buried) aspects of caring for human beings.

A more optimistic and broad-minded view may help nursing appreciate its strengths, including specifically how it contributes to the larger whole. Furthermore, acknowledging strengths (vs. limitations) may stimulate more innovative approaches to practice change. To reinforce and intensify human caring in health systems, this essential relational process of nursing must be valued, consistently applied, tied to outcomes, and rewarded.

In summary then, the term *quality* in the evolving QCM is viewed as a dynamic process of learning that is fully embedded in practice and is evidenced in the attainment of specific health goals. It uses qualitative and quantitative evaluative techniques to provide the data required for actionable practice changes. *Caring* is a seminal component of nursing practice that, together with continuous learning (and resultant practice improvement), facilitates *feeling cared for* and, ultimately, *self-advancing* individuals, communities, and health systems.

ASSUMPTIONS, MAJOR CONCEPTS, AND PROPOSITIONS OF THE QUALITY-CARING MODEL

Assumptions

Assumptions of a model include the underlying values and beliefs that are used as premises for its development. In the QCM, they include the following:

- Humans are multidimensional beings capable of growth and change.
- Humans exist in relationship with themselves, others, communities or groups, the environment (including the workplace), and the larger universe.

- Humans evolve in a dynamic and interconnected manner.
- Humans are inherently worthy.
- Caring relationships require intent, specialized knowledge, and deliberate use of time.
- Caring for self is a prerequisite for caring relationships with others, including patients.
- Caring relationships are naturally self-caring or self-healing.
- Caring consists of interpersonal processes that are used individually or in combination and often concurrently.
- Caring is a social process that is done "in relationship."
- Caring for self enhances caring for others.
- Caring relationships are protective.
- Caring is embedded in the daily work of professional nursing.
- Professional nursing work is done in the context of human relationships.
- The display of caring relationships varies.
- Caring is a tangible concept that can be measured.
- Caring relationships benefit both the carer and the one being cared for.
- Caring relationships benefit society.
- Feeling "cared for" is a positive emotion.
- Feeling "cared for" is adaptive for individuals, groups, and systems.
- Self-advancing systems evolve over time and in context.

Major Model Concepts

Major concepts are those ideas or components that form the essence of the model. In the QCM, the four major concepts are humans in relationship, relationship-centered professional encounters, feeling "cared for," and self-advancing systems (see Figure 3.2). Humans, with their unique beliefs, attitudes, behaviors, physical attributes, and life experiences, are holistic in nature and relate throughout their lives to others, including their families and communities, and the larger universe.

During illness or suffering, specific health characteristics (such as severity of illness, years living with a disease, social determinants of health, and number of comorbidities) and the aforementioned unique individual characteristics become important considerations since they may impact processes and outcomes of care. Through their many relationships, individuals live, work, and die, and if caring in nature, relationships enable individuals to persist, progress, evolve, achieve healthy states, and advance. If, however, those relationships are uncaring, individuals may respond by withdrawing or falling behind or even becoming ill.

In healthcare professional encounters, persons with health needs relate to healthcare providers who function independently and collaboratively with

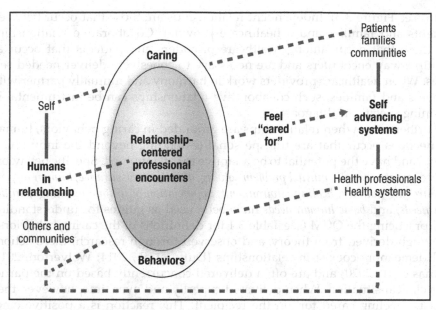

FIGURE 3.2 Quality-Caring Model©.

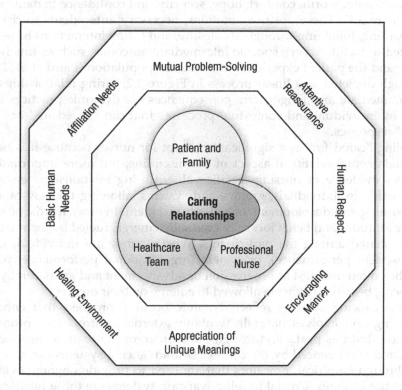

FIGURE 3.3 Caring relationship-centered professional encounters.

them (see Figure 3.3). Independent relationships are those that occur between patients and families and a healthcare provider. Collaborative relationships are those that occur among healthcare providers and patients that occur as multiple-way encounters and are necessary to cohesively deliver needed services. When healthcare providers work in harmony and mutually partner with patients and families, such collaborative relationships can be instrumental in attaining specific health goals.

Furthermore, when relationships are grounded in caring behaviors, human connections occur that are transpersonal (extending beyond the individuals alone) and have the potential to be adaptive for all involved. Specific behaviors or processes, namely, *mutual problem solving, attentive reassurance, human respect, encouraging manner, healing environment, appreciation of unique meanings, affiliation needs,* and *basic human needs* have been used as guides for understanding and practicing the QCM (see Table 3.1 for definitions of the caring behaviors). Although derived from theory, and observed through research, these actions and demeanors coexist in relationships (Duffy et al., 2014; Wolverton, 2018; Salinas et al., 2020) and are often delivered concurrently based on the particular clinical situation. When delivered expertly and over time, however, they lead to "feeling cared for" in the recipient. This reaction is a positive emotion generated as a result of the caring processes (Duffy, 2018) that leads to feelings of ease, worth, comfort, hope, security, and confidence to name a few (see Figure 3.4). These positive emotions, necessary antecedents to risk-taking, learning, following-through, disclosure, and future interactions have been reported to facilitate very specific intermediate outcomes such as timely discharge and the patient experience in the stroke population (Baird et al., 2016). Although depicted as a linear process in Figure 3.2, caring relationships and their immediate and longer term consequences are dynamic practices influenced by individual and contextual processes that can "speed up" or "slow down" responses.

Feeling "cared for" is a significant concept for nurses because it is tied to the fundamental relational aspect of the discipline; but more importantly, it provides evidence of nursing-specific value. Caring relationships engender this reaction in individuals, groups, and systems, allowing for new capabilities, learning and development, or self-advancement. In other words, new and unique attitudes and behaviors may gradually emerge, fueled by the relational energy shared among the participants. Whether they are individual, group (microsystem performance), or system (organizational performance) behaviors, they often manifest as progression or advancement and are naturally self-advancing because they were allowed to emerge on their own.

Self-advancing systems reflect dynamic positive progress that enhances well-being and evolves naturally without external control. This process is not linear, but has peaks and troughs, and emerges gradually over time and space, and is influenced by the context. Self-advancing systems can be evaluated through empirical indicators that are used to provide ongoing evidence for practice changes. Crucial to self-advancing systems are those relationship-centered professional encounters that are grounded in caring and enable attainment of feeling "cared for."

TABLE 3.1 Definitions of the Caring Behaviors

Caring Behaviors	Definitions
Mutual problem solving	Behaviors that help patients and caregivers understand how to confront, learn, think about, and act in relation to their health and illness. Providing information, reframing, facilitating learning, exploring alternatives, brainstorming together, deciding what questions to ask, validating, accepting feedback from patients, and experimenting with different approaches all involve mutual input and participation from *both* patients and health professionals. This factor implies that health professionals are informed, actively listen, are continuously learning, and engaged.
Attentive reassurance	Behaviors that assure patients that they can rely on health professionals. These include availability, displaying a hopeful outlook, exhibiting confidence, regular surveillance, conveying possibilities, being actively present, and paying attention. This factor implies that health professionals postpone action long enough to be authentically accessible to notice, actively listen, focus, and to concentrate fully on the patient in a particular moment.
Human respect	This behavior refers to honoring the worth of human persons through unconditional acceptance, kind and careful handling of the human body, recognition of rights and responsibilities, and appreciation of the *whole* human person (body, mind, and spirit). This involves performing holistic assessment and engaging the patient/family in planning, implementation, and evaluation of care. The health professional attends to the self, models self-caring, reflects on self as it relates to professional practice, and displays healthy lifestyle behaviors.
Encouraging manner	An affective behavior consisting of the demeanor or attitude of the health professional and expressed through verbal and nonverbal messages of support, positive thoughts and feelings, openness, belief in the patient and the health system, tolerance for both positive and negative feelings, creation of "safe space," reinforcement, and praise. Patient/family self-caring is supported.
Appreciation of unique meanings	Concerned with a person's context or worldview. Knowing what is important to patients, including their distinctive sociocultural connections; avoidance of assumptions; acknowledging the subjective value placed on persons, situations, or events; distinguishing how social determinants of health impact care received; inclusive; consider health literacy when designing plan of care, demonstrate cultural sensitivity; recognize the significance of the patient's frame of reference and using that in the provision of care.
Healing environment	Refers to the surroundings where care is taking place, including the setting, spaces, stressors (noise, lighting), just culture, workflow, and structures for maintaining privacy, safety, aesthetics, confidentiality, and quality; includes the context for learning, adapting, and improving practice.
Basic human needs	Recognizing and responding to the primacy of those needs identified by Maslow (1954): Physical needs, safety and security needs, social and relational needs, self-esteem, and self-actualization.
Affiliation needs	An individual's needs for belonging and membership in families or other social contexts (including the health system). Includes appreciation and engagement of the family/caregivers and employees in the healthcare situation, decision making, and participation in care.

Source: Maslow, A. (1954). *Motivation and personality*. Harper.

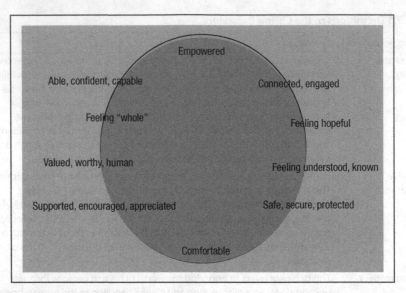

FIGURE 3.4 Feeling "cared for."

Propositions of the Quality-Caring Model

Propositions are those relational statements that tie model concepts to each other and in some instances can be the basis for hypothesis testing. Propositions of the QCM include the following:

- Human caring capacity can be improved.
- Caring relationships are composed of processes or behaviors that can be observed.
- Caring for self supports individual self-advancement
- Engagement in communities through caring relationships enhances self-caring.
- Independent caring relationships between patients and healthcare providers influence feeling "cared for."
- Collaborative caring relationships among nurses and members of the healthcare team enhance team cohesiveness.
- Caring relationships influence healthy behaviors.
- Caring relationships influence feeling "cared for" in the recipient.
- Caring relationships facilitate change.
- Feeling "cared for" facilitates cooperation, engagement, and disclosure in recipients.
- Feeling "cared for" is an antecedent to self-advancing systems.
- Feeling "cared for" contributes to individual, group, and system self-advancement.
- Caring relationships generate feeling "cared for."

■ Caring relationships influence advancement.

■ Feeling "cared for" positively influences self-advancing systems.

ROLE OF THE NURSE

The overall role of the professional nurse applying the QCM is to competently engage in caring relationships with self and others, enabling feelings of being "cared for" in recipients. Such actions are theorized to positively influence intermediate ("feeling cared for") and terminal health outcomes (self-advancing systems), including those that are nursing sensitive. Some specific examples of professional nursing responsibilities include the following:

■ Recognize and attend to the wholeness of human persons, including oneself, other health professionals, and the community served.

■ Apply knowledge of the QCM as the foundation for nursing practice.

■ Attain and continuously advance knowledge and competency in caring processes.

■ Articulate the unique contribution of nursing to patient outcomes

■ Initiate, cultivate, and sustain caring relationships (as evidenced by the caring behaviors) with patients and families, members of the healthcare team, and the community served.

■ Maintain an ongoing awareness of the patient's and the family's point of view.

■ Persist in self-caring activities, including personal and professional development.

■ Integrate caring relationships with specific evidence based nursing interventions to positively influence health outcomes.

■ Engage in continuous learning and practice improvement, using best available evidence.

■ Collaborate in a caring manner with interprofessional team members.

■ Use caring relationships to enhance the professional work environment.

■ Use the expertise of caring relationships embedded in nursing to actively participate in community groups.

■ Ensure safe, equitable, quality, and person-centered healthcare.

■ Exhibit accountability for safe, equitable, quality, and patient-centered care delivery.

■ Contribute to the knowledge of caring and, ultimately, to health systems using all forms of knowing, including research.

■ Maintain an open and flexible perspective.

■ Mentor others in caring professional practice.

■ Advocate for the inclusion of patients and their families in healthcare decisions.

■ Use measures of caring to evaluate professional practice.

This partial list of nursing responsibilities is presented as an example of quality caring professional nursing practice. Notice that it is written in a competency format that can be observed in practice and possibly leveled for career advancement programs. In health systems using the QCM as the foundation for their practice, the above list may provide the first step toward revising performance expectations, job descriptions, annual competency reviews, and promotions; distinguish among varying nursing roles; and serve as a resource for those interested in future nursing careers.

HOPEFUL INSIGHTS FOR A MORE CARING FUTURE

The complexity and uncertainty that currently characterizes the U.S. health system at the time of this writing appears gloomy and discouraging to some. For example, at present, many health professionals are leaving their employment, others are retiring early, and some are re-examining their "desire to serve" (Warden et al., 2021; Smiley et al., 2021). In light of this instability and unpredictability, many questions are emerging, such as:

- How will a new health system affect resources, including the healthcare workforce? How will healthcare be delivered in the face of financial instability, increased use of technology, and empowered consumers?
- How will the profession of nursing be situated in a post-pandemic health system?
- How will we best educate future nurses with less nursing faculty?
- How can we best optimize patient experience and reduce adverse events?
- How will health professionals be supported in the workplace of the future? What specifically will this look like?

These unanswered questions impact the unique cultures of health systems and give rise to an uneasiness that is palpable in the workplace. Health professionals and their leaders are tired, many are disengaged, leaders come and go, new gimmicks are tried each week in an effort to boost system outcomes, and there is a sense that healthcare may never be the same again. In fact, some have hinted that the "new normal" usually seen after crises will not be normal at all, but rather, merely "new"—something not seen before. Professional nurses report that time spent with patients and families has declined significantly relative to other demands during COVID-19, and this presents a source of concern that many find is tied to less meaningful work (Hoogendoorn et al., 2021). Patients and families are not consistently receiving the care they need and often report less than desirable hospital experiences (see Chapter 1). Sometimes, it seems as if the current status of health systems is losing ground.

BOX 3.2: It is precisely at these times of doubt that deeply held beliefs or philosophical values can provide direction. Rather than simply rearranging the deck chairs or removing oneself from the unpleasantness, being alert to and intentionally engaging disciplinary core beliefs productively, promotes the capacity to respond. Intentionally caring (for self and others) may, in fact, facilitate successful adaptations or adjustments that lead to the development of novel and innovative patterns of behavior. Practicing nursing's most deeply held values recovers and strengthens our soul!

Many nursing pioneers have espoused the relational aspect of nursing as the core or central most fundamental component of the discipline (King, 1981; Peplau, 1988; Travelbee, 1966; Watson, 1979, 1985, 2012), and patients consistently point out that it is important to them (Tuominen et al., 2020; Ng, 2020). The QCM is derived in part from those early pioneers in nursing who believed that while nursing draws on other disciplines, it is, by its very nature, an assistive and compassionate discipline that provides services in the context of relationships. The QCM is now 18 years old and has been used as the theoretical framework in many PhD dissertations and Doctor of Nursing Practice (DNP) scholarly projects, master's theory classes, as a guide for undergraduate students' honors' projects, as the framework for the development of nursing interventions, and to guide research studies. It has been used to develop measures of caring from the perspectives of patients, nurses, and students; some of these measures have been translated into Spanish and Japanese. Most notably, the model has been adopted in over 60 U.S. hospitals to guide professional practice. Several of these organizations have gone on to achieve Magnet® designation, while others have now changed their professional practice model to incorporate the QCM *after* initial Magnet designation. The QCM has undergone some expected revisions and much more work needs to be done relative to its validation, but there are promising signs of its adoption among many nurses and health systems.

Many organizations (community hospitals, academic medical centers, and educational institutions) and countless health professionals who have integrated or are in the process of adopting a more relationship-centric approach to practice have shared their experiences with this author. The common thread was that systematic integration of the QCM demonstrated increased benefit to patients and families, health professionals, and health systems.

Below are some examples:

- In one mid-Atlantic academic medical center that has adopted the QCM, integration of model components into nurses' clinical workflow is beginning to show positive improvement in patients' experiences of care (as evidenced by HCAHPS scores) (Centers for Medicare and Medicaid Services, 2014).

- In another hospital, nurse researchers are using the model to evaluate "feeling cared for" in the workplace. Specifically, they are evaluating the perceptions of staff nurses of their leaders' use of caring behaviors; analysis will drive performance improvement plans.

- Another large academic health system is using a systematic pre-post assessment strategy to assess patients' perceptions of "feeling cared for" followed by specific integration approaches. Their findings will provide very useful guidance for future integration of professional practice models into health systems.

- Interestingly, clinical nurses who provide care for specific populations are beginning to examine how caring behaviors are manifested in their work. In one such example, a secondary analysis of data from guided interviews was performed to validate whether discrete behaviors described by stroke patients as generating the emotion of "feeling cared for" were consistent with the theory. In most instances, there was agreement with some overlap among the behaviors (Salinas et al., 2020).

- A shining example of consistent Quality-Caring Professional Practice is evident at the MD Anderson Cancer Center in Houston, Texas, where, since 2001, the nursing organization has earned five consecutive Magnet redesignations, making it one of only 20 organizations nationwide to achieve this status. The QCM undergirds its professional practice model and Quality Caring excellence awards have been accepted by nurses annually for the last 15 years! During this time, MD Anderson has received national awards from Press Ganey for excellence in patient and ambulatory patient experience. Remarkably, the model remains in place after 18 years, even after a major nursing leadership transition, pointing to its hold on patient care delivery.

- Two large nursing organizations, namely the Association of Women's Health, Obstetric and Neonatal Nurses (AWHONN) and the International Association of Forensic Nurses (IAFN) have adopted the QCM to guide practice and evaluation of care (AWHONN, 2014; IAFN, 2021). The National TeleNursing Center (NTC) associated with IAFN's Sexual Assault Nurse Examiner (SANE) Program in Massachusetts recently completed a demonstration project in which the NTC integrated the QCM to support the delivery of teleSANE services (US Department of Justice [DOJ]) (Meunier-Sham et al., 2019). Based on their successful outcomes, the DOJ implemented another funding opportunity in four states to continue the program with the NTC as a consultant (Office for Victims of Crime, 2021; United States Office of Justice Programs, 2017). The use of the QCM was a criteria for the award!

- A recently published report used a cross-sectional, correlational design to examine the relationship between staff nurses' perceptions of nurse manager caring behaviors and patient experience. Although limited by the sample size, the results showed that in hospital departments where staff nurses rated their manager higher in caring, better overall HCAHPS scores were reported. Furthermore, the more staff nurses reported actually interacting with their nurse manager during a shift, the more they perceived their nurse manager as caring (Kostich et al., 2021).

- Another recently published article by staff nurses working in a community hospital examined nurses' self-caring practices. Using a convenient online survey, findings showed that nurses rarely rated their own self-caring at the highest levels; however, older registered nurses (RNs) reported more self-caring practices (Davis et al., 2022). More work is being done in relation to this finding.

Of note in these examples is the mounting evidence reporting (albeit preliminary) by several clinical nurses. Many organizations using the QCM as the foundation for practice have clinical nurses who are leading members of their communities serving on local boards and nonprofit agencies. Furthermore, professional nurses at these organizations have been engaged in leading the dissemination of results of their work with the model and creatively designing programs and interventions that promote relationship-centered practice. Daisy awards (The Daisy Foundation, 2012) abound in organizations that use the QCM, with nurses who relate to patients and families in a caring manner being recognized most often . One medical center so embraces the model that it has become the basis for all health professionals' practice. Another academic medical center has provided funding to create an endowed professorship to advance the use of the QCM, including its contributions to research and evidence-based practice.

Health systems use the caring assessment tool (CAT; Duffy et al., 2014) to evaluate feeling "cared for" during hospitalization and at discharge are using these results to improve nursing practice. Some even use the tool in nursing portfolios designed for clinical advancement, and one large well-known academic medical center has consistently used the CAT—Admin Version (CAT-adm; Duffy, 2008; Wolverton, 2018) annually for the last 10 years to evaluate the caring behaviors of the leadership team.

These successful health systems are only a few of the many that are leading the way to a "new" relationship-centric future, one that is optimistic and offers promising practice revisions that if evidenced as beneficial, may reshape the larger health system.

SUMMARY

The QCM has evolved as expected since its introduction over 18 years ago, more recently influenced by complexity science and sociological structures. The terms *quality* and *caring* are redefined as dynamic *processes*, with caring relationships remaining the central, organizing component of nursing work. Relationship-centered professional encounters are situated within larger health systems and are influenced by this ever-changing context. Some revisions have been made to model assumptions and propositional statements and the concept, feeling "cared for," and its consequences are explained. Examples of potential roles of nursing are highlighted and instances from health systems using the QCM as the foundation for professional practice are revealed.

CALL TO ACTION

Complex health systems demand caring relationships. **Notice** what you are doing and what you are **not doing**. Caring for patients and families is a complex social process that remains the foundation of nursing work. Appreciating the impact of health and illness on patients' holistic nature is an underlying premise of caring relationships. **Observe** how illness is affecting the physical, emotional, social, cultural, and spiritual dimensions of both yourself and your next patient. Reliably implementing caring interpersonal relationships with members of the health team is a nursing responsibility according to the QCM. Practicing this upholds each health team member's unique contribution and enhances the meaning of professional nurse work. **Appraise** the consistency of your own interprofessional behavior. **Attend** to caring relationships by making them the central, organizing aspect of your practice.

REFLECTIVE QUESTIONS/APPLICATIONS

For Professional Nurses in Clinical Practice:

■ Discuss whether aspects of the QCM are visible in your healthcare institution.

■ Are nurses' relationship oriented or task oriented? Does it matter?

■ What avenues exist at your institution for nurses to adopt a professional practice model?

■ What specific health outcomes may be advanced as a result of implementing a more relational approach to care?

■ What is your assessment of the examples provided in this chapter that many nursing departments have implemented? Do they seem feasible?

■ How do you envision the future of nursing?

For Professional Nurses in Educational Practice:

■ Is middle range theory presented to students at your institution? If so, how and at which levels of education? If not, should it be? What learning strategies are used to help students translate them into practice?

■ Reflect on the QCM—its foundation, evolution, major concepts, and propositional statements. How do students best demonstrate competency in these phenomena? What new knowledge and skills are required to help students learn the value of nursing theory?

■ How will you integrate competency-based examples of quality caring behaviors into the classroom? In clinical settings?

■ What avenues exist to help students realize the power of relationships between patients and nurses? Among healthcare professionals? Is this a necessary aspect of undergraduate learning? Of graduate learning?

For Professional Nurses in Leadership Practice:

■ Describe how complexity science has influenced leadership practice.

■ How is professional nursing organized at your institution? Is it based on nursing theory? If not, should it be?

■ Reflect on the network of relationships at your institution. Are they facilitated by the nursing leadership to be of a caring nature? If so, how are they demonstrated?

■ Are you leading a continuous learning organization? How would you demonstrate it?

■ In what innovative ways do nurses at your facility demonstrate caring relationships? How often are these approaches disseminated to the larger nursing community?

PRACTICE ANALYSIS

XYZ Health is a nonprofit community-based healthcare system located in a rural, semi-mountainous area of the mid-Atlantic region of the United States. Its mission is to improve the health of the communities it serves with a special focus on wellness and preventative care. XYZ Health has 604 licensed inpatient beds, 166 long-term care beds, 5,300 employees, and a medical staff exceeding 500 professionals. There are over 500,000 residents in its primary service area, of whom 7% are older than 65 years, with a projected growth in older adults and non-White populations. A high percentage of individuals are uninsured, and mental and behavioral health issues were recently cited as the secondmost frequent health concern, with access to primary care cited as first. Chronic disease and substance abuse are ongoing health challenges.

Often individuals in outlying counties who need acute care services are transported via ambulance to the flagship hospital. Due to the rural nature of the community, it sometimes takes 2 hours for an ambulance to get from the originating site to the larger hospital. Emergency department (ED) nurses in the larger hospital complain that patients often arrive in unstable condition with little information about their past and present health conditions. At least six times in the last month, a patient transported from an outlying hospital presented to the ED unstable and either needed resuscitation in the ED or needed immediate admission to the ICU. This was overwhelming during the COVID-19 pandemic when the ICU was already engulfed with acutely ill patients on ventilators. In one instance, a 49-year-old male who was transferred and admitted to a medical–surgical unit, experienced cardiac arrest, could not be resuscitated, and died.

The Director of Performance Improvement has directed his team to create a database that will track all transfers so that analysis could be performed to better understand and prevent such experiences. However, defining what should be included in the database, identifying specific sources of data, and how to capture them among system hospitals has become a nightmare. Some of the hospitals say they have no data, others are reluctant to share, and still others, while willing to comply, do not have competent staff to facilitate the process. Eight months later, the project has stalled, and relationships among personnel at the various hospitals are tense.

- What aspects of the above scenario reflect a CAS?
- How do collective relationships among the agents in this CAS contribute to the natural feature of emergence in this health system? How is the system coevolving over time?
- How can knowledge of complexity science inform ongoing behavioral adaptations in this large health system?
- What suggestions do you have for helping the system move toward a more responsive approach?

REFERENCES

American Nurses Association. (2021). Nursing: Scope and standards of practice (4th ed). Washington, DC: Author.

Association of Women's Health, Obstetric and Neonatal Nursesl. (2014). AWHONN position statement: Nursing care quality measurement. *Journal of Obstetric, Gynecologic, and Neonatal Nursing, 43*(1), 132–133. https://doi.org/10.1111/1552-6909.12276

Baird, J., Rehm, R. S., Hinds, P. S., Baggott, C., & Davies, B. (2016). Do you know my child? Continuity of nursing care in the pediatric intensive care unit. *Nursing Research, 65*(2), 142–150. https://doi.org/10.1097/NNR.0000000000000135

Begun, J., & Jiang, H. J. (2020). Health care management during Covid-19: Insights from complexity science. *NEJM Catalyst Innovations in Care Delivery.* https://doi.org/10.1056/CAT.20.0541

Carmichael, T., & Hadžikadić, M. (2019). The fundamentals of complex adaptive systems. In T. Carmichael, A. Collins, & M. Hadžikadić (Eds.), *Complex adaptive systems: Understanding complex systems.* Springer. https://doi.org/10.1007/978-3-030-20309-2_1

Carthon, J. M. B., Hatfield, L., Brom, H., Houton, M., Kelly-Hellyer, E., Schlak, A., & Aiken, L. H. (2021). System-level improvements in work environments lead to lower nurse burnout and higher patient satisfaction. *Journal of Nursing Care Quality, 36*(1), 7–13. https://doi.org/10.1097/NCQ.0000000000000475

Centers for Medicare and Medicaid Services. (2014). HCAHPS: Patients' perspectives of care survey. https://www.cms.gov/medicare/quality-initiatives-patient-assessment-instruments/hospitalqualityinits/hospitalhcahps.html

Cunningham, F. C., Ranmuthugala, G., Plumb, J., Georgiou, A., West brook, J. I., & Braithwaite, J. (2012). Health professional networks as a vector for improving health quality and safety: A systematic review. *BMJ Quality and Safety, 21*, 239–249. https://doi.org/10.1136/bmjqs-2011-000187

Davis, K., Duffy, J., Marchessault, P., & Miles, D. (2022). Self-caring practices among nurses: Findings from an online survey of registered nurses. *Holistic Nursing Practice, 36*(1):7–14. https://doi.org/ 10.1097/HNP.0000000000000490.

Dieppe, P., Fussell, I., & Warber, S. L. (2020). The power of caring in clinical encounters. *British Medical Journal, 371*, m4100. https://doi.org/10.1136/bmj.m4100

Donabedian, A. (1966). Evaluating the quality of medical care. *Milbank Memorial Fund Quarterly, 44*, 166–206. https://doi.org/10.1111/j.1468-0009.2005.00397.x

Duffy, J. (2008). The caring assessment tools—Administrative version. In J. Watson (Ed.), *Assessing and measuring caring in nursing* (2nd ed.). Springer Publishing Company.

Duffy, J. (2009). *Quality caring in nursing and health systems: Applying theory to clinical practice, education, and leadership.* Springer Publishing Company.

Duffy, J. (2018). *Quality caring in nursing and health systems: Implications for clinicians, educators, and leaders.* Springer Publishing Company.

Duffy, J., Brewer, B., & Weaver, M. (2014). Revision and psychometric properties of the caring assessment tool. *Clinical Nursing Research, 23*(1), 80–93. https://doi.org/10.1177/1054773810369827

Duffy, J., Kooken, W., Wolverton, C., & Weaver, M. (2012). Evaluating patient-centered care: Feasibility of electronic data collection in hospitalized older adults. *Journal of Nursing Care Quality, 27*(4), 307–315. https://doi.org/10.1097/NCQ.0b013e31825ba9d4

Freeman, L. C. (2004). *The development of social network analysis: A study in the sociology of science.* Empirical Press.

Haizlip, J., McCluney, C., Hernandez, M., Quatrara, B., & Brashers, V. (2020). Mattering: How organizations, patients, and peers can affect nurse burnout and engagement. *JONA: The Journal of Nursing Administration, 50*(5), 267–273. https://doi.org/10.1097/NNA.0000000000000882

Holland, J. H. (2006). Studying complex adaptive systems. *Journal of Systems Science and Complexity, 19*(1), 1–8. http://hdl.handle.net/2027.42/41486

Hoogendoorn, M. E., Brinkman, S., Bosman, R. J., Haringman, J., de Keizer, N. F., & Spijkstra, J. J. (2021). The impact of COVID-19 on nursing workload and planning of nursing staff on the intensive care: A prospective descriptive multicenter study. *International Journal of Nursing Studies, 121,* 104005.

Institute of Medicine. (2013). *Best care at lower cost: The path to continuously learning health care in America.* Washington, DC: Institute of Medicine.

Institute of Medicine. (2001). *Crossing the quality chasm: A new health system for the 21st century.* Washington, DC: National Academies Press.

International Association of Forensic Nurses. (2021). Sexual assault nurse examiners. https://www.forensicnurses.org/page/aboutSANE

Irvine, D. M., Sidani, S., & McGillis Hall, L. (1998). Linking outcomes to nurses' roles in health care. *Nursing Economics, 16*(2), 58–64.

King, I. M. (1981). *A theory for nursing: Systems, concepts, process.* Wiley.

Knoke, D., & Yang, S. (2020). *Social network analysis* (3rd ed.). Sage Publications.

Kostich, K., Lasiter, S., Duffy, J., & George, V. (2021). The relationship between staff nurses' perceptions of nurse manager caring behaviors and patient experience. *JONA: The Journal of Nursing Administration, 51*(9), 468–473. https://doi.org/10.1097/NNA.0000000000001047

Lasater, K. B., McHugh, M., Rosenbaum, P. R., Aiken, L. H., Smith, H., Reiter, J. G., Niknam, B. A., Hill, A. S., Hochman, L. L., Jain S., & Silber, J. H. (2020) Valuing hospital investments in nursing: Multistate matched-cohort study of surgical patients. *BMJ Quality & Safety, 30*(1). https://doi.org/10.1136/bmjqs-2019-010534

Lindberg, C., Nash, S., & Lindberg, C. (2008). *On the edge: Nursing in the age of complexity.* Plexus Press.

Mahajan, A., Islam, S. D., Schwartz, M. J., & Cannesson, M. (2017). A hospital is not just a factory, but a complex adaptive system-implications for perioperative care. *Anesthesia & Analgesia, 125*(1). 333–341. https://doi.org/10.1213/ANE.0000000000002144

Marshall, E. S., & Broome, M. E. (2016). Understanding contexts for transformational leadership: Complexity, change, and strategic planning. In *Transformational leadership in nursing: From expert clinician to influential leader* (2nd ed.). Springer Publishing Company.

Martin, C. M. (2018). Complex adaptive systems approaches in health care—A slow but real emergence? *Journal of Evaluation in Clinical Practice, 24,* 266–268. https://doi.org/10.1111/jep.12878

Maslow, A. (1954). *Motivation and personality.* Harper.

Meunier-Sham, J., Preiss, R. M., Petricone, R., Re, C., & Gillen, L. (2019). Laying the foundation for the national telenursing center: Integration of the quality-caring model into TeleSANE practice. *Journal of Forensic Nursing, 15*(3), 143–151. https://doi.org/10.1097/JFN.0000000000000252

Ng, L. K. (2020). The perceived importance of soft (service) skills in nursing care: A research study. *Nurse Education Today, 85*(2), 10430.

Peplau, H. (1988). *Interpersonal relations in nursing: A conceptual frame of reference for psychodynamic nursing.* Springer Publishing Company.

Pines, D. (2014). *Emergence: A unifying theme for 21st century science.* Satna Fe Institute. https://medium.com/sfi-30-foundations-frontiers/emergence-a-unifying-theme-for-21st-century-science-4324ac0f951e

Plsek, P. E., & Greenhalgh, T. (2001). Complexity science—The challenge of complexity in health care. *BMJ, 323*(7313), 625–628. https://doi.org/10.1136/bmj.323.7313.625

Ratnapalan, S. & Lang, D. (2020). Health care organizations as complex adaptive systems. *The Health Care Manager, 39*(1), 18–23. https://doi.org/10.1097/HCM.0000000000000284

Rosenkoetter, M. (2016). Overview and summary: Organizational outcomes for providers and patients. *OJIN: The Online Journal of Issues in Nursing, 21*(2), 1. https://doi.org/10.3912/OJIN.Vol21No02ManOS

Salinas, M., Salinas, N., Duffy, J. R., & Davidson, J. (2020). Do caring behaviors in the quality caring model promote the human emotion of feeling cared for in hospitalized stroke patients and their families? *Applied Nursing Research, 55*(15), 1299. https://doi.org/10.1016/j.apnr.2020.151299

Scott, J. (2000). *Social network analysis: A handbook* (2nd ed.). Sage.

Smiley, R. A., Ruttinger, C., Oliveira, C. M., Reneau, K. A., Silvestre, J. H., & Alexander, M. (2021). The 2020 National nursing workforce survey. *Journal of Nursing Regulation Supplement, 12*(1), S1–S96. https://doi.org/10.1016/S2155-8256(21)00027-2

Swanson, K. M. (1993). Nursing as informed caring for the well-being of others. *Image, 25*(4), 352–357. https://doi.org/10.1111/j.1547-5069.1993.tb00271.x

The Daisy Foundation. (2012). Daisy award. https://www.daisyfoundation.org/daisy-award

Travelbee, J. (1966). *Interpersonal aspects of nursing.* F. A. Davis.

Tuominen, L., Leino-Kilpi, H., & Meretoja, R. (2020). Expectations of patients with colorectal cancer towards nursing care: A thematic analysis. *European Journal of Oncology Nursing, 44*(10), 1699. https://doi.org/10.1016/j.ejon.2019.101699

Uhl-Bien, M., & Arena, M. (2017). Complexity leadership: Enabling people and organizations for adaptability. *Organizational Dynamics, 46*(1), 9–20. https://doi.org/10.1016/j.orgdyn.2016.12.001

United States Office of Justice Programs. (2017). Office for Victims of Crime. (2021). Building a theoretical framework for SANE practice. https://www.ovcttac.gov/sane-guide/introduction/building-a-theoretical-framework-for-sane-practice/

Valente, T. W., & Pitts, S. R. (2017). An appraisal of social network theory and analysis as applied to public health: Challenges and opportunities. *Annual Review of Public Health, 38*, 103–118. https://doi.org/10.1146/annurev-publhealth-031816-044528

Warden, D. H., Hughes, R. G., Probst, J. C., Warden, D. N., & Adams, S. A. (2021). Current turnover intention among nurse managers, directors, and executives. *Nursing Outlook, 69*(5):875–885. https://doi.org/10.1016/j.outlook.2021.04.006

Wasserman, S., & Faust, K. (1994). *Social network analysis: Methods and applications.* Cambridge University Press.

Watson, J. (1979). *Nursing: The philosophy and science of caring.* Little, Brown and Company.

Watson, J. (1985). *Nursing: Human science and human care.* Appleton-Century-Crofts.

Watson, J. (2012). *Human caring science.* Jones & Bartlett.

Wolverton, C. L., Lasiter, S., Duffy, J. R., Weaver, M. T., McDaniel, A. M. (2018). Psychometric testing of the caring assessment tool: Administration (CAT-adm©). *SAGE Open Medicine, 6*, 2050312118760739. https://doi.org/10.1177/2050312118760739

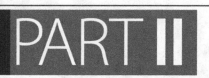

PART II Practicing in Quality-Caring Health Systems

CHAPTER 4

Humans in Relationship

"Human relationships help us to carry on because they always presuppose further developments, a future… "

—Albert Camus

CHAPTER OBJECTIVES:

1. Discuss how human relationships influence nursing work.
2. Describe at least three approaches to nurse self-caring.
3. Evaluate how the Quality-Caring Model guides interprofessional practice.
4. Explore the benefits of nursing engagement in the community.

THE RELATIONAL CONTEXT OF BEING HUMAN

Relationships are the context for human birth, living, working, growing, learning, advancing, and dying. As multidimensional beings, humans exist in relationship to others and their environment and, to a larger extent, the universe. Humans also exist as unique individuals, separate from other people, with varied characteristics and life experiences. Philosophically, human beings are differentiated from other forms of life by features such as consciousness, the ability to reason and move autonomously, and the capacity to use language. From most formal religious perspectives, such uniqueness confers respect, dignity, and value for human life.

Through relational life experiences and ordinary growth processes, humans develop biologically, cognitively (Piaget, 1972, 1990), psychosocially (Buhler & Allen, 1972; Buhler & Marschak, 1967; Erikson, 1964, 1968; Gould, 1978; Havighurst, 1953; Jung, 1933; Levinson, 1966; Levinson et al., 1978; Sheehy, 1976), morally (Kohlberg, 1986), and some would say spiritually, all influenced by specific contextual factors, such as gender, race, economics, and societal status throughout their life span.

In fact, the phrase, social determinants of health (SDOH), is often used to refer broadly to those non-medical factors that influence health, including health-related knowledge, attitudes, beliefs, or behaviors (such as smoking) (Braveman et al., 2011). However, these more overt health-related factors are often wrapped up in and influenced by complex underlying aspects embedded in sociocultural environments, such as living arrangements, working conditions, education and income levels, race and racism, family support, opportunities (or not), and healthcare access. Prior to COVID-19, a large and compelling body of evidence began to emerge that revealed the powerful influence of sociocultural factors on health (Braveman & Gottlieb, 2014). This evidence, together with various payment models, began to prompt interest in SDOH; and particular courses of action, including interventional research, were initiated by the healthcare community (Morgan, 2017). However, it wasn't until the COVID-19 pandemic was well underway that data began to amplify existing health disparities for marginalized populations in the United States (Dalsania et al., 2021). (See Chapters 1 and 2 for more detail on the impact of SDOH on health outcomes for persons with COVID-19.) These data showed the significant impact of sociocultural factors on individual and group behavior and health outcomes. New and important initiatives, for example, *The Future of Nursing Report: 2020 to 2030* (Institutes of Medicine, 2021) are now being instigated to facilitate health equity by identifying social needs and SDOH and addressing inequities. Furthermore, preparing and supporting health professionals to advance diverse and inclusive relationships in the populations/communities they serve may foster more *human* connections that matter. For, as Murthy (2020) states, "human relationships are as essential to our well-being as food and water" (p. 42).

The relational context associated with *being human* suggests a mutual connectedness among individuals that may facilitate or impede future attitudes and actions and ultimately influence progress or advancement. For example, in children, relationships that are reciprocal, attuned, culturally responsive, and trusting provide a positive basis for overall development (Bornstein & Leventhal, 2015). Others have hypothesized that *developmental* (or advancing) relationships are those characterized by attunement, social synchrony, compassionate communication, co-regulation, support, modeling, consistency, trustworthiness, cognitive stimulation, and a capacity to accurately perceive and respond to the other (Bergin & Bergin, 2009; Bornstein, 2015; Li & Julian, 2012; Osher et al., 2020). In contrast, relationships that are one-sided, domineering, inconsistent, insensitive, or are indifferent provide a negative basis for overall advancement and may impact long-term progress.

The complex blend of relational life experiences (including those experienced in healthcare) shapes the *whole* person (Serlin & DiCowden, 2007). When relationships are good, people feel reassured, safe, and are likely to advance. When, however, relationships are flawed or conflicted, individuals feel isolated, distressed, or even sick. Thus, relationships have a profound influence on human behavior, interpersonal interactions, health, longevity, and overall development. At the core of relationships, however, are the interactions that take place between persons—these interactions are influential to all and take place in a context that is ever-changing. Importantly, the quality of relationships impacts health (Allen et al., 2017; Feeney & Collins, 2015; Hall et al., 2016). In fact, some have suggested that strong and supportive social relationships result in better health and longer life (Howick et al., 2019).

Early transpersonal psychologists were concerned with understanding the connectedness of individuals as well as the benefits of higher levels of consciousness (Jung, 1933; Maslow, 1966; Rogers, 1961). Some of these views were integrated with the spiritual disciplines, taking on a more holistic view of an individual as a being connected to the larger universe. Relationships grounded in this belief are nonjudgmental and most often meaningful (profound) for all participants. In this way of thinking, humans are viewed as capable of moving forward or advancing (growing as humans through all phases of life), which has implications for learning, performance, advancement, and optimum health.

Awareness of Meaningful Relationships

A key to enabling meaningful relationships is self-awareness or clarity about one's strengths, weaknesses, actions, emotions, and presence in both the larger world and with humankind. The process of being aware of the present moment (the "being" mode) is a contrast to much of what health professionals experience in their daily lives. In fact, unintentional acting without deliberate effort (the "doing" mode; automatic pilot) or repetitively pushing away negative thoughts is common in health professionals as they go about their busy tasks. In such a state, individuals tend to function more inattentively or mechanistically. Mindless working influences individuals (in this case health professionals) to act in habitual ways that may not be open to present-day possibilities. This often leads to unintentional rigidity or detachment, sometimes even robot-like behavior. How many of us have witnessed health professionals walk into a patient's room or enter an elevator and mindlessly ask, "How are you?" never really expecting to get a true answer? Likewise, how often do we observe some health professionals stuck in their old ways or even driving home after a long shift and missing their exit on the freeway? Unfortunately, not paying attention to what is observed and experienced, decreases focus, health, mood, and creativity, leading to burnout and even ineffective patient care. Thus, maintaining awareness (non-doing) is crucial for busy health professionals.

Awareness of *both* subjective and objective phenomena in life occurs on a continuum from being fully awake and aware of oneself to being asleep or unaware (Morin, 2011). Self-awareness grounds an individual to better see with clarity how life experiences (including those faced at work) shape thoughts and behaviors. Concepts such as the perception of the physical body or body image, self-concept, agency (one's capacity to act), social identity and even weaknesses are accepted without pressure to change, understood, and refined as self-awareness or consciousness is heightened. Such an appreciation of self suggests that a depth of understanding is possible that may empower one to self-monitor and regulate behaviors, advance his or her full potential, have meaningful relationships, heal, and achieve some form of contentment or peace (Crane et al., 2017; Kabat-Zinn, 2012). There is a sense of freedom and freshness as experiences evolve, with feelings of openness, calmness, and flexibility.

Regrettably, as humans (and in particular, nurses) go about relating, working, and caring for each other, the self is often forgotten or lost along the way. Disappointments, insecurities, losses, physical ailments, and the everyday fast-paced demands of life build up over time leaving many individuals stressed and exhausted. Furthermore, many aspects of workplace performance, such as attention, cognition, emotions, behavior, and even physiology can be interrupted or limited by the unnecessary demands and approaches to the work, ultimately impacting key workplace outcomes, individual and group performance, relationships, and well-being (Good et al., 2015). The 24/7 connectivity that has consumed humans' lives in the last decade has added to the inability to be in touch with ourselves. To make matters worse, learned ways of knowing (externally derived), such as formal education, religious training, or orientation programs may limit or constrain the view of oneself. In this restricted view of the world, individuals tend to be more reactive, feel separated or disjointed, and function under an individualistic or misplaced perspective.

Nurses and other health professionals, in particular, tend to get accustomed to multiple work demands and "run on adrenalin" to accomplish them. Nurses have been unknowingly taught "to do," both during their educational programs and later in health systems. Behaviors such as assisting others, collaborating, assessing, teaching, documenting, rounding, administering medications, and delegating are typical nursing actions (the "doing" mode). In fact, activity dominance (being observed as busy) is considered proper behavior for nurses! *Good* nurses are viewed as those who can perform certain skills, get all their work done in the shortest amount of time, document correctly, think on their feet, and make good decisions, usually on their own (doing). Professional nurses are proud of their multitasking abilities—and rightly so. However, being busy is not the same as being productive or available to others. *Some* multitasking is inherent in nursing work, but too much of it slows our ability to focus and accurately perceive situations and their meanings, decreases learning ability, and increases stress (and its consequences). But more importantly, failing to concentrate can significantly reduce the accuracy and appropriateness of patient care decisions and may present serious threats to patient safety (Fore & Sculli, 2013). Deliberate focusing, on the other hand, is tied to better patient outcomes.

Known as situational awareness, this phenomenon refers to the conscious awareness of the current situation in relation to one's environment (Orique & Despins, 2018). Balancing highly acute patient needs with limited resources, the physical demands of nurse work, and making life-and-death decisions according to the latest evidence, along with personal family responsibilities, annoyances like traffic, and information overload can affect nursing decision-making, leaving little time for meaningful relationships with patients and families. Such experiences may even generate intense emotions and symptoms in nurses themselves, such as defensiveness, making excuses, inability to keep on task, poor health choices, lower energy, problems interacting with one's own family members, workplace frustration, physical symptoms, and feelings of being drained and worn out. Importantly, failing to accurately perceive or understand healthcare phenomena can significantly reduce the quality of patient care decisions, affecting health outcomes. And the same is true for nurse educators and leaders. Unawareness (not being) interferes with teaching strategies, leadership decisions, and one's own health!

Prior to COVID-19, nurses and other health professionals were raising concerns about workforce shortages, workplace violence, lack of readily available supplies and equipment, documentation, inadequate teamwork, poor accountability among colleagues, disappointing leadership, and patient safety concerns (Halter et al., 2017; The Betsy Lehman Center for Patient Safety, 2019; Martinez, 2016). The doing mode of clinical work (getting things done) seemed endless. Increasingly, in the healthcare literature, professional burnout was being documented. For example, using a secondary data analysis, 687 direct care RNs (30%) in a total of 540 nursing homes across the US reported high levels of burnout, 31% were dissatisfied with their job, and 72% reported missing one or more necessary care tasks on their last shift due to lack of time or resources, even after controlling for RN and nursing home characteristics. In fact, RNs with burnout were five times more likely to leave necessary care undone (odds ratio [OR] = 4.97; 95% confidence interval [CI] = 2.56–9.66) than RNs without burnout. RNs who were dissatisfied were 2.6 times more likely to leave necessary care undone (OR = 2.56; 95% CI = 1.68–3.91) than RNs who were satisfied. In other healthcare settings, physician and nurse burnout was reported to be increasing and more importantly, contributed to negative clinical and organizational outcomes, not to mention those to the clinicians themselves! (Han et al., 2019; Zhang et al., 2018).

In 2016, the National Academy of Medicine responded to increased rates of burnout, depression, and suicide on clinician well-being and patient safety by launching the *Action Collaborative for Clinician Well-being and Resilience*. In 2019, they published a consensus report recommending action on clinician burnout. In this report, 35% to 54% of nurses and physicians as well as 45% to 60% of medical students and residents ("learners") indicated they experienced substantial symptoms of burnout. Several recommendations in the report were advised. They were:

1. Create positive work environments: Transform healthcare work systems by creating positive work environments that prevent and reduce burnout, foster professional well-being, and support quality care.

2. Create positive learning environments: Transform the education and training of health professions to optimize learning environments that prevent and reduce burnout and foster professional well-being.

3. Reduce administrative burden: Prevent and reduce the negative consequences on clinicians' professional well-being that result from laws, regulations, policies, and standards promulgated by the healthcare policy, regulatory, and standards-setting entities, including government agencies (federal, state, and local), professional organizations, and accreditors.

4. Enable technology solutions: Optimize the use of health information technologies to support clinicians in providing high quality patient care.

5. Provide support to clinicians and learners: Reduce the stigma and eliminate the barriers associated with obtaining the support and services needed to prevent and alleviate burnout symptoms, facilitate recovery from burnout, and foster professional well-being among learners and practicing clinicians.

6. Invest in research: Provide dedicated funding for research on clinician professional well-being (National Academies of Sciences, Engineering, and Medicine, 2019).

Again, in July 2019, The Joint Commission released a *Quick Safety Advisory of Combating Nurse Burnout Through Resilience* in response to recent studies on increasing burnout among nurses (Bronk, 2019). Their advisory highlighted that 15.6% of nurses reported burnout and that emergency room nurses were at a higher risk. Furthermore, nurses had reported in surveys that only 5% of healthcare organizations were assisting staff with burnout. The Joint Commission recommended that health systems remove barriers to nurses' work flow, staffing, and workplace environment concerns. All of these publications were offered *before* the onset of COVID-19, highlighting the nation's increasing evidence for healthcare workforce stress, burnout, dissatisfaction, and even depression and suicide.

The coronavirus pandemic exacerbated the situation as health professionals, in crisis mode, responded (in the *doing* mode) to shifting protocols, ethical challenges, shortages of resources, and the astonishing numbers of patients who required care in expedited conditions. As of this writing, the prior concern of burnout has been elevated somewhat to include moral distress, higher vacancy rates, early retirements, and even death, leading to even higher costs and reports of decreasing hospital quality (Fakih et al., 2021). On a positive note, however, there is increased attention being paid to prioritizing the well-being of the healthcare workforce by leading authorities, health systems, and healthcare professionals themselves (see more on this in the section on caring for self later in this chapter).

BOX 4.1: Integrating *being* (authentic awareness of self) along with *doing* (getting things done) contributes to a more fully functioning human being—a healthy self that is more available for patients and families.

Professional nurses and other health professionals interact and relate to patients and families with ease; yet, most have not traditionally been taught how to do this for themselves. In fact, personal observations and anecdotal reports suggest that integrating being and doing is not the norm for most health professionals (see Figure 4.1).

BOX 4.2: Learning how to reduce "doing" and heighten "being" for a while permits one to slow down enough to actually focus on one's inner thoughts and feelings and access new ways of seeing the whole. Once accessed, this attention to self helps one see his or her situation more clearly. In turn, such actions may help health professionals appreciate and honor the important work they do.

Integrating being and doing is believed to be so necessary to meaningful relationships and positive health outcomes that many centers have led efforts to help patients and health professionals learn better self-awareness practices. In fact, attention to the whole person or linking separate systems in humans, such as bodily sensations with emotions, for example, enables overall well-being by continually shaping connections in the brain. The empirical evidence beginning to emerge demonstrating connections between emotions and physiological

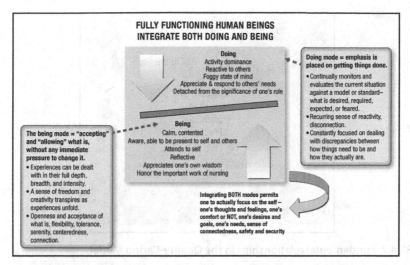

FIGURE 4.1 Fully functioning human beings.

processes is noteworthy (Siegel & Solomon, 2020). The relatively new field of interpersonal neurobiology integrates findings from recent brain research with human interactions and emphasizes the brain as a social organ developed over time and through experiences with others. Many in this field would argue that human relationships actually shape neural connections and modify how the brain develops and changes over time (Siegel, 2015). Programs of research on the effects of mindful awareness are increasing, including a number of randomized controlled trials. In general, studies have shown benefits; however, robust studies on patients with a few key conditions, such as depression, chronic pain, and anxiety have shown positive outcomes with effects similar to other existing treatments (Powell, 2018).

THE FUNDAMENTAL RELATIONSHIPS OF THE QUALITY-CARING MODEL©

Because of the interpersonal nature of humans as the primary focus of healthcare, the Quality-Caring Model© (QCM) relies on relationships to position itself. Four relationships (Figure 4.2), in particular, are considered foundational to the QCM and must be attended to in order to practice from this relationship-centered stance. Each will be described in the next few pages.

Relating to Self

Although connection with others is what exemplifies our humanness, the relationship with one's self influences how we think, feel, and interact with others. The way a person thinks and feels about his or her physical and emotional states, traits, abilities, beliefs, likes and dislikes, physical sensations, and motivation is dynamic and contributes to one's perception of his or her uniqueness

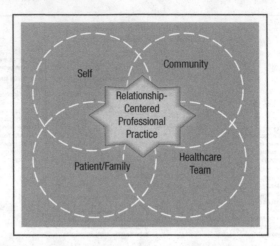

FIGURE 4.2 Fundamental relationships in the Quality-Caring Model.

as a person (Rasheed et al., 2019). Understanding oneself or having a sense of who one is allows one to recognize their purpose in the world, develop satisfying relationships, make beneficial choices, and accept one's entire self, physical and emotional (Carden et al., 2021). A strong sense of self is associated with the ability to align one's actions with his or her passions, manage emotions, decrease stress, and allow for a sense of pride (Rasheed et al., 2019). Put another way, a robust sense of self is that "continuous experience of being a complete and authentic person who feels in control of their own activities" (Basten & Touyz, 2020, p. 159).

Another aspect of knowing oneself is the ability to clearly grasp how others view us. Individuals who understand how others perceive them are typically more empathetic (Haley et al., 2017). An example of this includes recognizing that a particular co-worker often takes your feedback personally because of the pitch of your voice. Using that knowledge about yourself to purposefully alter the quality of your dialog during encounters with that co-worker may positively influence their perceptions. Or, realizing that a patient may be stressed about a certain lab report presented to him or her, you alter your style to accommodate and support them as they hear it for the first time. Having a good sense of how others perceive us allows us to accept or address areas of dissatisfaction more confidently and with a sense of calm. In essence, self-awareness not only benefits the self, but enables nurses and other health professionals to engage in therapeutic communication with patients and others and continuously improve their relationships and communication styles (Rasheed, 2015).

Being more aware (or present to self) is a particularly healthy way to work and deepens one's ability to be present for patients and their families. Mindfulness, fully attending to the present moment, has drawn the attention of health educators and health professionals and is the focus of current research. Mindfulness-based stress reduction developed by Kabat-Zinn (2012) is a program of class instruction and practice in mindfulness techniques, meditation, and Hatha yoga designed to promote physical and psychological well-being (Penque, 2019). Several studies have shown the benefits of this approach. Although limited by sample size and attrition, results suggest that mindfulness interventions promoted significant positive changes in outcome variables (Koren & Purohit, 2014).

Cultivating an innate understanding of the self helps one to identify what is valued, what brings joy, and ways to pursue it. Self-awareness is an essential nursing competency (Rasheed et al., 2021) that is incorporated in the new Essentials for Entry-Level (and above) Professional Nursing Education (American Association of Colleges of Nursing [AACN], 2021).

Lack of knowing the self (attributed to failure of prioritizing self-caring) can make one feel gloomy and unfulfilled, often uninterested in pursuing or improving professional goals. Moreover, it can lead to increased stress, anxiety, and even depression; poor health choices; and discontent (Andrews et al., 2020). Nurses' work environment, with the incessant background noise, competing priorities, uncertainty, ethical concerns, interruptions, and nonstop automatic doing is already stressful, unhealthy, and prone to error. It is easy in this context to remain in a task-oriented frame of mind without awareness of one's own health, patients' relational needs, co-workers' needs for help, or one's own feelings about certain situations encountered during the work day/night. This lack of awareness detracts from one's own personal development, decision-making, attention to the quality of one's practice, or generating meaningful relationships with patients and families. Prioritizing *caring for self* is the antidote to this feeling of discontent.

Caring for self is a comprehensive set of actions that includes the dedicated, intentional time one allocates to check in with the self, to focus on how one feels (physically and emotionally), to identify unsatisfactory feelings and resolve to improve them, to engage in healthy behaviors, and to acknowledge the impact of one's actions. Caring for self is not a simple one-time action; rather, it is an intentional lifestyle that recognizes one's worthiness, includes deliberate activities that influence well-being, solicits feedback from others, considers inspiring messages, and routinely practices the caring behaviors with self. It is also a time to reflect on nursing practice as well as personal and professional goals. It entails taking care of one's own physical and mental well-being, which ultimately allows us to best serve our patients.

The willingness to look deeply and reflectively at one's practice regardless of what it holds and in a spirit of acceptance and caring toward oneself helps us see possibilities and value in what we do. In the work environment, regular efforts to increase conscious awareness through reflection may help health professionals focus more attentively on the human person of the patient, holistically assess patients' needs, make better clinical judgments, and use best evidence to improve the quality of care. Creating the space to reflect (thinking analytically) on nursing practice, by yourself, with a colleague or as part of a group, can help one gain insight into the practice, recognize positive experiences, identify lessons learned that could be applied in similar situations in the future, and lead to innovative improvements. Structuring reflection offers a way to make sense of an experience, learn from it, and apply any changes needed to future actions that could improve the outcome. The well-known Gibbs' Reflective Cycle (Gibbs, 1988) offers a framework for examining experiences using six stages:

1. **Description of the experience**: Describe what happened, when and where it happened, who was involved, what did the individuals involved do, what were the outcomes, why were you there, and what did you want to happen.
2. **Feelings and thoughts about the experience**: Describe what feelings arose during the situation, what you felt before and after the situation, what other people thought about the situation, what you believe people think now, and what you currently think about the situation.
3. **Evaluate the experience**: Describe what was good and bad about the experience, what went well and what did not, and what did you and other people contribute to the situation (positively or negatively).
4. **Analysis**: Describe why you think things went well, and why they did not (if appropriate), what sense can you make of this, what knowledge is available to better help understand the situation.
5. **Conclusion**: Describe what you have learned from this situation, how could the situation have been more positive for everyone involved, what skills do you need to develop to handle a situation like this better, and what else could have been done.
6. **Action plan:** Describe how, if you had to do the same thing again, what you would do differently, how you would develop the required skills needed, and how you would deal with similar situations differently the next time.

(University of Edinburgh, 2020)

Using this format or other reflective models, reflection on practice can be done privately, used in a group dialog, written, or even videoed. Some have advocated that given the current pandemic circumstances, for nurses to go beyond reflection-on-action and also include reflection-in-action and reflection-for-action as a part of their practice is beneficial (Patel & Metersky, 2021). More formal reflection, such as regularly soliciting feedback from patients, families, supervisors, and co-workers can also be revealing. Reflective practice helps nurses learn about their own practice by examining who they are as nurses, questioning their place in or their view of the discipline, encouraging deep thoughts about certain encounters to come to the surface, and using these experiences to clarify and enhance the practice. To do this, one must be disciplined and willing to make the effort. Although somewhat threatening (to self), if taught to honor themselves this way early on, nurses may come to view such behaviors as less risky and be able to uncover the hidden meanings and learning opportunities embedded in clinical work and integrate them into future practice.

Other approaches to caring for self at work include taking short pauses between patient rooms, seizing brief time-outs to sit and reflect, and using routine tasks such as handwashing, documenting, or walking from room to room as opportunities to feel one's body and assess one's emotions. Such approaches may, in fact, be therapeutic for both the patient and the health professional.

Appreciating the fact that professional nurses and other health care professionals live and work in relationship to self and others, just as other humans do, acknowledges that caring for self is integral to caring for others. When relationships with self are honored and of a caring nature, they support integrated, fully functioning professional nurses who balance being and doing, who know and understand themselves, and attend to the present, enabling them to better engage in caring relationships with patients and others.

Practicing Caring for Self

In the literature, the term *self-care* is used frequently, confusing its intent. In fact, self-care is a noun and somehow has become associated with immediate stress relievers such as spa days and other treats, including new clothes or an evening out with friends. Although there is nothing inherently wrong with these examples, authentic self-caring is a verb, a living practice that is incorporated into one's regular behaviors. Self-caring manifests in the ways one shows respect and compassion for the self as a worthy human being. It fosters catching ourselves when we are judgmental or mean to ourselves or start comparing ourselves with others. It allows us time to check in with our feelings and physical sensations, as well as for being present with emotions without judgement. According to the American Nurses Association (ANA), self-caring refers to valuing oneself, continuously improving oneself, and regularly activating practices to improve physical, emotional, social, work-related, and spiritual aspects of being human (ANA, 2017). It is a holistic concept that supports effective clinical care (Hofmeyer et al., 2020). In fact, the regular practice of personal and professional self-caring sets up the conditions for helping others (ANA, 2015); thus, caring for oneself is necessary in order to provide safe and high quality care. The World Health Organization (WHO) has determined that self-caring helps establish and maintain health as well as prevent and manage illness (WHO, 2020). Components of self-caring include:

- **Physical self-care**: Includes diet and hydration, sleep hygiene, exercise, taking care of one's health by keeping doctor and dental appointments. Combined, caring for the physical self is one of the fastest and most effective ways to boost well-being.

- **Mental self-care**: Includes stimulating your mind by learning new skills, reading, problem-solving, being conscious of the media you consume, not overworking, and listening to music.

- **Emotional self-care**: Practicing emotional relaxation (allowing difficult emotions to surface), regular reflection, using mindfulness to cultivate positive emotions such as compassion, joy, and flow, *understanding triggers, setting boundaries, practicing gratitude, and nurturing passions.*

- **Social self-care**: Socially connecting with others, including cultivating intimate relationships, joining interesting groups, networking, becoming part of a community, staying in touch (reaching out to others), listening, volunteering, taking up a hobby, and staying away from relationships that are unhealthy.

- **Spiritual self-care**: Focuses on the deeper themes of life, including meaning, purpose, and connection to the earth and the wider universe. Practices such as meditation, quiet time, gratitude, compassion, prayer, time in nature, worship, and service all fall into this category.

Nurses know how to care for others, yet focusing on caring for oneself is often difficult for them and other health professionals (Drick, 2016). The literature is replete with descriptions of RNs' lack of self-caring practices. In fact, the ANA has reported that registered nurses are less healthy than many Americans and tend to be overweight, overstressed, and suffer from lack of sleep (ANA, 2020). Prior to COVID-19, RNs were reported to be particularly vulnerable to compassion fatigue, burnout, moral distress, and unhealthy physical and emotional practices (Thacker et al., 2016). Dyrbye et al., (2017) reported that lack of self-caring among RNs was an international phenomenon associated with adverse outcomes. These outcomes included serious safety and cost/reimbursement implications that can affect nurses, their patients, and health systems. For this reason, maintaining physical, mental, and spiritual health through self-caring practices was recommended to be a priority that supports nurses' well-being, as well as the health outcomes of their patients (p. 77).

The COVID-19 pandemic, however, has intensified nurses' reported levels of stress, anxiety, and depression, particularly among those with the greatest amount of patient contact and interaction (Shechter et al., 2020). These emotions and others became labeled, the "second pandemic" (Borges et al., 2020), and may have affected not only individual nurses, but also their families, personal and work relationships, as well as their work experience itself. For some nurses and other health professionals, the experience of this significant (hopefully once-in-a-lifetime) event inflicted overwhelming trauma, often labelled moral injury. Moral injury was a term developed in military medicine to describe soldiers' long-lasting emotional, psychological, social, and spiritual effect from actions taken that run contrary to one's moral values (Greenberg et al., 2020). It was and continues to be used to describe what occurred in working personnel when individuals or systems carried out, failed to prevent, or became aware of human actions that violated deep moral commitments. As a consequence of COVID-19, a variety of mental health problems in health professionals began to surface, leading many to seek counseling and support services, others to resign or retire, and still others to exhibit unhealthy behaviors. As of this writing, most health systems are establishing major adjustments to employee wellness programs with special attention to frontline nurses (Chipps et al., 2021; Teall & Melnyk, 2021).

In fact, adequate self-caring is a shared responsibility between health professionals and the systems they work in. A nurse's obligation to self-care is made explicit in the competencies listed in the *Core Competencies for Professional Nursing Education* (AACN, 2021). The Code of Ethics for Nurses with Interpretive Statements (ANA, 2015) states explicitly that nurses must adopt self-caring as a duty to self in addition to their duty to provide care to patients. ANA's *Scope and Standards of Practice* 4th edition (2021) suggests that the moral respect that nurses extend to all human beings "extends to oneself as well: the same duties that we owe to others we owe to ourselves" (p. 14). These duties include the responsibility to:

- promote health and safety
- preserve wholeness of character and integrity

- maintain competence
- continue personal and professional growth

(ANA, 2021)

In terms of evidence on the benefits of nurse self-caring, older preliminary research (discussed in the 3rd edition of this book) showed that yoga, mindfulness, and/or educational interventions were helpful. More recently, published research reports of RNs, nursing faculty, and student nurses' self-caring practices revealed that most still suffered from small sample sizes, non-probability samples, poor explanation of the actual interventions or their consistent administration, and limited use of valid and reliable instruments. However, one integrative review of interventions to improve *spiritual* self-caring found that mindfulness was the most often used intervention. Ten of the 15 studies reviewed applied some form of mindfulness intervention with durations ranging from one day to as long as 15 weeks. Although limited by sample sizes and attrition, results suggest that mindfulness interventions showed significant positive changes in outcome variables (Koren & Purohit, 2014). Another small pilot randomized clinical trial ($N = 40$; 20 in each group) examined an 8-week yoga intervention on participants' self-caring. Participants in the intervention group reported significantly less emotional exhaustion and depersonalization upon completion (Alexander et al., 2015). Other quasi-experimental studies showed benefit as reported by nurses after mindfulness practices (Bronson, 2017: Farina et al., 2018), stress reduction techniques (Thacker et al., 2016), and yoga practice (Anderson et al., 2017). Overall, mindfulness practices and yoga interventions showed some promise to improve RNs' self-caring or health promoting lifestyles. The limited studies available and their weaknesses, however, identified the need for more robust foundational research to quantify the nature of self-caring among RNs, the demographic factors that influence it, and which interventions most benefit RNs.

Regardless of the lack of robust research, regular attention to the self seems to help one see situations more clearly and over time, may generate wisdom (Levey & Levey, 2019). Taking the time to look back (reflect), clarify, and become aware of where one is (in relation to one's practice) is liberating and helps to remind us of the important work we do. Making time to "be with" oneself, gaining insight into emotions, thoughts, bodily sensations, and other feelings contributes to well-being (Kushlev et al., 2017; Wilson et al., 2021). Health professionals need to acknowledge and allow themselves to feel the meanings associated with their work, including suffering.

Prioritizing time for true relaxation—not just time off from work, but authentic quiet time by oneself—is essential. Nursing is so people oriented and other-focused that time alone is often not seen as valuable. Yet, alone time can become a practice that enhances self-caring. In the nursing culture of self-sacrifice and adrenalin-induced nervous energy, creating balance through regular private time is meaningful. For example, a few minutes alone practicing deep breathing or taking a leisurely walk by oneself can promote insight and help one reframe a situation or experience differently, not to mention the physiologic benefits! Committing to private time each day (even if it is short) is a requisite for quality nursing care. Similar to physical exercise, obligating oneself to quiet time requires altering of daily habits. Waking up 15 minutes early or creating an evening ritual of quiet time or just sitting quietly with oneself is essential to nurses' well-being. For some, walking, rehearsing a song, even service itself— when performed in a conscious manner—can be relaxing. These kinds of experiences help one become attuned to the larger whole, allowing connections to surface that might otherwise remain buried. The key word here is *practice*; a verb, practice requires application or use of a concept, repeatedly in order to sustain and improve performance. Much like an athlete or a musician, regular connection to the self requires intention and follow-through or commitment. Repetition of this relaxation time relating to self reinforces the habit. Deeper relaxation techniques such as meditation practices, yoga and tai chi, or contemplative prayer are also ways to care for self (Nilsson, 2021).

Expression of oneself through artistic or creative pursuits, such as music, painting, sewing, quilting, gardening, woodworking, or non-competitive sports, when consciously pursued, can also raise awareness. These activities keep us "in the moment" and, although considered recreational, with the right intent, attention, repetition, and guidance, they can provide the same accessibility to the self as more traditional practices. In the case of music and/or dance, there is some evidence that it may even be physically and emotionally therapeutic (Sheppard & Broughton, 2020; Bilgiç & Acaroğlu, 2017; Gallagher et al., 2018).

BOX 4.3: In the personal practice of deep relaxation, making the commitment (intent) to devote the necessary time as well as focused attention to breathing or other bodily functions, and repeating the practice in the same way and at the same time each day (repetition) enable self-caring. Furthermore, reading about or taking a class on relaxation techniques (receiving guidance) reinforces and may even improve the practice.

Another way to access the inner self is to spend time in nature. Professional nurses are most often found working in drab, enclosed environments with artificial lighting and limited temperature controls. Often, there are no windows or opportunities to even see the outside surroundings. Being in the natural environment and using the experience to appreciate its mystery provides a reflective way to ponder and even dream. In this way, one can learn to quiet the self and see the sacred in everyday life. Taking a walk around the building at lunchtime or sitting near a window while eating in the cafeteria may help assist nurses to recharge during their working hours; but regular exercise outside is a key action geared to self-caring. Taking care of the body through regular exercise and healthy eating are self-caring acts that many nurses forget to do for themselves as they take care of others. However, caring for the physical body is crucial to quality nursing practice and promotes effective modeling for patients and families. The ANA has reported that nurses "are less healthy than the average American…and are more likely to be overweight, have higher levels of stress and get less sleep" (2020).

The serious nature of healthcare often diminishes opportunities to see some of the lighter sides of human nature. The use of humor, particularly in the workplace, can be a source of joy even in the most difficult of circumstances (Mesmer-Magnus et al., 2012). Establishing a support network or taking classes that reinforce and help perfect awareness practices enhances one's performance. Monitoring oneself during working hours by regularly observing one's behavior and asking, "Am I stressed or at ease?" or "Am I busy doing or am I present to myself, my coworkers, and my patients?" keeps one alert and in the moment. Regular reminders to practice attending to self, such as listening to relaxation techniques in the car and pictures or other symbols in the workplace, may assist health professionals to practice self-caring daily.

Another factor that facilitates self-caring in many health professionals is the feedback they receive from patients and families in terms of their progression towards health and healing. After all, this is the purpose of our work! However, many nurses work in environments where regular patient feedback is not the norm; for example, operating rooms, emergency departments, procedural areas, and critical care units. In these areas, the outcomes of patients cared for are not known, limiting important positive inspiration.

Consider this example:

We experience suffering and death very frequently but rarely get to share in the joy of positive outcomes in our patient population. Because of this missing piece in our profession, many on the intensive care unit have started the work to connect with more positive outcomes. We are calling it "success stories."

Recently, a pulmonologist, who currently runs a post-ICU clinic in addition to her other work, has taken the time to ask patients if they would consider talking or even visiting with their former nurses and physicians. This physician is using these "success stories" for inclusion in burnout education with the fellows in training and is ultimately considering research. After some time observing the benefits of this approach, a nursing arm of this effort began. So far, we have had two former patients join our monthly Unit Based Practice Council meetings to simply check in and share how they are doing. If the patients are comfortable, we do ask about their experience and how we can improve as a unit. Now we are integrating the transplant team social workers as well (they often keep in close contact with former patients as this unit is involved very closely with transplant patients).

The "success stories" center around the hope that sharing experiences of our patients outside the hospital brings a sense of fulfillment to the nurses. Hopefully, connecting how their extraordinary efforts actually help people survive and meet their health goals provides encouragement and meaning to the work. We have more plans for these success stories. For example, we are hoping to make this a more formal process and easier for more patients to connect if they desire. Practice council interviews, short videos, huddle integration, and messages and photos on our bulletin boards are all part of the future plan.

So far, seeing some familiar faces that were former patients has done a lot to personally encourage me. Often, especially considering the difficulties our unit experienced with COVID-19, it can feel quite gloomy on the unit. Intensive care nursing is an intense practice; seeing former patients who are now at home, happy and offering thanks to us is incredibly encouraging. The patients receive the opportunity to reconnect and share gratitude, and the experience appears healing for them as well. Success stories offer welcome conclusions to our practice that we would otherwise never realize.

—Stacy Street, BSN, RN, CCRN, Clinical Nurse II

Regularly reflecting on the significant, good work that we do is a needed component of self-caring for those in clinical work.

BOX 4.4: Recommendations for Practicing Caring for Self

- Self-awareness techniques, including how we are perceived by others
- Caring for the physical, emotional, social, and spiritual self
- Reflection on practice
- Relaxation
- Creative expression of the self
- Access to the natural environment
- Healthy caring for the physical body—exercise, health eating, and sleep
- Use of humor
- Regular self-monitoring

As humans have the capacity to continuously learn and grow, it follows that caring for self both personally and professionally may have the potential to positively influence lives—both our own and those we care for.

BOX 4.5: Caring for self by allowing oneself to feel physical as well as emotional sensations, reflecting on them slowly, making meaning of them, and using this introspection to relate to others in a continual pattern of action and inaction keeps one balanced and more "in tune" with the world's energy. Practicing personal and professional self-caring regularly sets up the conditions for self-knowing, a prerequisite for helping others.

Using the caring behaviors to care for self is a good way to integrate being and doing. The QCM provides the foundation for self-caring. See Figure 4.3.

Using the QCM, and the caring behaviors in particular, see Box 4.6 for suggestions on how individual nurses might use the caring behaviors to care for self:

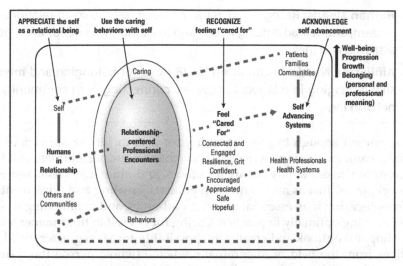

FIGURE 4.3 How does the Quality Model guide nurses' own well-being?

BOX 4.6: Intentionally Using the Caring Behaviors to Care for Self

- **Human Respect**: Recognizing *your* worthiness, use of a whole-person approach (biopsychosociculturalspiritual), careful handling of your body, acceptance of duty to self, preserving your autonomy, making contact with self (know thyself), and treating yourself with dignity.

- **Mutual Problem solving:** Regular reflection, information-seeking, using your strengths, clarifying misperceptions, accepting feedback, listening to self, assessing impact of work-life on health, adaption, finding ways to integrate being and doing, and seeking out new learnings.

- **Attentive Reassurance:** Paying attention to yourself, being accessible to yourself repeatedly, checking in with yourself (consistent availability to self), and reassuring yourself for a hopeful outlook.

- **Encouraging Manner:** Talking to self in a supportive manner, using encouraging behaviors related to lifestyle management, decreasing negative self-talk, reading inspiring stories, and spending time in nature.

- **Appreciation of Unique Meanings**: Personal "knowing" of self, including values and preferences, honoring your work experiences and intuitive knowledge; and appreciating and practicing within your sociocultural background.

- **Healing Environment:** Establishing a safe environment at work and home, creating aesthetically-pleasing surroundings, assembling "time-out" rooms at work, using appropriate apps, maintaining privacy/confidentiality/fidelity as appropriate, and using current evidence.

■ **Human Needs:** Recognizing YOUR physical, safety, socio-relational, self esteem, and self-advancing needs and assuring these needs are regularly assessed and met.

■ **Affiliation Needs:** Recognizing YOUR need for belonging and membership, engaging in relational activities, connecting with community, and networking

Valuing oneself enough to practice caring for self, including appreciating the internal meanings of our experiences, may change our perceptions, build confidence, optimize our ability to care for others, and ultimately create more positive workplaces. Just as nurses do with patients, creating and implementing a plan for self-caring is an essential aspect for attaining and maintaining wellness and performing optimally in practice. Caring for oneself in this manner leads to a more hopeful outlook and creates the possibility for even greater well-being. Initiatives from the field of integrative medicine (whole person [body–mind–spirit] health) are beginning to show some positive outcomes. For example, the state of North Carolina is developing a unique infrastructure to support integrated physical, behavioral, and social healthcare. The North Carolina Department of Health and Human Services, the Foundation for Health Leadership & Innovation, Cone Health, Atrium Health, and the One Charlotte Health Alliance are working together to advance the operationalization and garner resources for the program. Reducing inefficiencies and disparities by bringing together teams of primary and behavioral healthcare providers, using shared tools, and evidence-based, innovative practices while documenting lessons learned, are drawing national attention (Tilson et al., 2020). Although limitations exist in studies, emerging evidence about whole person health is showing some positive results, potentially enabling the other three foundational relationships. (Dusek et al., 2018; Kotalczyk & Lip, 2021; Leach et al., 2019).

Relating to Vulnerable Patients and Families

Before engaging in relationships with patients and families, health professionals must be sensitive to and appreciate the illness experience, including the enormous uncertainty and vulnerabilities that accompany illness and suffering. As complex beings that are constantly changing and relating, humans have objective (physical), subjective (emotional, cultural, spiritual), social (family, role functions), and spiritual characteristics. During an illness, all these characteristics are affected, and the results can be profound. First, there is the emotional reaction and necessary adjustment to the illness itself. Illness represents a fundamental threat to one's basic sense of wholeness. Persons may form certain meanings about their illnesses based on the knowledge they have about their own bodies, what they have heard or read about others in similar situations, individual psychological traits, and societal/cultural points of view. During the early part of the COVID-19 pandemic, for example, fear and uncertainty were profound. Included were such fears as fear of infection, death, pain, and isolation. The uncertainties about treatments as well as work, caring for dependent children, and the government's response added stress, anxiety; and in some cases, these conditions evolved into moral distress, depression, substance use, and even anger (Roy et al., 2021).

The physiological changes associated with illness can create feelings of discomfort, vulnerability, and dependence that generate loss of self-confidence and create doubt. Ambitions or plans must be suspended, and communication patterns change. Fulfilling one's role as parent, grandparent, spouse, worker, or friend is often disrupted; and the psychological impact of being ill presents a threat to one's sense of wholeness. Over time, these emotions may vary and can be viewed on a continuum from courageous acceptance to specific self-destructive behaviors that can lead to personal and family turmoil. With this awareness of the illness experience, consider the additional burden of residing (temporarily) in a cold and rushed hospital environment where others have created the conditions under which one will live for a few days.

Early in the hospital admission process, for example, emphasis is placed on payment and consent to treatment versus the transition to a new living space. Once admitted, individuals must conform to the work habits of the employees, including their shift changes, their unique norms and behaviors (the culture of the department), and their disciplinary traditions; the environment, including the noise, lights, facilities, and conversations; and the organization, including its leadership practices, protocols/procedures, and resources (or lack thereof). The sudden dependency placed on formerly independent individuals is an uneasy, tenuous state that may interfere with normal human needs such as rest and sleep, mood, feelings of safety and security, dignity, mobility, nourishment and elimination, affiliation needs, and sociocultural—spiritual practices, and situate them at high risk for adverse outcomes.

BOX 4.7: Hospitalization unintentionally introduces nonstop invasion of patients' personal spaces by complete strangers, impersonalizes the care experience by labeling patients according to diagnoses, and allows little autonomy in terms of patients' personal routines. Thus, hospitalization itself poses significant risks that are not the result of the illness; in fact, many individuals leave the hospital in worse condition than when they entered!

Hospital-acquired infections, pressure ulcers, deconditioned limbs, development of delirium, falls, and other adverse errors, not to mention frustration, unnecessary anxiety, and embarrassment, are examples of the inadvertent consequences of hospitalization. Many of these situations have now been used to develop specific advice to patients and families regarding hospitalization. For example, the American Hospital Association publishes The Patient Care Partnership (2003) on their website. It explains what to expect, patient rights, and patient responsibilities (www.aha.org/other-resources/

patient-care-partnership). Individual health systems also offer patients and their families information on how to protect themselves during hospitalization such as pamphlets or television-based displays on how to prevent falls. However, central to providing quality caring is the ability of healthcare professionals to "experience the other person's private world and feelings and to communicate to the other person some significant degree of that understanding" (Watson, 1979, p. 28).

Consider this example:

I am an extracorporeal membrane oxygenation (ECMO) specialist, the charge nurse of a 24-bed unit, and a Code/Rapid Response team member. I became a nurse after a successful career as a respiratory therapist. But then, one day, I became a patient. After spending the day sick, locked in my bedroom, I chose to call my doctor, who advised me to call 911. I decided to have my youngest son drive me to the emergency department, arriving in my pajamas and slippers with a blanket wrapped around myself due to extreme chill tremors.

I walked up to admissions and could barely write due to the severity of my entire body shaking. The nurse sat me down, and they immediately took my vital signs. My heart rate was over 150, my systolic blood pressure was in the 70's, and I had an elevated temperature.

I was rushed back to a room where they began fluid resuscitation. After two hours and four liters of fluid, my blood pressure remained low. The physician informed me they would be inserting a central line, starting levophed, and that I was being admitted to the intensive care unit.

I arrived in the intensive care unit well after midnight. I had worked in this unit years ago. However, nothing appeared familiar. I spent four days in the unit but remembered very little of my stay. I have no idea who cared for me and only remembered the frightening parts of my stay. The nurses woke me up and placed ice packs to bring down my fever. A young nurse changed the dressing on my peripherally inserted central catheter (PICC) line, ripping my skin off. The uncontrollable tremors would not stop. I was frightened and could not believe I was on the other side of the hospital bed. It was terrifying not knowing what was going to happen next. I just wanted the nurses to "care for me and help me recover" so I could go home and resume my everyday life.

Did the nurses appreciate the awful experience of this patient and how vulnerable she felt or did they "brush it off" since she "was an ICU nurse and should know?" Thankfully, this example has a positive ending:

My experience of being a patient in the intensive care unit was life changing. For example, during my ICU stay, the unit educator introduced me to journaling and highlighted the importance of this practice. Journaling, she said, could help me remember my stay and put my life back together once discharged from the hospital.

Once discharged, my primary care doctor informed me I would never work again as a critical care nurse. She felt the high-dose steroids and the long, 12-hour shifts would impair my capabilities. I was devastated! I could not imagine doing anything other than being a critical care nurse.

Thankfully, I was able to return to work with the support of my manager and the educator. They allowed me to ease back into 12-hour shifts. My coworkers were fantastic in ensuring I was supported during my transition back to work, always there to lend a helping hand.

A few months after my return, the educator asked me if I would like to participate in an 18-month project to develop intensive care unit diaries. I felt this was a perfect opportunity for me due to my experience of being a patient in an intensive care unit. I knew the importance of journaling and putting the puzzle of life back together after a critical illness.

My journey began through the development and implementation of the ICU diaries. Over the past few years, I have worked diligently to implement the ICU diaries in the cardiovascular ICU. The project originated as an evidence-based practice change supported by the healthcare facility in which I am employed.

The use of ICU diaries helps reduce patient and family member anxiety, depression, and post-traumatic stress. The concept of diaries as a potential vehicle for balancing the physical and psychological complications due to complex ICU patients is now a recommended standard practice (Davidson et al., 2017). The diary can explain what happened to the patient in the ICU, thus assisting patients to fill in any significant gaps, put any delusional memories into context, and aid physical and psychological recovery (Jones et al., 2012). "Intensive care diaries have been developed as a tool to improve factual memory of time spent in intensive care, with an aim to improve recovery from critical illness" Ulllman et al., 2015). They also are known to reduce post-intensive care syndrome in ICU survivors and families.

I then continued my research about how writing in diaries can affect nurses. Although the original diaries were written for the patient, writing by nurses may help them as well. Even though patients are not awake, the nurse sustains a conversation via diary writing. There is a temporal lag before the message reaches its destination, but delivering the message might offer nurses a sense of caring, comfort, and closure.

Understanding more about nurses' experiences while writing in diaries will help researchers develop the best methods of implementing diary programs and may improve communication and family satisfaction.

—Tamara Norton BSN, RN, CCRN

Or, consider this new grandmother's experience whose 1-year-old grandson was transferred from a rural hospital to a specialized children's hospital with a high fever and no urine output:

The first few days that he was in the hospital, it was my observation that he wasn't a priority or that he was receiving substandard care. I envisioned he would be transported quickly and received by a team of experts who were ready to treat him immediately. Rather, after the 5 hours it took for the transport service to coordinate and drive through traffic, he was finally admitted. Although a young doctor saw him in the first few hours after admission, his parents were left alone for the next 7 hours with no feedback on a plan of care. After a myriad of interviews with various doctors, a flurry of activity ensued to place a dialysis catheter. No further communication occurred during the first 2 days, so the mother called a hotline number she saw on a hospital pamphlet; and finally, a hospital administrator appeared to play the role of mediator between the parents, doctors, and nurses. The baby was moved to the pediatric intensive care unit (PICU) where he got better attention, but his fever climbed and complicated treatment. Both sets of grandparents and the parents lost confidence in the care provided and began to feel "he wouldn't make it." As the paternal grandmother stated, "I didn't want to insert myself between the parents and the staff—I felt terribly helpless—it was so hard to watch it all unfold. In observing the staff work, there were tremendous delays from when a decision was made to delivering the care—for example, 6 hours from the ordering of an important antibiotic medication to administration. In this case, although there were a whole slew of people involved in decision making and checking and rechecking, the patient paid a high price in delayed care. And yet, mistakes were made… several. The excuses we received several times were that there were more patients than usual. Don't they routinely plan for higher volumes of patients? However, sometimes I'd go out to the nurses' station and see nurses sitting at the station clearly not talking about work! Watching this play out and assuming most hospitals run this way, I have to say they are much worse than any environment I have ever worked in—so I would NEVER want to work in a hospital. It's too bad the cost of this hospital stay will be the same whether the care was excellent or not. I don't know of another industry or service where this is the case.

"On a positive note, a male nurse in the PICU was exceptional. He went out of his way to coordinate with the doctor to advocate for the baby to have more feedings while being held by his parents since that was the only thing that comforted him. This particular nurse went to the trouble to analyze his treatment plan and spent time with me explaining in detail the rationale for how much and what kinds of fluids the baby could have."

The child received multiple dialysis treatments and eventually got well enough to go home. However, six family members (two parents and four grandparents) were anxious, fearful, and received inadequate communication. The child experienced multiple delays in treatment that contributed to a longer length of stay. Why was only one nurse attuned to the needs of the patient and family? What could have been done differently?

BOX 4.8: As patients and families present to the health system for needed care, they are already compromised from their illness or situation, but they are further burdened by well-intentioned health professionals and health systems that are not designed to relate. In fact, this ability to authentically relate in a caring manner is essential to high quality.

The patient experience is an independent and reimbursable outcome measure that is routinely used as one indicator of healthcare excellence (Agency for Healthcare Research and Quality, 2021). Interestingly, when many patients are asked about their hospital experiences, most discuss their interactions with staff members and talk about issues such as communication patterns, how safe they felt, whether they were treated with respect and included in decision-making, and whether "people knew what they were doing" (personal experience). Just as relationships are an important aspect of human living, they are just as important during illness and hospitalization (maybe more so). In fact, relationships with health professionals play an important role in shaping patient experiences and other health outcomes.

Practicing Caring for Patients and Families

The patient–clinician relationship is central to the provision of high-quality care; ensuring it is authentically caring, however, is the cornerstone of practicing according to the QCM. The word, therapeutic, has been used to denote characteristics of high-quality relationships between patients and clinicians. Also known as the therapeutic alliance, therapeutic relationships have been described as beneficial, satisfying, healing, and restorative. Often, therapeutic relationships have been recognized as essential for positive patient outcomes (Pratt et al., 2021). Nevertheless, therapeutic relationships are often incomplete, not valued in the overall scheme of healthcare, or simply overlooked by some. Even more disappointing is the fact that that they are not routinely assessed or modified as a part of ongoing performance improvement efforts. Preliminary evidence, however, reveals that positive patient-clinician relationships positively influences health outcomes (Allen et al., 2017; Tavakoly Sany et al., 2020).

Several healthcare theorists have documented certain factors as necessary for therapeutic relationships (Rogers, 1961; Yalom, 1975). Nursing theorists such as King (1981) discussed "perceptual accuracy;" Watson (1979, 1985) identified 10 factors, also known as clinical caritas processes (Watson, 2008); Peplau (1952) described orientation, identification, development, and conclusion of patient–nurse relationships; and Travelbee (1966) discussed the humanistic processes of original encounter, emerging identities, empathy, and sympathy. In general, these authors refer to the demeanor, communication style (verbal and nonverbal), and presence, along with the specific behaviors of health professionals that are engaging, assistive, and supportive. This relationship is considered therapeutic, healing, or caring when recipients feel affirmed, understood, and somewhat equal. In reality both the carer and the one being cared for benefit from therapeutic relationships in terms of the shared process and the attainment of something valuable.

BOX 4.9: When nurses (and other health professionals) attentively look patients in the eye, understand their discomfort and worries, and help mutually solve them, caring relationships are revealed, and through the experience, great pride is perceived.

More recently, a scoping review of the authenticity (the process of engaging genuinely) was undertaken. The authors used thematic analysis of 21 studies to reveal four patient and nurse-related themes common to authentic relationships. They were getting to know the patient as a person, the complexity of relationship building, the nurse characteristics and behaviors that support the relationship, and the patient's voice (Pratt et al., 2021).

According to Pratt et al., (2021), knowing the patient as person requires interaction that eventually deepens through ongoing engagement into a genuine connection. Attentive listening to patients and families over time enabled them to feel as if they "mattered" and consequently were more able to trust and disclose. Nurses and patients both benefitted from authentically relating, feeling valued and experiencing greater satisfaction. However, cultivating these relational aspects of professional practice requires interaction, knowledge, skills, and presence (time). Experienced health professionals know this and are able to integrate this relational component with the more instrumental activities associated with professional practice. Finally, the patients' voice is central to authentic engagement. Working in this manner is somewhat countercultural in this day of fast-paced, highly intense health systems. As such, it requires the ability to tolerate some uncertainty or ambiguity and remain attentive and open minded. Use of oneself in this way honors the individual patient and the health professional as life-giving energy sources. Specific processes of relating during relationship-centered professional encounters will be described in Chapter 5.

BOX 4.10: A key aspect of *therapeutic* relating is the recognition that patients' experiences and concerns, versus their diagnosis or procedure, are primary and then responding in a timely and caring manner. Recognizing patient problems, anticipating patient experiences, being (relating) and doing (acting) together, monitoring how patients change in response to clinical practice, and appropriately revising care represent caring practice.

Relating to Each Other

Health professionals today are a multigenerational, diverse working group with individual psychosociocultural, spiritual, and life experience characteristics that shape their performance. In addition, many are caring for the most complex, diverse, acute, and chronically ill population this nation has ever seen. Professional nurses supervise unlicensed personnel, provide care 24/7, chase down equipment and supplies, coordinate healthcare teams, participate in shared governance councils and performance improvement meetings, assist in the implementation and evaluation of electronic health records, and many are pursuing advanced education. Meanwhile, the pandemic-related and economic constraints of the last few years have forced hospitals and other healthcare agencies to concentrate on cost containment and restructuring efforts, many of which have not been evaluated in terms of their consequences to patients and employees. Health professionals today are frequently working at the interface between the efficiency and resource needs of the health system and the human caring needs of patients and families.

In this environment, there is enormous responsibility, high intensity, and workplace tension. Complicating these system difficulties are future unknowns concerning the workforce, long-term employment, reimbursement, and retirement, all contributing to perceived insensitivities in the workplace. Horizontal violence among peers is sadly prevalent, and interprofessional collaboration has not been optimized. However, creating a therapeutic context in which healing can occur relies not just on the caring dispositions of individual clinicians but also on the collective relational capacities of interprofessional healthcare teams (Lee et al., 2021; Pascucci et al., 2020).

Although colleagues typically are associated through common work, *being collaborative* has a stronger meaning. It denotes a commitment to working together by sharing knowledge and power, appreciating each other as role models, making decisions together, relying on each other, and rooting for one another—all of which are ways that health professionals demonstrate a collaborative nature. *Being collaborative* suggests a higher form of relating to another that assumes sharing of information followed by collective action so that mutual goals are attained (in this case, what is in the best interest of the patient and family). Furthermore, interprofessional collaborative practice (IPCP) is a dynamic process that is interpersonal and interdependent (e.g., two or more disciplines interacting in a trusting manner with patients and families) and is characterized as an alliance or partnership (World Health Professions Alliance, 2010). In other words, practicing interprofessionally involves a combination of attitudes, thoughts, and actions that characterize IPCP. Interestingly, in a small qualitative study ($N = 36$), the perspectives of healthcare professionals on ways to promote IPCP was investigated. Using face-to-face in-depth interviews, findings indicated that the underlying facilitator of IPCP was a culture of caring—human connections among interprofessional team members. Building caring relationships, developing an ownership mentality, providing constructive feedback, applying strengths-based practice, and acting as the first and last lines of defense were recommended as strategies for promoting IPCP (Wei et al., 2020).

The term, *Interprofessional Education Collaborative (ICPC)*, has been reported in the past to be related to groups of health professionals working "in relationship" (Mathewson, 1955). However, a more precise direction for IPCP is now available. For example, The World Health Organization (WHO, 2010) has published a framework for action on collaboration and interprofessional education (IPE) and practice, core competencies have been established (AACN, 2011), and centers for IPCP research (e.g., National Center for Interprofessional Practice and Education, 2021, https://nexusipe.org/) has been established at the University of Minnesota in the hopes of offering evaluation, research, data, and evidence supporting IPCP. Interprofessional research is well underway with multiple universities establishing programs and websites promoting IPCP training and research.

The National Center for Advancing Translational Sciences at the National Institutes of Health has built a systems approach enabling effective team science to assist in their own efforts to facilitate cross-disciplinary team science to advance translation of findings into practice (Vogel et al., 2021). During the COVID-19 pandemic, healthcare teams necessarily practiced with greater flexibility and adapted rapidly to shifting situations and circumstances. In turn, the pandemic heightened team-based care, including interprofessional values and practices and may even have diluted hierarchies within healthcare practice and delivery (Michalec & Lamb, 2020). Using this opportunity to accelerate IPE and IPCP research provides an opportunity for advancing the understanding of core team phenomena. However, truly "placing the patient at the center of care"

(p. 1) seems to be the core of IPCP with benefits reported to health systems and patient and job satisfaction realized as well (Flood et al., 2021).

Although advances have been made in IPE, true IPCP (especially in the hospital setting) remains developmental. Past reports of discrepancies in nurse and physician perceptions of IPCP have accumulated, particularly in specialty areas (Makary et al., 2006; Thomas et al., 2003; Sexton et al., 2006). However, a more recent multisite study of interprofessional teamwork and collaboration on medical units using 420 participants, found significant differences in perceptions of teamwork climate across sites and in collaboration across professional categories on general medical services (O'Leary et al., 2020). Although limitations were present, these findings are consistent with research in other settings, with physicians perceiving collaboration with nurses as more favorable than nurses perceived collaboration with physicians. Thus, true IPCP may remain more of an ideal rather than a real practice, especially in the hospital setting where competing priorities are constantly changing.

Although team science and particular funding mechanisms demonstrate the importance of interprofessional collaboration to advancing knowledge, ongoing research related to maximizing IPCP practice, and the lessons learned about teamwork during COVID-19 may help reduce the time required to transition from observations made through the research process into real world interventions that can improve the health of individuals and the American public. Key to all these initiatives is the collaborative (caring) relationships established and cultivated between two or more health professionals with the patient as a participating partner, and mutual goals (as established by the patient) are shared (see Figure 4.4).

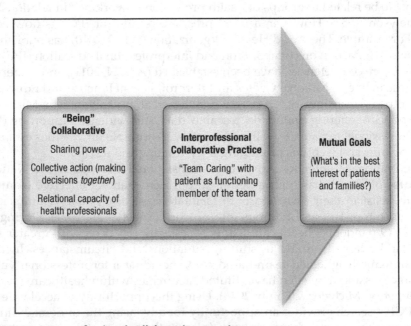

FIGURE 4.4 Interprofessional collaborative practice.

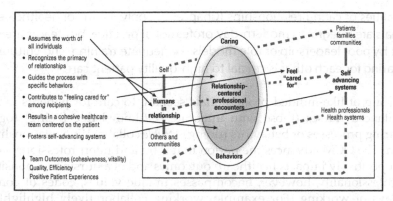

FIGURE 4.5 **How does the Quality-Caring Model guide interprofessional collaborative practice?**

Practicing Caring for Each Other

IPCP involves the integration of different disciplinary perspectives to better understand and treat complex patient conditions. Solutions created this way could not be accomplished by a single person or organization alone. Rather, IPCP requires continuous interaction and knowledge sharing, reconciliation of differences and sometimes opposing views among multiple health professionals. Resolving and/or exploring a variety of care issues taps relational processes that optimize team and patients' participation, that is, the *caring behaviors*. In this way, various health professionals and patients are driven by patient needs, but function interdependently, and are simultaneously active members of the team and recipients of the process. In other words, health professionals who use the caring behaviors to work interprofessionally not only help patients achieve their health goals, but also benefit from the process. Caring for each other, nurse to nurse and interprofessionally, is essential to quality health outcomes. IPCP is situated in the QCM as an integral relationship and has benefits not only for the patient and family but for healthcare providers as well. See Figure 4.5.

In health systems where IPCP is optimized, communication, shared decision-making, respect, excellence, altruism, and caring are typical characteristics of the practice environment.

Organizational leadership is crucial to the success of IPCP as is initial and ongoing education. IPE competencies (i.e., values/ethics for IPE, roles and responsibilities, interprofessional communication, and teams and teamwork) are foundational for ICPC (2016). The revised *Essentials: Core Competencies for Professional Nursing Education* (AACN, 2021) contains an entire standard centered on "intentional collaboration across professions and with care team members, patients, families, communities, and other stakeholders to optimize care, enhance the healthcare experience, and strengthen outcomes" (p. 42).

BOX 4.11: Such collaborative relationships, when optimized, become meaningful—beyond disciplinary boundaries—with the patient as a functioning participant. Thus, true collaborative relationships are often referred to as team-based care or team care; in the QCM, a more appropriate term may be *team caring*, as the qualities of caring relationships (Chapter 5) apply. Teams of healthcare professionals are integral to modern-day professional practice, but teams are easily broken by poor leadership or role models, inadequate training, and cultural barriers. Caring for each other is crucial to high-quality patient care.

As a group of like-minded professionals seeking to care for patients in need, well-balanced nurses (those who integrate self-knowledge [being] together with caring processes or behaviors (doing), *enable* collaborative relationships to flourish. The QCM advances the notion that intra and interprofessional collaboration positively impacts healthcare outcomes and is a nursing responsibility. Interprofessionality, however, encompasses unique values, codes of conduct, and ways of working. For example, working collaboratively highlights the patient/client as central to the process with health professionals and patients/families relating interdependently. Patients' needs in this case determine the interactions between professionals. IPCP recognizes and honors the diverse interests and uneven power among the care team as well as the bonds that develop between team members. Finally, taking the time to "know" team members in terms of understanding, at least conceptually, each other's frame of reference and roles and responsibilities helps to move the team from individual exclusive professional "turfs" to sharing a common professional space. Using caring relationships in day-to-day interactions with colleagues fosters this common professional space (i.e., healthy work environments) that may contribute to improved quality of work life, engaged employees, more opportunities for shared clinical research, and improved and more efficient patient outcomes.

Relating to the Community Served

Just as caring for self, patients and families, and other health professionals, caring for communities is a foundational relationship in the QCM. Communities are associated with groups of people with diverse characteristics who are linked by various factors such as geographic location, social ties, or demographics and often share common perspectives. Just as individuals are multidimensional, so too are communities. In fact, communities are complex entities that have specific features such as size, density, spacing, demographics, and industry and, when considering healthcare, life expectancy, health status, and SDOH. Understanding and using these features in care delivery optimizes self-advancing systems.

On the other hand, today's communities are facing tremendous pressures. Members of growing communities are living with shifting crime rates, economics, environmental issues, health and health equity, literacy, activism, differing faith/s and other changes, often without supportive extended families. Some commute long distances to work, while others work from home or are unemployed. Geographic areas are evolving. For example, some rural environments are expanding, whereas other cosmopolitan areas are downsizing without real solutions for the interruptions that these alterations prompt. Functions of communities are transforming as workplaces change or are deleted, families leave or move in, tax rates increase, school problems occur, and public policy varies.

Such stressors sometimes lead to less engagement in community service and eventual frustration, apathy, and stagnation as community members begin to feel powerless over their changing circumstances.

For example, the acceleration of COVID-19 and its negative consequences have had grave consequences in certain American communities. The COVID-19 pandemic affected marriages, childcare, and employment. Furthermore, implications for schools and universities, local police departments, and hospital emergency rooms drove some communities to despair. Others were mobilized—some communities, for example, joined forces to immunize persons in large geographic areas, and others created communities of learning for children who could not attend school in person. Community challenges can be problematic while at the same time energizing as citizens decide whether to engage.

Nurses and other health professionals can augment community engagement by using their relationship-centric approach to participate. Healthy communities are dependent on individuals who are committed to healthy environments and who can communicate and drive needed change. For example, health professionals can help drive agendas for neighborhood or community group meetings, share their knowledge of more healthful approaches, help adequately disseminate research, and most importantly, participate through caring relationships in decision making and implementation of local projects. In this way, communities can make more healthy decisions, informed by expert members who share an identity.

Many have suggested that community engagement benefits health professionals as well. For example, playing a meaningful role in the deliberations and decision-making about community projects or programs creates opportunities for health professionals to link with schools and other public services, gain access to community personnel and resources, obtain expert recognition, and learn while increasing the likelihood that effective solutions may be realized. The Centers for Disease Control and Prevention (CDC) views community engagement as necessary for health and equity (CDC, 2021). Thus, commitment of time and energy in true community partnership is a form of caring that is beneficial for healthcare professionals as well as their communities. Using their unique relational strengths outside of the normal work environment, health professionals who are engaged in their communities, provide needed expertise in support of health and health equity in the larger population served.

While health professionals who work in other environments are often involved in geographically based groups or populations with similar sociocultural features, the use of the term *community* varies. In reality, it has also come to mean a group of people who share something in common (regardless of where they live). This definition expands the notion of a geographic community to one where connection or belonging to a group becomes associated with ongoing support, promotion of resilience, and sustainability. For example, communities of practice (CoP) are groups of people who share a common interest or concern or a passion for a topic, and who deepen their knowledge and experience in the topic by interacting on a regular basis (Wenger et al., 2002). Common characteristics in CoPs are interaction, collaboration to share and create knowledge, and the promotion of a shared identity among its members. As a process, one of the key elements of a CoP is mutual engagement (Delgado et al., 2021). Likewise, learning communities, often used in higher education, are associated with higher student engagement and academic achievement. As members of practice or learning communities, health professionals use their relational skills to mutually interact, advancing the collective aims of the group.

Practicing Caring for Communities

Caring for communities can take many forms. A fundamental principle of caring is *enabling others* through the various caring behaviors. Facilitating community members to "feel cared for" provides the glue to ongoing engagement. The key to caring for communities is building a network of relationships among members and the informal day-to-day exchanges that occur among them. When individual relationships among members are of a caring nature, they feel safe and dignified, resulting in richer collective participation. Because most community involvement is voluntary, it is important that members see the value of their participation so that continued engagement and resulting human advancement is possible. As professionals who deliver care to community members, better understanding of their unique characteristics helps target health services to their particular needs. Thus, really understanding the "community served" is a responsibility of health professionals who use the QCM as the foundation of their practice.

Many initiatives in healthcare are ongoing to increase participation by health care professionals in larger community groups. For example, an organization in the northeast has collaborated with a community group to develop and obtain funding to increase breastfeeding rates among the diverse community they serve. Emergency department nurses at a hospital in the middle Atlantic region that uses the QCM as the basis for practice engaged with the local regional committee on substance use to develop a comprehensive prevention program. Nursing students and their faculty members led immunization clinics all over the United States during the COVID-19 pandemic. Many nurses are participants in regional disaster teams and respond to natural disasters; regularly provide education to community groups, including schools; facilitate wellness clinics; and raise money for research and other community health initiatives. A large national demonstration project, namely the Massachusetts Department of Public Health's (MDPH) National TeleNursing Center (NTC) has integrated the QCM into the NTC's Professional TeleSANE Practice Model to provide a quality, trauma-informed patient experience (Meunier-Sham et al. 2019). Consider the following example.

Since Sexual Assault Nurse Examiners (SANE) have been shown to improve the experience of sexual assault survivors in many perspectives (Shaw & Coates, 2021; Shaw et al., 2017), access to their expertise is important. Unfortunately, such expertise is not equitable across the nation. Telehealth has provided an important opportunity to expand SANE access to underserved communities by adding remote TeleSANE practice so that expert TeleSANEs are virtually side-by-side with a Remote Site Clinician (RSC) throughout a 3 to 4-hour sexual assault examination that includes forensic evidence collection. In this practice, the QCM Caring Behaviors, modeled by the TeleSANE, are foundational to the sexual assault patient's experience. The application of the Caring Behaviors is critical to building the TeleSANE/RSC relationship, which helps ensure respectful teamwork during all three phases of the NTC's model (PreEncounter, Encounter, Post-Encounter). During the PreEncounter (outside of the patient's presence), the two clinicians discuss the RSC's experience with conducting forensic exams, what concerns the RSC may have (Appreciation of Unique Meanings), if there is patient or case specific information that could provide a challenge, and what approaches might be helpful to mitigate negative outcomes (Mutual Problem Solving). The Pre-Encounter phase gives the teleSANE time to acknowledge and appreciate the RSC's prior experience (Human Respect), demonstrates a supportive approach, and reassures the RSC that she will be "by their side" throughout the entire patient encounter (Encouraging Manner). A critical component of the Pre-Encounter is to establish a negotiated "gentle interruption" a key phrase or signal that either party can use if the RSC requires additional assistance (Attentive Reassurance). Negotiating the interruption prior to the patient interaction assures the RSC that the TeleSANE's presence is to provide guidance and support not to undermine the RSC's role with the patient (Human Respect). During the Pre-Encounter, the TeleSANE also discusses ways to ensure that the patient's requests, such as food, drink, and toileting are met (Basic Needs) while also maintaining privacy and confidentiality (Healing Environment).

While patient care, the forensic exam, and forensic evidence collection are the major components of the Encounter phase, the trust and rapport that the nurses establish during the Pre-Encounter is pivotal to a successful patient experience. During the Encounter, the TeleSANE's "birds eye view" of the room allows for assessment of verbal and non-verbal cues from the RSC, providing input, encouragement, and feedback to the RSC (Attentive Reassurance). The Post-Encounter begins after the patient has been discharged and provides an opportunity for the TeleSANE and RSC to review documentation, packaging of evidence and chain of custody. Together they discuss what went well and what could be improved upon (Mutual Problem Solving), and debrief about the emotional impact of the case (Appreciation of Unique Meaning). If needed, the TeleSANE reviews vicarious trauma and self-Care resources available through the NTC. It is also a time for the TeleSANE to acknowledge the RSC's ability to provide excellent care during what may be a stressful experience (Affiliation Needs). The QCM model has now proven helpful in over 560 Encounters and Consultations that the NTC has provided to support/mentor less experienced SANEs, as well in situations in which RSCs have previously received limited to no training in caring for patients who are reporting a sexual assault (Walsh et al., 2019).

—Randi Petricone MSN, CNP, RN, WHNP-BC,
SANE
Associate Director, NationalTelenursing Center,
TeleSANE Services, and
Joan Meunier-Sham RN, MS,
Director—MA SANE Program,
National Nursing TeleNursing Program,
Massachusetts Department of Public Health

It is obvious in this example that the remote TeleSANE's use of the caring behaviors facilitates the RSC's ability to "feel cared for," reducing anxiety and providing the motivation for ongoing interaction and disclosure, and ultimately, to increase equitable services particularly in remote communities throughout the United States.

Health educators regularly use service-learning concepts as strategies to bridge the gap between classroom and community. Most universities have formal service-learning curricula that generate genuine linkages among the university, its students, and the community that positively affect student learning and overall community health. Engaging members of the local community by offering information and education assists students in expanding their knowledge of healthcare and appreciation of cultural diversity by participating directly in the community in which they live.

At the graduate level, examples of community-based health professions programs are plentiful. Many health researchers routinely partner with community agencies to consider interventions that may enhance the health of the community. Connecting to the larger community in which one lives provides unique experiences for health professionals to improve the health of that community.

For example, assisting communities to improve their capacity for change in a specific geographic area is necessary to tackle their ongoing problems, while preserving their unique sociocultural ties. Without regular interaction among citizens, communities are unable to move forward, ensure social justice, build collective resilience (needed in times of disasters or great change), and promote the common good; in other words, they become unhealthy. Healthy communities, on the other hand, provide opportunities for authentic citizen participation in which old and new ideas are included. Building community capacity is a civic duty to which healthcare providers can greatly contribute. Healthy communities are fundamental to the health and safety of citizens and allow citizens to have a voice, promote quality of life and economic opportunity, and raise hope for the future. In healthy communities, there is a noticeable collaboration between private and governmental services and attractive and clean surroundings. These outcomes are of special interest to health professionals who are advocates for good health. Actively community-engaged health professionals will not only realize great personal benefits, but will ensure the ongoing vitality of the communities they serve. See Figure 4.6.

IMPORTANCE OF RELATIONSHIPS IN HEALTH SYSTEMS

The primacy of relationships among health professionals and those they interact with on a daily basis must be acknowledged as fundamental to the QCM. In fact, Relational Coordination Theory (Bolton et al., 2021) focuses on the interdependency of health systems and the high-quality relationships that are necessary for quality outcomes. The focus on communication, building shared goals and knowledge, and mutual respect across boundaries (e.g., among departments and communities) aligns well with the QCM and reinforces the power of relationships to effectively coordinate the work. The importance of meaningful relationships in healthcare cannot be underestimated. With increasing

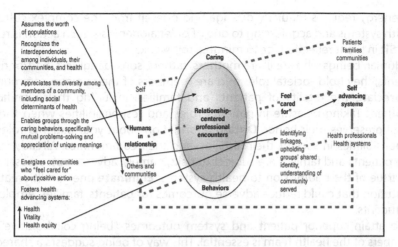

FIGURE 4.6 How does the Quality-Caring Model guide caring for communities?

evidence that building and maintaining strong caring relationships is a process for change in itself, health professionals must recognize their role in cultivating caring relationships with self, patients and families, with other health professionals, and in communities, ultimately facilitating the generative force necessary to advance positive health outcomes.

SUMMARY

The focus of this chapter centered on the four relationships foundational to the QCM—relating to self, to patients and families, to each other, and to the community served. These four relationships form the basic underpinnings for quality caring professional practice; some evidence links them to improved patient and health professional outcomes. Relationships that are of a caring nature are meaningful or therapeutic (healing or caring) and induce empowerment, a sense of belonging and well-being. Furthermore, they may generate positive energy that fuels new or sustained healthy behaviors. Finally, caring relationships with self are explored in depth as foundational to caring relationships with others.

CALL TO ACTION

Relationships are central to the human condition; **reflect** on the beauty of the human person as he or she lives in relation to the universe. Slowing down enough to contact one's inner world—thoughts, desires, feelings—permits one to gain access to his or her own realty. Linking to this valuable resource of self helps one remember what he or she already knows—the powerful impact of one's work. **Recognize** nursing's power. The duality of doing (actions) and being (authentic use of self in the moment) simultaneously is crucial to quality patient care. Nurses who integrate the two behaviors create meaning, are comforting, and affirm human dignity. **Practice** being and doing together. Balancing external and internal energy requires regularly disengaging oneself from the complex culture of health systems and acquiescing to one of quiet aloneness—such action is renewing. **Sit** in silent reflection for 15 minutes this week.

Human beings who are ill are mothers, fathers, sons, daughters, and/or grandparents; they hold societal roles and are members of their unique communities. **Appreciate** the totality of patients and families, including their significance to others. Taking pleasure in patients' roles and responsibilities when they are not ill preserves their honor. **Obtain** information about your patients' roles and responsibilities in society, their families, and their communities. Already vulnerable patients and families are subject to risks, namely, adverse outcomes, merely by virtue of their admission to health systems. **Eliminate** one condition at your institution that could reduce adverse outcomes for patients, families, employees, or students.

To attain superior patient and system outcomes, "being collaborative" with members of the health team is essential. This way of being suggests a shared and reciprocal relationship that is focused on the common goal of "what is best for patients and families." **Share** your true self with the health team. Reaching out to health team members to actively listen, being accessible to energetically dialogue about clinical issues, providing encouragement and enthusiasm, reinforcing one's importance to the health team, respecting privacy and safety, and acknowledging the team member's human and affiliation needs set the tone for future interactions and generates ease in the workplace. **Choose** to be caring with the health team.

Healthy communities are enhanced by caring relationships. **Join** a community group today. Caring relationships are essential for safe and quality health systems. **Practice** caring for self, for patients and families, for each other, and for communities served.

REFLECTIVE QUESTIONS/APPLICATIONS

For Professional Nurses in Clinical Practice:

- Are self-caring practices among nurses visible in your institution? What are they? Are they routinely used?
- What avenues exist at your institution for nurses to integrate mindful practice into the workflow?
- Name three things you do to care for your physical self.
- What specific adverse outcomes occur at your health system as a consequence of the hospitalization itself?
- What routine interprofessional collaboration occurs in your department? Do you participate? Why or why not?
- How do you capture the patient's unique situation during the admission assessment? Is it necessary?
- What community-based activities are you engaged in? How does your expertise benefit your community?

For Professional Nurses in Educational Practice:

- How would you assist students to learn the four foundational relationships? How would it differ by program or level?
- Reflect on IPCP, including the revised AACN competencies. How would you ensure that undergraduate students are competent in these behaviors? What new learning strategies would you employ to help students attain competence in IPCP? How would you evaluate attainment of IPCP competencies at graduation?
- How do you practice holistic self-caring? Are your students aware of it? Why or why not?
- What avenues exist to help students realize the personal benefits of caring for communities? What about understanding the vulnerabilities associated with hospitalization?

For Professional Nurses in Leadership Practice:

- What new relationship insights from this chapter will inform your leadership?
- What environmental reminders could you create to prompt professional nurses at your institution to be mindful of the important work they do?
- Reflect on the four relationships discussed in this chapter. At what level are they being performed at your institution? How could they be strengthened?
- Are you leading a relationship-centered organization? How do you know?
- Describe the innovative ways in which nurses at your facility care for the community they serve. How often are these activities disseminated to a wider audience?
- How do you specifically care for yourself?
- Give specific examples of tangible ways in which the organizational culture at your institution demonstrates support for IPCP.

PRACTICE ANALYSIS

Outside the door of a patient's room on an inpatient unit at a prominent academic health center, five individuals were observed shouting, one was crying, and two more were sitting on the ground. As it turns out, all were family members of a woman in her 40s who had been healthy prior to admission. Apparently, she had a partial colectomy for a benign mass and was post-op for 2 days when she starting spiking fevers up to 103°F and 104°F. Over several days, it was determined that she had a widespread abdominal infection and needed IV antibiotics. The nurses asked her to call them when she needed to use the bathroom because she had been unstable on her feet. However, early the day before, she got up by herself and fell. A head CT scan and vital signs were negative.

Over the course of the next 24 hours, the nurses observed that she appeared a little lethargic and did not seem able to do her own activities of daily living (ADLs). Nevertheless, she was recovering from the infection nicely, and the patient's surgeon (who did not see the patient in person) informed the family of this via telephone prior to their arrival. They expected to see a woman well on her way to recovery. In fact, many of them had skipped work that day to be with her. What they saw when they arrived was a huge surprise and not a positive one! They immediately acted out and demanded to see the "head nurse" who came to the bedside and explained that her slight change in status had not yet been communicated to the surgeon who had been in the OR all morning. She assured them that the patient was being well monitored and asked them to please "quiet down" so other patients could rest. This only enraged the family more, and they continued to shout loudly, demanding to speak to the doctor and the hospital administration. The patient died 2 days later from a cerebral hemorrhage due to the fall.

- How attuned were the health professionals in this case to the family's experience of hospitalization?
- What could have helped them better appreciate the family's view?
- How did the "head nurse" relate to the family members? What would you have done differently?
- Were the surgeon and nurses collaborating on this patient's care? Why or why not? What would you have done differently, if anything?

REFERENCES

Agency for Healthcare Research and Quality. (2021). What is patient experience? Available at: https://www.ahrq.gov/cahps/index.html

Alexander, G., Rollins, K., Walker, D., Wong, L., & Pennings, J. (2015). Yoga for self-care and burnout prevention among nurses. *Workplace Health & Safety, 63*(10), 462–470. https://doi.org/10.1177/2165079915596102

Allen, M. L., Lê Cook, B., Carson, N., Interian, A., La Roche, M., & Alegría, M. (2017). Patient-provider therapeutic alliance contributes to patient activation in community mental health clinics. *Administration and Policy in Mental Health and Mental Health Services Research, 44*(4), 431–440. https://doi.org/10.1007/s10488-015-0655-8

American Association of Colleges of Nursing. (2011). *Core competencies for interprofessional collaborative practice*. Washington, DC: Author.

American Association of Colleges of Nursing. (2021). *The essentials: Core competencies for professional nursing education*. Washington, DC: Author.

American Hospital Association. (2003). The patient care partnership. Available at: https://www.aha.org/other-resources/patient-care-partnership

American Nurses Association. (2015). Code of ethics for nurses with interpretive statements. Available at: https://nursingworld.org/coe-view-only

American Nurses Association Enterprise. (2020). *What is the Healthy Nurse, Healthy Nation Grand Challenge? Healthy Nurse, Healthy Nation*. Available at: https://www.healthy-nursehealthynation.org/

American Nurses Association. (2021). *Nursing: Scope and standards of practice* (4th ed.). Author.

American Nurses Association and American Holistic Nurses Association. (2017). *Holistic nursing: Scope and standards of practice* (2nd ed.). Author.

Anderson, R., Mammen, K., Paul, P., Pletch, A., & Pulia, K. N. (2017). Using yoga to improve stress in psychiatric nurses in a pilot study. *Journal of Alternative and Complementary Medicine, 23*(6), 494–495.

Andrews, H., Tierney, S., & Seers, K. (2020). Needing permission: The experience of self-care and self-compassion in nursing: A constructivist grounded theory study. *International Journal of Nursing Studies, 101,* 103436. https://doi.org/ijnurstu2019.103436

Basten, C., & Touyz, S. (2020). Sense of self: Its place in personality disturbance, psychopathology, and normal experience. *Review of General Psychology, 24*(2), 159–171. https://doi.org/10.1177/1089268019880884

Bergin, C., & Bergin, D. (2009). Attachment in the classroom. *Educational Psychology Review, 21,* 141–170.

The Betsy Lehman Center for Patient Safety. (2019). The financial and human cost of medical error. Available at: https://betsylehmancenterma.gov/assets/uploads/Cost-of-Medical-Error-Report-2019.pdf

Bilgiç, S., & Acaroğlu, R. (2017). Effects of listening to music on the comfort of chemotherapy patients. *Western Journal of Nursing Research, 39*(6), 745–762. https://doi.org/10.1177/0193945916660527

Bolton, R., Logan, C., & Gittell, J. H. (2021). Revisiting relational coordination: A systematic review. *The Journal of Applied Behavioral Science, 57*(3), 290–322. https://doi.org/10.1177/0021886321991597

Borges, L. M., Barnes, S. M., Farnsworth, J. K., Drescher, K. C., & Walser, R. D. (2020). A contextual behavioral approach for responding to moral dilemma as in the age of COVID-19. *Journal of Contextual Behavioral Science, 17,* 95–101.

Bornstein, M. H. (2015). Children's parents. In R. M. Lerner (Ed.), Handbook of child psychology and developmental science, Vol. 4, ecological settings and processes (7th ed., pp. 55–132). Wiley.

Bornstein, M. H., & Leventhal, T. (2015). Children in bioecological landscapes of development. In R. M. Lerner (Ed.), Handbook of child psychology and developmental science. Vol. 4. Ecological settings and processes (7th ed., pp. 1–5). Wiley.

Braveman, P., & Gottlieb, L., (2014). The social determinants of health: It's time to consider the causes of the causes. *Public Health Reports, 129*(1 suppl 2), 19–31. https://doi.org/10.1177/00333549141291S206

Braveman, P., Egerter, S., & Williams, D. R. (2011). The social determinants of health: Coming of age. *Annual Review of Public Health, 32,* 381–98.

Bronk, K. (2019). The joint commission issues quick safety advisory on combating nurse burnout through resilience. The Joint Commission. Available at: https://www.jointcommission.org/resources/news-and-multimedia/newsletters/newsletters/quick-safety/quick-safety-50-developing-resilience-to-combat-nurse-burnout/

Bronson, K. (2017). Using mindfulness to decrease burnout and stress among nurses working in high intensity areas. [Doctoral dissertation, University of North Carolina—Chapel Hill]. https://doi.org/10.17615/t94t-ak26

Buhler, C., & Allen, M. (1972). *Introduction to humanistic psychology.* Brooks/Cole.

Buhler, C., & Marschak, M. (1967). Basic tendencies of human life. In C. Buhler & F. Massarik (Eds.). *The course of human life* (pp. 92–102). Springer Publishing Company.

Carden, J., Jones, R. J., & Passmore, J. (2021). Defining self-awareness in the context of adult development: A systematic literature review. *Journal of Management Education, 46*(1), 140–177. https://doi.org/10.1177/1052562921990065

Centers for Disease Control and Prevention. (2021). Meaningful community engagement for health and equity. Available at: https://www.cdc.gov/nccdphp/dnpao/state-local-programs/health-equity-guide/pdf/health-equity-guide/Health-Equity-Guide-sect-1-2.pdf

Chipps, E. M., Joseph, M. L., Alexander, C., et al. (2021). Setting the research agenda for nursing administration and leadership science: A Delphi study. *Journal of Nursing Administration, 51*(9), 430–438. https://doi.org/10.1097/NNA.0000000000001042

Crane, R. S., Brewer, J., Feldman, C., et al. (2017). What defines mindfulness-based programs? The warp and the weft. *Psychological Medicine, 47*(6), 990–999. https://doi.org/10.1017/S0033291716003317

Dalsania, A. K., Fastiggi, M. J., Kahlam, A., et al. (2022). The relationship between social determinants of health and racial disparities in COVID-19 mortality. *Journal of Racial and Ethnic Health Disparities 9*(1), 288–295. https://doi.org/10.1007/s40615-020-00952-y

Davidson, J. E., Aslakson, R. A., Long, A. C., et al. (2017). Guidelines for family-centered care in the neonatal, pediatric, and adult ICU. *Critical Care Medicine, 45*(1), 103–128. https://doi.org/10.1097/CCM.0000000000002169

Delgado, J., Siow, S., De Groot, J., et al. (2021). Towards collective moral resilience: The potential of communities of practice during the COVID-19 pandemic and beyond. *Journal of Medical Ethics, 47*, 374–382.

Drick, C. (2016). Self-care: A busy person's guide for finding time and balance. *Beginnings, 36*(4), 6–7.

Dusek, J. A., Griffin, K. H., Finch, M. D., Rivard, R. L., & Watson, D. (2018). Cost savings from reducing pain through the delivery of integrative medicine program to hospitalized patients. *Journal of Alternative and Complementary Medicine, 24*(6), 557–563. https://doi.org/10.1089/acm.2017.0203

Dyrbye, L., Shanafelt, T., Sinsky, C., et al. (2017). Burnout among health care professionals: A call to explore and address this under recognized threat to safe, high quality care. *National Academy Perspectives, 2017*, 1–11. https://iuhcpe.org/file_manager/1501524077-Burnout-Among-Health-Care-Professionals-A-Call-to-Explore-and-Address-This-Underrecognized-Threat.pdf

Erikson, E. H. (1964). *Insight and responsibility*. Norton.

Erikson, E. H. (1968). *Identity: Youth and crisis*. Norton.

Fakih, M., Bufalino, A., Sturm, L., et al. (2021). Coronavirus disease 2019 (COVID-19) pandemic, central-line–associated bloodstream infection (CLABSI), and catheter-associated urinary tract infection (CAUTI): The urgent need to refocus on hardwiring prevention efforts. *Infection Control & Hospital Epidemiology, 43*(1), 26–31. https://doi.org/10.1017/ice.2021.70

Farina, S., Minerva, E., & Bernardo, L. (2018). Introducing mindfulness practices for self-care. *Journal of Nurses in Professional Development, 34*(4), 194–198.

Feeney, B. C., & Collins, N. L. (2015). A new look at social support: A theoretical perspective on thriving through relationships. *Personality and Social Psychology Review, 19*(2), 113–147. https://doi.org/10.1177/1088868314544222

Flood, B., Smythe, L., Hocking, C., et al. (2021). Interprofessional practice: The path toward openness. *Journal of Interprofessional Care, 26*, 1–8. https://doi.org/10.1080/13561820.2021.1981264

Fore, A. M., & Sculli, G. L. (2013). A concept analysis of situational awareness in nursing. *Journal of Advanced Nursing, 69*(12), 2613–2621. https://doi.org/10.1111/jan.12130

Gallagher, L. M., Lagman, R., & Rybicki, L. (2018). Outcomes of music therapy interventions on symptom management in palliative medicine patients. *American Journal of Hospice and Palliative Care, 35*(2), 250–257. https://doi.org/10.1177/1049909117696723

Gibbs, G. (1988). *Learning by doing: A guide to teaching and learning methods: Further education unit*. Oxford Polytechnic.

Good, D. J., Lyddy, C. J., Glomb, T. M., et al. (2015). Contemplating mindfulness at work. *Journal of Management, 42*(1), 114–142. https://doi.org/10.1177/0149206315617003

Gould, R. (1978). *Transformations: Growth and change in adult life*. Simon & Schuster.

Greenberg, N., Docherty, M., Gnanapragasam, S., et al. (2020). Managing mental health challenges faced by healthcare workers during covid-19 pandemic. *British Medical Journal, 368,* m1211.

Haley, B., Heo, S., Wright, P., et al. (2017). Relationships among active listening, self-awareness, empathy, and patient-centered care in associate and baccalaureate degree nursing students. *NursingPlus Open, 3,* 11–16, https://doi.org/10.1016/j.npls.2017.05.001

Hall, L. H., Johnson, J., Watt, I., et al. (2016). Healthcare staff wellbeing, burnout, and patient safety: A systematic review. *PLoS One, 11*(7):e0159015. https://doi.org/10.1371/journal.pone.0159015

Halter, M., Boiko, O., Pelone, F., et al. (2017). The determinants and consequences of adult nursing staff turnover: A systematic review of systematic reviews. *BMC Health Services Research, 17*(1), 824, https://doi.org/10.1186/s12913-017-2707-0

Han, S., Shanafelt, T. D., Sinsky, C. A., et al. (2019). Estimating the attributable cost of physician burnout in the United States. *Annals of Internal Medicine, 170,* 784–790. https://doi.org/10.7326/M18-1422

Havighurst, R. (1953). *Human development and education.* McKay.

Hofmeyer, A., Taylor, R., & Kennedy, K. (2020). Knowledge for nurses to better care for themselves so they can better care for others during the Covid-19 pandemic and beyond. *Nurse Education Today, 94,* 104503. https://doi.org/10.1016/j.nedt.2020.104503

Howick, J., Kelly, P., & Kelly, M. (2019). Establishing a causal link between social relationships and health using the Bradford Hill guidelines. *SSM—Population Health, 8,* 100402, https://doi.org/10.1016/j.ssmph.2019.100402

Interprofessional Education Collaborative. (2016). *Core competencies for interprofessional collaborative practice: 2016 update.* Washington, DC: Interprofessional Education Collaborative. Available at: https://hsc.unm.edu/ipe/resources/ipec-2016-core-competencies.pdf

Jones, C., Bäckman, C., & Griffith, C. (2012). Intensive care diaries reduce PTSD-related symptoms in relatives following critical illness. *American Journal of Critical Care, 21*(3), 172–176.

Jung, C. (1933). *Modern man in search of a soul.* Harcourt, Brace.

Kabat-Zinn, J. (2012). *Mindfulness for beginners: Reclaiming the present moment—and your life.* Sounds True.

King, I. M. (1981). *A theory for nursing: Systems, concepts, process.* Wiley.

Kohlberg, L. (1986). *The philosophy of moral development.* Harper and Row.

Koren, M., & Purohit, S. (2014). Interventional studies to support the spiritual self-care of health care practitioners. *Holistic Nursing Practice, 28*(5), 291–300. https://doi.org/10.1097/hnp.0000000000000044

Kotalczyk, A., & Lip, G. (2021). Disparities in atrial fibrillation: A call for holistic care. *The Lancet Regional Health Europe, 7,* 100160. https://doi.org/10.1016/j.lanepe.2021.100160

Kushlev, K., Heintzelman, S. J., Lutes, L. D., et al. (2017). ENHANCE: Design and rationale of a randomized controlled trial for promoting enduring happiness & well-being. *Contemporary Clinical Trials, 52,* 62–74. https://doi.org/10.1016/j.cct.2016.11.003

Leach, M. J., Eaton, H., Agnew, T., et al. (2019). The effectiveness of integrative healthcare for chronic disease: A systematic review. *International Journal of Clinical Practice, 73,* e13321. https://doi.org/10.1111/ijcp.13321

Lee, J. K., McCutcheon, L. R. M., Fazel, M. T., et al. (2021). Assessment of interprofessional collaborative practices and outcomes in adults with diabetes and hypertension in primary care: A systematic review and meta-analysis. *JAMA Network Open, 4*(2), e2036725. https://doi.org/10.1001/jamanetworkopen.2020.36725

Levey, J., & Levey, M. (2019). Mindful leadership for personal and organisational resilience. *Clinical Radiology, 74*(10), 739–745. https://doi.org/10.1016/j.crad.2019.06.026

Levinson, D. J. (1966). *Seasons of a woman's life*. Alfred A. Knopf.

Levinson, D. J., Darrow, C. N., & Klein, E. B. (1978). *Seasons of a man's life*. Random House.

Li, J., & Julian, M. M. (2012). Developmental relationships as the active ingredient: A unifying working hypothesis of "what works" across intervention settings. *The American Journal of Orthopsychiatry, 82*(2), 157–166. https://doi.org/10.1111/j.1939-0025.2012.01151.x

Makary, M. A., Sexton, J. B., Freischlag, J. A., et al. (2006). Operating room teamwork among physicians and nurses: Teamwork in the eye of the beholder. *Journal of the American College of Surgeons, 202*(5), 746–752. https://doi.org/10.1016/j.jamcoll-surg.2006.01.017

Martinez, A. J. (2016). Managing workplace violence with evidence-based interventions: A literature review. *Journal of Psychosocial Nursing and Mental Health Services, 54*(9), 31–36. https://doi.org/10.3928/02793695-20160817-05

Maslow, A. (1966). *Psychology of science*. Maurice Bassett.

Mathewson, R. H. (1955). Symposium on interprofessional relations: Essential conditions for improvement of interprofessional relations. *Journal of Counseling Psychology, 2*(3), 196. https://doi.org/10.1037/h0045267

Mesmer-Magnus, J., Glew, D. J., & Viswesvaran, C. (2012). A meta-analysis of positive humor in the workplace. *Journal of Managerial Psychology, 27*(2), 155–190. https://doi.org/10.1108/02683941211199554

Meunier-Sham, J., Preiss, R. M., Petricone, R., Re, C., & Gillen, L. (2019). Laying the foundation for the National teleNursing center: Integration of the quality-caring model into TeleSANE practice. *Journal of Forensic Nursing, 15*(3):143–151. https://doi.org/10.1097/JFN.0000000000000252

Michalec, B., & Lamb G. (2020). COVID-19 and team-based healthcare: The essentiality of theory-driven research. *Journal of Interprofessional Care, 34*(5), 593–599. https://doi.org/10.1080/13561820.2020.1801613

Morgan, S. (2017). Social determinants of health 101 for health care. *National Academy of Medicine/Perspectives*, Available at: https://nam.edu/wp-content/uploads/2017/10/Social-Determinants-of-Health-101.pdf

Morin, A. (2011). Self-awareness Part 1: Definition, measures, effects, functions, and antecedents. *Social and Personality Psychology Compass, 5*(10), 807–823. https://doi.org/10.1111/j.1751-9004.2011.00387.x

Murthy, V. H. (2020). *Together: The healing power of human connection in a sometimes lonely world*. Harper Collins.

National Academies of Sciences, Engineering, and Medicine. (2019). *Taking act ion against clinician burnout: A systems approach to professional well-being*. Washington, DC: The National Academies Press. https://doi.org/10.17226/25521

National Academies of Sciences, Engineering, and Medicine. (2021). *The future of nursing 2020–2030: Charting a path to achieve health equity*. The National Academies Press. https://doi.org/10.17226/25982

National Center for Interprofessional Practice and Education. (2021). Critical events of interprofessional practice and education (IPE). Available at: https://nexusipe.org/advancing/ipe-critical-events

Nilsson, H. (2021). Spiritual self-care management for nursing professionals: A holistic approach. *Journal of Holistic Nursing, 40*(1), 64–73. https://doi.org/10.1177/08980101211034341

O'Leary, K. J., Manojlovich, M., Johnson, J. K., et al. (2020). A multisite study of interprofessional teamwork and collaboration on general medical services. *Joint Commission Journal on Quality & Patient Safety, 46*(12), 667–672. https://doi-org.proxy.ulib.uits.iu.edu/10.1016/j.jcjq.2020.09.009

Orique, S. B., & Despins, L. (2018). Evaluating situation awareness: An integrative review. *Western Journal of Nursing Research, 40*(3), 388–424. https://doi.org/10.1177/0193945917697230

Osher, D., Cantor, P., Berg, J., Steyer, L., & Rose, T. (2020). Drivers of human development: How relationships and context shape learning and development. *Applied Developmental Science, 24*(1), 6–36, https://doi.org/10.1080/10888691.2017.1398650

Pascucci, D. M. T., Riccardi, M., Sapienza, M. C., et al. (2020). Interprofessional collaboration and chronicity management: A systematic review of clinical trials, *European Journal of Public Health, 30*(suppl 5), ckaa166.495, https://doi.org/10.1093/eurpub/ckaa166.495

Patel, K. M., & Metersky, K. (2021). Reflective practice in nursing: A concept analysis. *International Journal of Nursing Knowledge, 33*(3), 180–187. https://doi.org/10.1111/2047-3095.12350

Penque, S. (2019). Mindfulness to promote nurses' well-being. *Nursing Management, 50*(5), 38–44. https://doi.org/10.1097/01.NUMA.0000557621.42684.c4

Peplau, H. E. (1952). Interpersonal relations in nursing. *American Journal of Nursing, 52*(6), 765. https://doi.org/10.1097/00000446-195206000-00062

Piaget, J. (1972). *The psychology of the child*. Basic Books.

Piaget, J. (1990). *The child's conception of the world*. Littlefield Adams.

Powell, A (2018). When science meets mindfulness: Researchers study how it seems to change the brain in depressed patients. The Harvard Gazette. Available at: https://news.harvard.edu/gazette/story/2018/04/harvard-researchers-study-how-mindfulness-may-change-the-brain-in-depressed-patients/

Pratt, H., Moroney, T., & Middleton, R. (2021). The influence of engaging authentic ally on nurse–patient relationships: A scoping review. *Nursing Inquiry, 28*, e12388. https://doi.org/10.1111/nin.12388

Rasheed, S. P. (2015). Self-awareness as a therapeutic tool for nurse/client relationship. *International Journal of Caring Sciences, 8*(1), 211.

Rasheed, S. P., Sundus, A., Younas, A., et al. (2021). Development and testing of a measure of self-awareness among nurses. *Western Journal of Nursing Research, 43*(1), 36–44. https://doi-org.proxy.ulib.uits.iu.edu/10.1177/0193945920923079

Rasheed, S. P., Younas, A., & Sundus, A. (2019). Self-awareness in nursing: A scoping review. *Journal of Clinical Nursing (John Wiley & Sons, Inc.), 28*(5/6), 762–774. https://doi-org.proxy.ulib.uits.iu.edu/10.1111/jocn.14708

Rogers, C. (1961). On becoming a person: A therapist's view of psychotherapy. *Archives of General Psychiatry, 62*, 1377–1384. https://doi.org/10.1002/jpoc.20072.95

Roy, A., Singh, A. K., Mishra, S., et al. (2021). Mental health implications of COVID-19 pandemic and its response in India. *The International Journal of Social Psychiatry, 67*(5), 587–600. https://doi.org/10.1177/0020764020950769

Serlin, I. A., & DiCowden, M. A. (Eds.) (2007). *Whole person healthcare Vol. 1: Humanizing healthcare*. Praeger.

Sexton, J. B., Holzmueller, C. G., Pronovost, P. J., et al. (2006). Variation in caregiver perceptions of teamwork climate in labor and delivery units. *Journal of Perinatology, 26*(8), 463–470. https://doi.org/10.1038/sj.jp.7211556

Shaw, J., Campbell, R., Cain, D., & Feeney, H. (2017). Beyond surveys and scales: How rape myths manifest in sexual assault police records. *Psychology of Violence, 7*(4), 602. https://doi.org/10.1037/vio0000072

Shaw, J., & Coates, V. (2021). Emergency contraception administration, toxicology kit use, and postassault reporting: A comparison of sexual assault nurse examiner (SANE) and non-SANE medical providers. *Journal of Forensic Nursing, 17*(3), 146–153. https://doi.org/10.1097/JFN.0000000000000320

Shechter, A., Diaz, F., Moise, N., et al. (2020). Psychological distress, coping behaveors, and preferences for support among New York healthcare workers during the COVID-19 pandemic. *General Hospital Psychiatry, 66,* 1–8. https://doi.org/10.1016/j.genhosppsych.2020.06.007

Sheehy, G. (1976). *Passages: Predictable crises of adult life.* E. P. Dutton.

Sheppard, A., & Broughton, M. C. (2020). Promoting wellbeing and health through active participation in music and dance: A systematic review. *International Journal of Qualitative Studies on Health and Wellbeing, 15*(1), 1732526, https://doi.org/10.1080/1 7482631.2020.1732526

Siegel, D. F., & Solomon, M. F. (2020). *Mind, consciousness, and well-being.* W.W. Norton & Co.

Siegel, D. J. (2015). *The developing mind: How relationships and the brain interact to shape who we are.* Guilford.

Tavakoly Sany, S., Behzhad, F., Ferns, G., et al. (2020). Communication skills training for physicians improves health literacy and medical outcomes among patients with hypertension: A randomized controlled trial. *BMC Health Services Research, 20,* 60. https://doi.org/10.1186/s12913-020-901-8

Teall, A., & Melnyk, B. M. (2021). Innovative wellness partner program to support the health and well-being of nurses during the COVID-19 pandemic. *Nursing Administration Quarterly, 45*(2), 169–174. https://doi.org/10.1097/NAQ.0000000000000457

Thacker, K., Stavarski, D., Brancato, V., et al. (2016). An investigation into the health-promoting lifestyle practices of RNs. *American Journal of Nursing, 116*(4), 24–30.

Thomas, E. J., Sexton, J. B., & Helmreich, R. L. (2003). Discrepant attitudes about teamwork among critical care nurses and physicians. *Critical Care Medicine, 31,* 956–959.

Tilson, E. C., Muse, A., Colville, K., et al. (2020). Investing in whole person health working toward an integration of physical, behavioral, and social health. *North Carolina Medical Journal, 81*(3), 177–180. https://doi.org/10.18043/ncm.81.3.177

Travelbee, J. (1966). *Interpersonal aspects of nursing.* F. A. Davis.

University of Edinburgh. (2020). *Reflection toolkit.* Available at: https://www.ed.ac.uk/reflection/reflectors-toolkit/reflecting-on-experience/gibbs-reflective-cycleG

Vogel, A., Knebel, A., Faupel-Badger, J., et al. (2021). A systems approach to enable effective team science from the internal research program of the National Center for Advancing Translational Sciences. *Journal of Clinical and Translational Science, 5*(1), E163. https://doi.org/10.1017/cts.2021.811

Walsh, W. A., Meunier-Sham, J., & Re, C. (2019). Using telehealth for sexual assault forensic examinations: A process evaluation of a national pilot project. *Journal of Forensic Nursing, 15*(3), 152–162.

Watson, J. (1979). *Nursing: The philosophy and science of caring.* Little, Brown and Company.

Watson, J. (1985). *Nursing: Human science and human care.* Appleton-Century-Crofts.

Watson, J. (2008). *Assessing and measuring caring in nursing and health sciences* (2nd ed.). Springer Publishing Company.

Wei, H., Corbett, R. W., Ray, J., & Wei, T. L. (2020). A culture of caring: The essence of healthcare interprofessional collaboration. *Journal of Interprofessional Care, 34*(3), 324–331. https://doi.org/10.1080/13561820.2019.1641476

Wenger, E., McDermott, R., & Snyder, W. M. (2002). *Cultivating communities of practice.* Harvard Business School Press.

Wilson, V., Donsante, J., Pai, P., et al. (2021). Building workforce well-being capability: The findings of a wellness self-care programme. *Jouranl of Nursing Management, 29,* 1742–1751. https://doi.org/10.1111/jonm.13280

World Health Organization. (2010). *Framework for action on interprofessional education and collaborative practice.* Author.

World Health Organization. (2020). *Self-care interventions*. Available at: https://www. who.int/news-room/fact-sheets/detail/self-care-health-interventions

World Health Professions Alliance. (2010). *Interprofessional collaborative practice*. Available at: https://www.whpa.org/activities/interprofessional-collaborative-practice

Yalom, I. D. (1975). *The theory and practice of group psychotherapy*. Basic Books.

Zhang, Y.-Y, Han, W.-L, Qin, W., et al. (2018). Extent of compassion satisfaction, compassion fatigue and burnout in nursing: A meta-analysis. *Journal of Nursing Management, 26*, 10–819. https://doi.org/10.1111/jonm.12589

CHAPTER 5

Relationship-Centered Professional Encounters

"Never forget that it is not a pneumonia, but a pneumonic person who is your patient."

—William Withey Gull

CHAPTER OBJECTIVES:

1. Compare the similarities and differences among patient-centered, family-centered, and person-centered care.
2. State three benefits of relationship-centered care.
3. Describe the meanings associated with nurses'"being and doing."

WHAT PATIENTS AND FAMILIES WANT FROM HEALTH PROFESSIONALS

Sick and vulnerable individuals in strange places (doctors' offices, outpatient clinics, nursing homes, or hospitals) and their family members often assume that health professionals "know what they are doing" (personal conversations with countless patients). What they expect, however, is another story.

"Patients and families want their healthcare to be delivered by healthcare providers that are both competent and compassionate" (Sinclair et al., 2021, p. 1). Since 1993, when the Picker Institute study was first published, characteristics of healthcare professionals and systems that were important to patients and families known as patient-centered care (PCC), have been known (Gerteis, 1993). Again, in 2001, the "ten rules for redesigning and improving care" that were part of the Institute of Medicine's (IOM, 2001) report, Crossing the Quality Chasm reintroduced PCC characteristics for health systems. According to recommendation four:

- Care should be based on continuous healing relationships that are available to patients and families wherever they are 24/7.
- Care should be customized based on the patient's needs and values (e.g., designed to respond to patients' needs).

- The patient should be in control.

- The system should encourage shared knowledge and free flow of information, including patients' access to their respective records.

- The system should anticipate patients' needs. Such care requires partnering with patients and families in designing, implementing, and evaluating care systems (IOM, 2001, p. 8).

Aspects of PCC were seen in several of the other five rules as well. For example, the rule "the system should constantly strive to decrease waste" included not wasting patients' time (IOM, 2001, p. 3). The IOM has defined PCC as "care that is respectful of and responsive to individual patient preferences, needs, and values" and ensures "that patient values guide all clinical decisions" (p. 3).

Definitions of PCC have varied over the years, complicating its theoretical clarity. From a clinical perspective, PCC has been defined as understanding the patient as a unique human being (Balint, 1969; Shaller, 2007) and promoting the trust, confidence, and clarification of their concerns by clinicians who have specific knowledge, attitudes, and skills (Lipkin et al., 1984). A literature review in 2000 revealed five domains of PCC: a biopsychosocial perspective, understanding the patient as person, sharing power and responsibility, building a therapeutic alliance (relationship), and understanding the clinician as a person (Kaba & Sooriakumaran, 2007).

Over time, the hospitalized patient's perspective of PCC emerged as a unique and important point of view and now embraces understanding and responding to "what matters" to patients and families (Schall et al., 2009). In fact, the patient's perspective, particularly at the point of care, is now considered crucial in the evaluation of PCC (Wasson & Baker, 2009). In 2010, PCC was defined as "healing relationships between providers and patients" (Epstein et al., 2010, p. 1489) and "a quality of personal, professional, and organizational relationships" (Epstein & Street, 2011, p. 100). Furthermore, based on a literature review, Sidani & Fox (2014) reported three specific elements that represented PCC: holistic, collaborative, and responsive care.

During the last fifteen plus years, PCC has become a worthy goal for healthcare systems as evidenced by federal investment in studying how best to measure and ensure it (Patient-Centered Outcomes Research Institute [2021] and the Patient Protection and Affordable Care Act [2010]). This legislation tied federal reimbursement rates to reported patient experience (an indicator used to measure the patient's perspective, otherwise known as Hospital Consumer Assessment of Healthcare Providers and Systems [HCAHPS]) (Goldstein et al., 2005). Yet, many health systems tackled this reporting obligation from a consumer-driven approach, similar to conventional competitive markets. Evidence for this includes many hospital CEOs continued inability to define PCC (personal observations and anecdotal reports), the building of "patient-centered" hospital spaces (hotel-like environments), and services (e.g., valet services, kiosks), and countless educational hours spent on customer service principles or scripting patient-health professional interactions. Furthermore, a whole new health professional, the patient experience officer, has arisen, along with supportive patient experience departments!

Fueled by the ongoing and pervasive safety and quality problems in health systems, feverish efforts have been undertaken by accrediting organizations, payers, and health systems to embrace PCC as a means of improving safety and quality, while meeting the needs of diverse patient populations. Stakeholders in all health systems—professional organizations, public policy groups, hospital administration, health professional school leadership, insurance carriers, and health professionals themselves—have welcomed the focus on PCC. However, although the healthcare community universally endorses the ideal of PCC, many health systems are still struggling to understand what PCC truly means, how it is displayed, the obligations it entails, and how best to evaluate it.

Fast forward to 2021. After several years of trying to deliver PCC, many American patients remain dissatisfied with it and are still struggling to influence healthcare decisions and policies that shape their lives (Gusmano et al., 2019; Reinhart, 2018). For example, at the National Research Corporation (NRC), a peer network focused on helping healthcare organizations understand what matters most to the people they serve, a recent report related to gathering patient history revealed that patients often feel vulnerable, anxious, and do not understand what is discussed during healthcare encounters. Active engagement in the process seems to alleviate some of these concerns. According to the report, patients want their providers to:

- review their medical history before seeing them in person;
- show personal knowledge of them and their history; and
- ask questions and offer solutions.

Furthermore, listening without interruption, staying present in the dialogue, and offering options empowers patients and assures them that their choices are wise (Volland, 2020).

In another small qualitative study in Canada, participants expressed "caring about me" as the overarching need when describing interactions with health professionals. In addition, they desired health professionals to collaborate with them, help them understand and self-manage their care, and personalize care to address their needs (Youssef et al., 2020). Interestingly, even artificial intelligence (AI) has recently emerged to assess care experiences. Using short phrases from diverse patient populations, findings from one study showed that physician respect and courtesy was a primary driver of positive care experiences. However, empathy, compassion, patience, kindness, helpfulness and attentiveness were also implicated in positive care experiences (Guney & Gandhi, 2022). In this study, differences among racial and ethnic groups were also identified. Studies from England have suggested that empathy and patient satisfaction is decreasing (Smith et al., 2020). In reality, most U.S. patients who have procedures or are hospitalized today are bombarded with surveys, post-discharge phone calls, and opportunities to share compliments and concerns, and yet hospitals are still struggling to increase their patient experience scores.

Unfortunately, throughout this time, health systems have unknowingly created barriers to PCC that challenge its consistent delivery. For example, several obstacles to PCC have been identified, including the lack of information and a way to measure PCC from the patients' perspective; lack of respect and trust between patients and providers; racial, ethnic, or religious discordance between patients and providers; organizational culture and clinicians' training and beliefs; inadequate alignment of incentives, including access, costs, and community factors (Sinaiko et al., 2019). Hence, consumer-oriented approaches to PCC appear to be superficial fixes that do not address the core ethical and relational obligations inherent in professional interactions between healthcare providers and patients.

PCC affirms the ethical principles of respect for individuals (autonomy), beneficience, maleficence, and justice which provide the foundation of the ANA Code for Nurses (2015). Furthermore, its intent focuses on healthcare professionals' centering their work on the whole person, including emotional, mental, spiritual, social, and financial perspectives (NEJM Catalyst, 2017). These attributes of PCC are consistent with and are a central component of health professional work. It stands to reason then that to authentically deliver PCC, the emphasis should be placed on what and how health professionals interact with and provide care to patients and families—that is, the processes of care. Furthermore, as PCC is frequently stated in health systems' mission statements or promises, authentic delivery of it must be connected to whether health professionals and the culture they practice in are aligned with their respective organizational values and mission. With all the focus on PCC encompassing over two decades, continuing system challenges beg the questions: Why has the definition of PCC been so elusive? Why is the delivery of PCC so varied? Are health systems *really* centered on the patient? Are health professionals?

Recently, the term "person-centered" care has emerged as a more individualistic approach to healthcare that concerns "what matters most" to patients and families. It encompasses the entirety of a person's needs and preferences, beyond just the clinical or medical (American Geriatrics Society Expert Panel on Person-Centered Care, 2016). Some health professionals are moving toward this term because it seems to be more wholistic, shifting the focus beyond the disease state and supporting patients' choice and autonomy in healthcare decision-making. Ekman et al. (2011) viewed the patient as a capable human being who, together with the healthcare provider/s, is seen as a partner in care and a co-creator of the healthcare plan. Listening to patients by taking into careful consideration their experiences, conditions, and individual expectations results in a mutually derived health plan that is agreed upon and updated continuously. According to the American Geriatrics Society (2016) Expert Panel on Person-Centered Care, person-centered care espouses that "individuals' values and preferences are elicited and, once expressed, guide all aspects of healthcare, supporting realistic health and life goals" (p. 16). A thematic analysis that examined the differences between PCC and person-centered care indicated that the goal of patient-centered care is a *functional* life for the patient, whereas the goal of person-centered care is a *meaningful* life for the person (Eklund et al., 2019). The authors concluded that the concepts were similar but had subtle differences that were important to acknowledge. Both terms, however, embrace the moral and professional obligations of health professionals.

Finally, the term, family-centered care (FCC) entered the scene in the 1990s after considerable family advocacy group work. FCC, expands and deepens the meaning of PCC to include families, partnerships, collaboration, engagement, information-sharing, mutual respect, and trust (Kuo et al., 2012; Jafarpoor et al., 2020; Johnson, 2000). It is commonly used to describe optimal healthcare as experienced by families and is frequently accompanied by terms such as "partnership," "collaboration," and families as "experts" to describe the process of care delivery (American Academy of Pediatrics, 2003; Antonelli et al., 2009; Kuo et al., 2012). FCC honors the social, ethnic, cultural, and socioeconomic diversity of the family and is viewed as a primary source of strength and support for children (American Academy of Pediatrics, 2003). Enhanced outcomes have been observed (Goldfarb et al., 2017) and FCC is considered empowering for children and parents alike.

PATIENT-CENTERED, FAMILY-CENTERED, OR PERSON-CENTERED: IS IT REALLY RELATIONSHIP-CENTERED?

PCC is a dynamic, multidimensional construct comprised of characteristics and behaviors that are meant to shift the focus of healthcare from a clinical or disease-driven process to one that is patient driven. In health systems that are patient-centric, the attitudes and activities of the workforce are grounded in the needs and preferences of patients. Unfortunately, as noted in the previous section, not all health systems or health professionals practice PCC. Despite health professionals' ethical imperatives for PCC, the subtle but hidden power imbalances between patients, individual healthcare professionals, and healthcare systems often affect relationship quality, a necessary component of PCC. It turns out that realizing the promise of PCC is easier to articulate than to implement (Stollenwerk et al., 2019).

Variation in the definitions and ultimate delivery of PCC has important implications for health professionals, health systems, patients/families, and health policy. Because of these differences in definitions and related responses, the impact of PCC on health outcomes remains under-evidenced, leading to confusion regarding how best to deliver it or report on its benefits. "PCC remains one of the most-used and least-understood terms in healthcare" (Weissman et al., 2017, p. 1). Adding to this confusion is the use of the aforementioned similar phrases, "person-centered care" and "family-centered care."

BOX 5.1: Despite the complexity in defining, delivering, and evaluating PCC , person-centered care, or FCC, an obvious similarity among these phrases is the consistent emphasis on human relationships. Aspects such as the uniqueness of patient needs, human respect, active participation, collaboration, mutuality, and shared decision-making all take place in the context of relationships. It appears that the quality of human relationships, the fundamental connection used by health professionals and persons seeking healthcare, is the common denominator. It is through such intimate relationships that personal information is shared, emotions are identified, symptoms are analyzed, physical assessments are performed, counseling and education is offered, and expectations for health outcomes are expressed. Attending to the quality of this special relationship is the foundation for safe and high-quality healthcare.

Although not labeled PCC, FCC, or person-centered care per se, registered nurses (RNs) have consistently embraced human persons as the primary focus of their practice and the essence of their work (Mitchell, 2008). In fact, one of the four metaparadigm concepts (person) (Fawcett, 1984) represents a crucial phenomenon of interest to nursing, that has consistently centered nursing work on the "humanness" of persons, including their wholeness and unique perspectives and preferences. As nurses connect with human persons during healthcare encounters, they interdependently and dynamically relate, opening up new possibilities for understanding, discovery, healing, and advancement. Furthermore, the remaining metaparadigm concepts, namely *nursing, environment, and health*, represent how the work of the nursing honors patients' diversity, empowers them to participate in their care, attends to their surroundings, and is oriented towards health. The Quality-Caring Model©'s (QCM) four assumed relationships describing human persons, together with the concept of relationship-centered professional encounters is congruent with contemporary notions of PCC, FCC, and person-centered care (see Table 5.1).

Elements of the whole person of the patient, the works of the pioneering nurse theorists of the 1950s, 1960s, and the 1970s, and the terms *meeting patient needs, interpersonal relationships between patients and nurses, keeping patients safe*, and *family presence* are also common in most nursing curricula. Yet, we rarely acknowledge their importance in everyday practice! How ironic is it that such longstanding and fundamental principles of nursing are now part of the national agenda? And sadly, how is it that nursing still is not driving this work?

Unfortunately, although patients have reported a need for authentic connections with healthcare providers as well as the authority to be drivers of their healthcare, practicing clinicians have difficulty relating to and granting them this role. Furthermore, health systems unknowingly create barriers to it, and interventions to improve it, although apparent in peer-reviewed literature, are not yet fully adopted.

EVIDENCE OF THE BENEFITS OF RELATIONSHIP-CENTERED (PCC, FCC, OR PERSON-CENTERED) CARE

Although earlier versions of this text reported on studies that have demonstrated positive associations between aspects of PCC and improved outcomes (including clinical outcomes, decreased utilization, lower costs, and fewer lawsuits), newer studies consistently show benefits. For example, orthopedic surgical patients (knee, hip, and back) who participated in patient-centered informed decisions showed better overall quality of life, higher satisfaction levels, and less regret (Sepucha et al., 2018). Similarly, poorly rated shared

TABLE 5.1 Congruence of Nursing Metaparadigm Concepts with Characteristics of Patient-Centered Care, Family-Centered Care, Person-Centered Care, and the Quality-Caring Model

Nursing Concepts*	Patient-Centered Care	Family-Centered Care	Person-Centered Care	Quality-Caring Model©
Human beings	Patient as person (Mead & Bower, 2000) worthy of respect (IOM, 2001; Epstein et al., 2010).	Family is the primary source of strength and support for a child (American Academy of Pediatrics, 2003).	The patient is viewed as a capable human being (Ekman et al., 2011) Encompasses the entirety of a person's needs and preferences, beyond just the clinical or medical (American Geriatrics Society Expert Panel on Person-Centered Care, 2016).	Humans are inherently worthy and exist in relationship to themselves, others, communities or groups, and the larger universe. Humans are multidimensional beings capable of growth and change. Humans evolve in a dynamic, interconnected manner.
Environment	A quality of personal, professional, and organizational relationships (Epstein & Street, 2011).	Honors social, ethnic, cultural, and socioeconomic diversity of the family (American Academy of Pediatrics, 2003).	Considers peoples' desires, values, family situations, social circumstances, and lifestyles (American Geriatrics Society Expert Panel on Person-Centered Care, 2015).	Specific contextual characteristics (including social determinants of health) that may impact processes and outcomes of care. Complex nature and social structures of health systems affect individuals, including the quality of their relationships. Interactions among agents in health systems functions interdependent, dynamic, and are continuously evolving.

(continued)

TABLE 5.1 Congruence of Nursing Metaparadigm Concepts with Characteristics of Patient-Centered Care, Family-Centered Care, Person-Centered Care, and the Quality-Caring Model (*continued*)

Nursing Concepts*	Patient-Centered Care	Family-Centered Care	Person-Centered Care	Quality-Caring Model©
Health	The goal of patient-centered healthcare is to empower patients to become active participants in their care (Reynolds, 2009). Responsiveness to patients' expressed needs, preferences, and values (IOM, 2001; Radwin, 2003).	Improved patient and staff outcomes such as decreased anxiety, increased recovery, increased parent confidence, and decreased length of stay. Increased staff satisfaction and positive work environments (Goldfarb et al., 2017).	Holistic, individualized, respectful, and empowering (Morgan & Yoder, 2012). Personalized, coordinated, and enabling (Ahmad et al., 2014). Individualized, goal-oriented care plan based on the person's preferences (Zhao et al., 2016).	The goal of the Quality-Caring Model is to facilitate "feeling cared for," allowing for the emergence of individual, organizational, and community growth, change, health, learning, and development, in short self-advancement. Benefit is received by both the caregiver and the one being cared for.
Nursing (care delivery)	Individualized care (Mead & Bower, 2000). Therapeutic relationship (healing relationship), therapeutic engagement, caring presence (Epstein et al., 2010; Epstein & Street, 2011; Mead & Bower, 2000; Stewart et al., 2003). Includes education, information, and support (Epstein et al., 2010; Hobbs, 2009; Shaller, 2007).	Mutually beneficial partnerships between healthcare providers, patients, and families in healthcare planning, delivery, and evaluation (Johnson & Abraham, 2012). Collaboration for empowering children and family, sharing information, providing parental support, holistic approach allowing for negotiation, choice, therapeutic relationship (Morgan & Yoder, 2012).	Recognizing and maintaining selfhood (Fazio et al., 2018) Individual values and preferences are elicited (Brummel et al., 2016). Dynamic relationships among individuals, others who are important to them, and all relevant providers(Brummel et al., 2016).	The overall role of the nurse is to engage in expert caring relationships with self, others, and communities enabling feelings of being "cared for" in recipients. Recognize and attend to the holistic needs of self, patients, peers, and the community served through expert use of the caring behaviors. Maintain an ongoing awareness of the patient's and family's point of view. Carry on self-caring activities, including personal and professional development. Integrate caring relationships with specific evidence-based nursing interventions to positively influence health outcomes.

decision-making was associated with worse patient-reported health outcomes, worse established quality indicators, and higher healthcare utilization (Hughes et al., 2018). A literature review on PCC revealed that this approach leads to better management and improved patient satisfaction. Implied in this finding is that better treatment adherence, better health outcomes, and better perceived quality of healthcare services were apparent (Chandra et al., 2018).

An older Cochrane Review of 17 educational intervention studies targeting PCC demonstrated greater patient satisfaction, well-being, and communication (Lewin et al., 2001). A more recent meta-analysis of 30 studies in the geriatric population revealed that person-centered interventions showed reduced behavioral and psychological symptoms in dementia (BPSD) and improved cognitive function, but effect size differed by intervention type. Specifically, reminiscence therapy showed a moderate effect size, while music therapy and multisensory stimulation had a small effect size. Moreover, the results emphasized that music and reminiscence therapies were effective in improving Mini-Mental Status Exam (MMSE) scores, namely cognitive function (Lee et al., 2020). Additionally, some nurse studies were found examining relationships and patient outcomes, albeit limited.

For example, a nurse-led patient-centered self-management support intervention showed significantly lowered HbA1c among patients with type 2 diabetes compared to a control group (Jutterström et al., 2016). In this study, using PCC as the conceptual framework, 182 patients were randomized into intervention or control groups. The participatory intervention consisted of six sessions related to patients' illness experiences. After baseline adjustment of HbA1c levels, there was a significant difference between the groups. Nurse caring has also been linked to missed nursing care, specifically whether it influenced nurses' decisions to omit or provide care as well as reducing adverse events and promoting quality nursing care (Labrague et al., 2020). In an acute psychiatric setting, positive associations were found between perceived nurse caring and satisfaction with care, based on treating patient information confidentially, giving treatments and medications on time, and helping patients feel safe (King et al., 2019). Finally, as the Patient-Centered Outcomes Research Institute (PCORI) was created in 2012 as a result of the Affordable Care Act, many studies have been completed that bring healthcare stakeholders together—with patients at the center—to set research priorities and evaluate applications. You can view the accumulating evidence at www.pcori.org/impact/evidence-updates.

Despite the emerging and important evidence linking PCC, FCC, and person-centered care to improved patient and health system outcomes, many existing studies have important limitations. For example, the majority were observational and correlational studies with small, nonprobability samples and did not examine outcomes over time. Fewer studies led by nurses were found, and measures used to operationalize PCC, FCC, or person-centered care were varied. More robust research is needed to evidence actionable findings that matter to patients and families.

Although the meaning and evidence for PCC, FCC, and person-centered care are emerging, the competencies and moral implications (or accountability) for delivering them are less often stated. In the new AACN (2021) *Essentials: Core*

Competencies for Professional Nursing Practice, person-centered care and professionalism are listed as two of the 10 essential domains of nursing competence. In the document, person-centered care is described as "the core purpose of nursing as a discipline" (p. 29). Several sub-competencies such as exhibiting respect, empathy, compassion, and relationship-centered care (RCC); effective communication, development of plans of care; and accountability for care delivery, including coordination of care are included. In competency 9: *Professionalism,* demonstration of ethical comportment, a participatory approach, accountability, compliance with legal aspects of nursing, professional identity as a nurse, including the integration of diversity, equity, inclusion, and social justice are listed. The document further describes professionalism as "encompassing the development of a nursing identity embracing the values of integrity, altruism, inclusivity, compassion, courage, humility, advocacy, caring, autonomy, humanity, and social justice ... with nursing professionalism, requiring a continuous process of socialization that requires the nurse to give back to the profession through the mentorship and development of others (p. 49). As the new competencies become integrated into the curricula at schools of nursing during the next few years, opportunities for demonstrating them will abound.

BOX 5.2: Since PCC, FCC, and person-centered care are based on a deep respect for patients as worthy human beings who live in unique relational contexts, the professional obligations to care for patients and families in this fashion are readily apparent—they are disciplinary values. A growing body of knowledge suggests an association between them, particularly the quality of patient–clinician relationships and improved short and long-term quality indicators across healthcare settings. Respect for and appreciation for the uniqueness of human persons together with the mounting evidence base provide the foundation for professional obligations and health system actions to measure, improve, and consistently deliver RCC.

Such obligations and actions include consistently offering respect and attention; appreciating and incorporating patients' unique values and preferences; mutually helping patients solve their health problems, including providing information/ education; being optimistic and supportive; ensuring that human and affiliation needs are met; and guaranteeing patient safety (also known as caring behaviors). These duties and responsibilities are enmeshed in the Quality-Caring concept, relationship-centered professional encounters.

RELATIONSHIP-CENTERED PROFESSIONAL ENCOUNTERS

In healthcare situations, persons with health needs meet in relationship with health professionals who function independently and collaboratively with them. Independent relationships are those carried out between patients and their families and one health professional. Collaborative relationships are those interactions performed among multiple health professionals who work in a complementary nature to cohesively provide coordinated services to patients and families. These three-way encounters (see Chapter 3) are relationship-centered when they are grounded in caring processes or behaviors.

BOX 5.3: Caring relationships are healing or healthy for both patients and health professionals. Moreover, caring relationships (when cultivated and sustained) generate human connections that transcend the individuals alone and result in an understanding of others that anticipates, guides, provides for, teaches and learns, protects, and advocates. This form of relationship trumps the traditional diagnostic, procedural, disease-based care that usually occurs during an illness because it protects the overall health and well-being of whole individuals (not just the treatment of disease) and has the potential to be transforming.

Relationship-centered professional encounters begin between health professionals and potential patients in communities and primary care settings and hopefully follow individuals during episodes of acute illness and beyond. Characteristics of relationship-centered professional encounters include the caring processes or behaviors (see Table 5.2) that shift the focus from instrumental or "doing" activities to those that are more in line with "being" or "authentic presence." This is hard to practice for busy healthcare professionals who typically define their identities in terms of action: helping, assisting, fixing, or resolving problems. Creating a safe space for the disclosure of patients' feelings and emotions or mutually deciding the "right" course of action requires that health professionals redefine their practice and self-image from primarily "do-ers" to *both* "do-ers and "be-ers" (listeners and responders with relational knowledge who attend to the quality of the patient–provider relationship as the primary context for care).

Interestingly, authentic presence extends to non-person environments where care is taking place, such as telehealth or remote (virtual) care delivery. In fact, Groom et al. (2021) used a dimensional analysis to describe "telepresence" as patients, caregivers, and clinicians' experiences of realism during telehealth encounters. They further described a connection and collaborative experience founded on trust, support, and mediation that may enhance future telehealth implementation. Thus, caring behaviors used during care delivery in multiple venues spread quality patient–provider relationships across settings.

The eight caring behaviors or processes are multifaceted; and although comprised of both being and doing, the emphasis is on the genuine caring nature of the relationship that undergirds the activities. The caring behaviors are the basis for relationship-centered professional encounters—both those with patients and families and those among health professionals. These reciprocal relationships influence not only patients and families but health professionals as well. Hence, although the relationship with patients and families is primary, relationships with self, communities served, and other health professionals should also be based on the caring behaviors. Thus, the *quality* of relationships between health professionals, patients, and their families influences the overall quality care. When enacted in a caring manner, relationship-centered

TABLE 5.2 Caring Behaviors, Definitions, Required Competencies, Knowledge, and Attitudes

Caring Behavior	Definition	Required Professional Competencies	Required Knowledge and Attitudes
Mutual problem solving	Professional behaviors that help patients and families understand how to confront, learn, and think about their health and illness; involves a reciprocal, shared approach with resulting decisions acceptable to both.	Provide individualized information Reframe patients' concerns Deliver learning opportunities that engage patients in their care Exploring alternative options for dealing with health problems Respect individuals and families' choices in their healthcare decisions. Collaborate with others across health systems to address patient-defined health problems Brainstorm together Assist patients in figuring out questions to ask other health professionals Validate what patients already know Use culturally and linguistically sensitive communication strategies. Accept feedback from patients Experiment with different ways of providing care Adopt patients' ideas Use active listening Foster patient's preferred role in decision making Help patients reflect on and assess the impact of alternative health decisions on lifestyle Ensure access to understandable information Assess and use patients' competencies, problem-solving skills, including health literacy	Informed, up-to-date on the literature Knowledge of searchable databases Comfortable "in relationship" Skilled in multiple learning approaches Engaging approach Communication and active listening Cognizant of health literacy

Attentive reassurance	Reliability of health professionals to exhibit availability, a hopeful outlook, even when the future is not promising (in terms of a cure), and convey possibilities	Demonstrate optimism; convey possibilities Exhibit accessibility Repeatedly confirm availability Display confidence Clarify misperceptions Display consistent actions Pay attention to patients and families; postpone doing long enough to notice, actively listen, and be intentionally present in the moment	Knowledge of self Human awareness Understanding self as a resource to others Self-reliance Positive attitude Assertiveness knowledge
Human respect	Honoring the worth of human persons	Provide unconditional acceptance Demonstrate careful handling of the body Recognize human rights and responsibilities Appreciate the integrity of the patient (biopsychosociocultural or "whole person" approach) Elicit and call patient by preferred name Make eye and physical contact Active listening Preserve patient autonomy Understand the patient as a unique individual in relation to others	Knowledge of ethical principles Autonomy Beneficence Non-maleficence Justice and social justice Understanding of human persons' dignity Knowledge of patients' self-determination Active listening Partnership and mutuality of interactions
Encouraging manner	Affective dimension of behavior associated with demeanor/attitude	Use supportive verbal demeanor Display supportive nonverbal demeanor Show enthusiasm for the work Provide positive feedback Share a supportive view of the system Use approaches that empower and inspire	Knowledge of therapeutic communication techniques Knowledge of constructive feedback techniques Skillful therapeutic communication Positive attitudes

(continued)

TABLE 5.2 Caring Behaviors, Definitions, Required Competencies, Knowledge, and Attitudes (*continued*)

Caring Behavior	Definition	Required Professional Competencies	Required Knowledge and Attitudes
Appreciation of unique meanings	Knowing the patient's context and worldview; discerning and then acknowledging the subjective inner value attached to a situation, person, or event; knowing what is important to patients and families, including distinctive sociocultural connections	Demonstrate active listening Use nonjudgmental attitudes and behaviors Show tolerance for both positive and negative ideas or expressions Provide flexibility Elicit patient values and preferences Use patient values and preferences when designing and delivering care Appreciate differences of opinion and cultural diversity Appreciate social determinants of health	Knowledge of and appreciation for the whole person, including his/her life story and the meaning of the health-illness condition Personal "knowing" of patient (developed in relationship and over time) Cultural diversity Social determinants of health
Healing environment	Safe and aesthetically pleasing surroundings	Identify risks to patient safety Establish safe environment; use guidelines and EBP as appropriate Make frequent checks/surveillance Provides safety information and associated teach-back methods Ensures call systems in place Safeguard privacy, confidentiality, and autonomy in all interactions Perform accurate, timely, and comprehensive handoffs Maintain privacy and confidentiality of patient information Ensure clean and pleasant surroundings	Knowledge of safety standards, benefits, and limitations of selected safety-enhancing technologies Cultures of safety and high reliability Knowledge of the ethical standards, fidelity Knowledge of current evidence related to prevention of adverse outcomes

Basic human needs	Physical, safety, social/relational, self-esteem, and self-actualization needs	Demonstrate consistent attention to airway, intake, elimination, sleep and rest, mobility, and hygiene needs Attend to emotional, social, and self-esteem needs Regularly assess and maintain patient comfort	Knowledge of basic physiology and pathophysiology Knowledge of human emotions during health and illness Knowledge of human development across the life span Knowledge of pain and suffering, pain interventions, and pain/comfort theories
Affiliation needs	An individual's need for belonging and membership in families or other social contexts	Responds to families/significant others (SO) Engage family members in health decisions per the patient's wishes Allow family members' presence Involve family/significant other (SO) in care Conduct routine family meetings Provide resources to families	Knowledge of family theories Knowledge of individual patient's family situation and routines

professional encounters induce positive emotions and intermediate outcomes in recipients (Chapter 6) that guide the accuracy and efficiency of ongoing interactions, future use of the healthcare system, and ultimately healthy outcomes.

Kathleen's Story **(narrated here) illustrates the human experience of a postop patient as she was recovering from lung surgery in a step-down unit:**

Kathleen is a 62-year old woman who is married with no children. She is college educated, overweight, and a type II diabetic, controlled medically, who had a previous bout of thyroid cancer. On x-ray, it was noted that she had a small lesion on the lower lobe of the right lung. After a bronchoscopy and diagnosis of adenocarcinoma of the lung, her physician performed a video-assisted thoracoscopic surgery (VATS) procedure with partial removal of the right lower lobe. Immediately postop on the step-down unit, she was in a significant degree of pain from the position of the chest tube (high up on her back) and appeared quite anxious. Several nurses came in and out over the course of several hours. Most hurriedly completed their "tasks" and then moved on to the next patient. There was little interest or interaction with Kathleen. However, after 7 p.m., the night nurse came in to administer insulin. Because she did not take insulin, she questioned the nurse about her need for it, and she was pretty harsh in her questioning! The nurse, who was only 6 months out of school, sat down on the edge of the bed and shared with Kathleen how the surgery and her NPO status had temporarily altered her glucose levels. Kathleen was still wary of taking insulin, so the nurse used the computer in the room to pull up recent articles on glucose responses during and after surgery. The nurse sat with her and answered questions related to the articles. Kathleen, although still in pain, understood and agreed to take the insulin.

Because of the relationship she had established with Kathleen, when it was time to get up and walk, the nurse observed that Kathleen was still in pain. Her doctor did not want her to receive any more pain medication, so the nurse came to Kathleen's room once an hour and walked with her, using humor to encourage her despite her pain. This nurse was different. She reappeared multiple times during the evening with a calm demeanor and a smile, gently reminding Kathleen of the need to move and walk so she could go home quickly. Although other nurses had attended to some of her needs, this nurse emphasized caring and relationship over task completion. In so doing, Kathleen was able to be discharged the following day. It is important to point out that this type of care was significant to the patient and did not take too much time; however, what the nurse did with the moments she had made all the difference. Of all of the nurses Kathleen encountered, why was only one practicing caring? It leads one to wonder if other patients could benefit from a shorter length of stay if the caring behaviors of nurses were more apparent?

What caring behaviors were displayed by the "different" nurse? How would you teach the first group of nurses to "see" and attend to the family in this situation?

Contrast the story above with the following exemplar relayed by a nursing unit manager:

A 70-year-old male was admitted for syncopal episodes and frequent falling; this was thought to be related to cardiac arrhythmias and later confirmed to be so. The patient was alert and oriented throughout his 13-day hospital stay, but complained of ankle pain periodically with some swelling and bruising beginning on day 3. On the sixth day of his admission, an orthopedic consult was obtained after x-rays revealed a medial malleolus fracture in his left ankle. He was taken to surgery the following day and had an open reduction and internal fixation.

Since admission, the patient had been voiding in a urinal without difficulties and on day 6, the day it was discovered that the patient had a fracture, he attempted to walk across the room to get his urinal to void. He was in too much pain and returned to his bed and called his nurse. No one came. He continued to call the nurse for 30 minutes without success and eventually became incontinent. His nurse placed a diaper on him due to his incontinence and he was told he had to wear them throughout the rest of this stay. Afraid to speak up or cause any problems, he complied.

On the day of discharge, he shared this information with his son-in-law, also a nurse and visiting from another state. Immediately, his son-in-law contacted administration and voiced a complaint. "Administration" (including this nurse manager) visited the patient and heard the heart-breaking story from the voice of the 70-year-old man, who explained that even though he was 70 and wrinkled, "he was still a man and had been humiliated and stripped of his dignity from the moment the diapers were placed on him." It was his perception that his nurse that day was irritated that he messed his bed and assumed he was too lazy to retrieve his urinal. He also shared that when the same nurse would come and change his diaper, she would have him stand, holding onto the bed and yank his diaper to his knees while he was standing—naked, exposed, and humiliated.

Tears poured from this gentleman's eyes as he told the story and from mine as I held his hand and apologized for the lack of human respect shown by his nurse, the lack of mutual problem solving by not exploring alternate ways of assuring his basic human needs were met, the lack of attentive reassurance by not being available to him when he needed to urinate, and reassurance that it was not his fault, the lack of an encouraging manner by not helping him deal with bad feelings that he had become incontinent, the lack of appreciation of unique meanings by not knowing what was important to this man, the lack of a healing environment by not checking on him or ensuring a safe environment (urinal within reach), and the lack of affiliation needs by not encouraging family participation in care.

How did this man's experiences affect his outcomes? What could have been done to avoid this occurrence? How should this be addressed with the nurse, if at all?

Often, based on the work environment or an individual's own characteristics, an overreliance on objective clinical or technical skills can mimic "good" practice. However, without the integration of *both* the technical aspects of care with the appreciation of the wholeness of humans engaged in a healthcare encounter, the ability to co-produce healthcare is unintentionally thwarted. Relational comportment (embodying caring) (Maycut & Wild, 2019) refers to the personal demeanor of health professionals who assimilate caring behaviors into their performance. The nurse, the patient, and the healthcare team are the beneficiaries of nurses who demonstrate relational comportment.

Through the ongoing processes of interaction and mutual relating, patients and health professionals come together, communicate, express their views, and over time, develop a connection based on caring. This connection deepens the relationship and if sustained, leads to knowing who the other is and what matters to them. Sometimes, as the relationship intensifies, one can almost foresee the needs of the other. Knowing another in this way provides the insight needed to detect problems early, to protect, to provide anticipatory guidance and creative problem solving, and to facilitate healthy future behaviors. Thus, knowing another is dependent on ongoing caring interactions and resultant connections, and this is an important aim for professional practice.

Using the caring relationship to really understand how another perceives his/her situation and then jointly working together to develop individualized processes of care continues the connection. Effective use of the caring behaviors is central to relationship-centered professional encounters (and the delivery of RCC) and requires relational comportment, the behavioral integration of a health professional's external knowledge and skills with the more internal self-knowledge, beliefs, and attitudes.

BOX 5.4: Relationship-centered professional encounters require the ability to remain authentically present and attentive to relationships amid the everyday demands of the clinical environment. Such a stance entails courage on the part of health professionals to advocate for the importance of and expression of caring behaviors as crucial elements of safe and quality care.

RELATIONSHIP-CENTERED CARE AND QUALITY CARING

The QCM is aligned with current definitions of PCC, FCC, and person-centered care as depicted in Table 5.1 as well as the AACN's *The Essentials: Core Competencies for Professional Nursing Education* (2021). The model concept, relationship-centered professional encounters, is particularly suited for promoting RCC as it specifies explicit processes (caring behaviors) required for caring (or healing) relationships, a core aspect of all approaches. As such, it assists health professionals to see, to understand, and then actually interact in a way that matters to patients and families and others, versus the more current notion of caring relationships as intangible professional ideals. RCC contrasts with health professional or system-centered care that typically revolves around the health professional and his/her disciplinary orientation or the organization. In a relationship-centered health system, health professionals and patients/families coexist in relationships characterized as caring, where mutuality, shared decision making, and health services are performed with the patient as the authority for care delivered. Thus, the patient's health and the health professional's well-being and work satisfaction are dependent on reciprocal caring relationships, in which different perspectives are heard, understood, and honored. From this caring foundation, health services are provided that preserve the dignity and needs of patients and families while meeting professional standards and guidelines that define health professionals' work.

In spite of the challenges of delivering health care in this manner, some visionaries have attempted to incorporate aspects of RCC into some models of care, such as those for older adults (the Chronic Care Model [Wagner, 1998]), Nurses Improving Care for Healthsystem Elders (NICHE) (Mezey et al., 2004), primary care, transitional care (Naylor et al., 1999), and the medical home (National Committee for Quality Assurance, n.d.). Viewed by the general public, healthcare systems, and funding/licensing agencies as an essential component of high-quality healthcare (Patient Protection and Affordable Care Act, 2010; Price et al., 2015), PCC has been touted as a central aim for the nation's health system since 1999. It remains to be seen whether PCC, FCC, or person-centered care, that is, RCC , persists as a health system ideal or becomes a real, tangible process that can facilitate individual and health system advancement.

BOX 5.5: The QCM, with its emphasis on the caring nature of human relationships, may offer some hope in terms of authentic implementation of RCC in health systems. Its very nature is patient, person, and family-centered as it is founded on beliefs about the worth of human persons and their co-existing contexts.

The QCM has well-defined assumptions and concepts that can be learned, measured, and improved. It is centered on patients and families, but speaks to health professionals' individual and collective relationships and the community served, which are necessary components of quality care. The model proposes intermediate and terminal outcomes that are testable, both in the practice setting and through more rigorous research. Furthermore, it can serve as a unifying approach for health systems in which individual health professionals are oftenlocked in their own worldview. For those organizations currently and consistently using this middle range theory as a foundation for professional practice, it has become an energizing force for sustainable change.

SUMMARY

The history and characteristics of and evidence for PCC, FCC, and person-centered care are described and examined in relationship to the current healthcare system. Elements of the QCM, specifically the concept of relationship-centered professional encounters, are compared to these approaches and similarities are shown. The eight caring behaviors essential to relationship-centered professional encounters are defined and associated with specific behaviors, required knowledge, and competencies. The caring relationships among patients and health professionals, central to the QCM, are linked to the reality of a true relationship-centric health system.

CALL TO ACTION

The *quality* of relationship-centered professional encounters provides the foundational context for all healthcare actions. **Adopt** the caring behaviors as the grounding approach for healthcare delivery.

REFLECTIVE QUESTIONS/APPLICATIONS

For Professional Nurses in Clinical Practice:

- Discuss the delivery of authentic RCC in your healthcare institution.
- Are patients the drivers of healthcare delivery in your organization? Should they be and, if so, how can it be evaluated?
- Is there an expectation that the caring behaviors are a significant component of an RN's work? If so, how are they evaluated?
- Reflect on your own practice. Is RCC being practiced every day in every patient encounter? If not, what would it take to deliver it?
- What health outcomes could be enhanced with the delivery of genuine RCC in your institution?
- What organizing framework or professional practice model ensures the delivery of PCC on your unit? What are its essential components?
- How do you hold yourself and fellow nurses accountable for the delivery of RCC?

For Professional Nurses in Educational Practice:

- What specific curricular revisions have you developed that address PCC? What evidence did you use to shape them? What teaching/learning strategies will you use to help undergraduate and graduate students learn how to care?
- Reflect on today's practice environments. How do you think your educational program helps graduates stay focused on relationship-centered professional encounters? In what specific ways does your program build relational skills among the students? How do you know students are competent in these skills at graduation?
- What are the necessary thinking patterns that will have to occur in undergraduate and graduate faculty to meet the challenges of PCC?
- How might you suggest using PCORI and its website to educate today's health professional students?

■ Examine Table 5.2. Provide some suggestions for teaching/learning strategies to meet the behavioral skills and knowledge requirements.

For Professional Nurses in Leadership Practice:

■ How has patient or person-centered care improved/worsened over the past 3 years at your institution?

■ How have you specifically articulated and championed PCC at your institution? Is it working?

■ Reflect on the developmental activities in place at your institution. Do they include aspects of relationship building? How do you ensure that professionals are competent in caring relationships?

■ How is PCC monitored and measured to revise practice at your institution? What could you do to enhance this process?

■ How do you help health professionals to stay focused on caring relationships as the foundational basis of professional practice?

■ Does your leadership team embrace PCC? If not, how will you deal with them?

■ Create a plan for dramatically altering RN work such that the patient is truly at the center. Who should be involved? What methodology should be used? How long would it take? What are its implications for RN practice? How would you ensure that the plan is enacted as developed? How would you evaluate its implementation?

PRACTICE ANALYSIS

The COVID-19 pandemic brought with it many unique challenges to healthcare systems. Most organizations implemented strict visitation policies, limiting the ability for family to visit with individuals diagnosed with and on contact precautions for the coronavirus. Consider this instance:

Katherine (Katie) Siciliano, an RN , was caring for a patient in a step-down unit who was recovering from COVID-19. While caring for this patient, Katie identified that her patient was experiencing a great deal of distress related to the fact that her husband was in the intensive care unit, intubated, and not expected to survive. Katie also learned that her patient's entire family was ill and that her mother had succumbed to COVID-19 just days prior. During morning rounds, the interdisciplinary team discussed the plan to discharge this patient to a long-term acute care hospital (LTACH) the following day. Knowing that her patient was unaware of the plan, Katie understood the potential implications and went into action. She advocated for the patient by consulting with the primary team and Psychiatry to ensure that the patient was adequately treated for her anxiety and depressive symptoms. Katie also understood that given the discharge disposition to an LTACH and the patient's own medical needs, it would be extremely difficult, if at all possible, for this patient to return to the hospital to see her husband once she was discharged.

Understanding that a visit between this patient and her husband was technically "out of policy," Katie dedicated herself to finding a way to make this visit happen. She reached out to her unit leadership team, the ICU leadership team, hospital risk management, respiratory therapy, the infection control prevention team, and the medical team, explaining why this visit was imperative and how meaningful it would be for both patients. After hours of conversations and championing for the patient, Katie was able to secure approval from all necessary parties for a visit the following morning. The visit between these patients would require a multidisciplinary team and much coordination, all of which Katie arranged during her shift. The visit was scheduled for the following morning, which happened to be a scheduled day off for Katie; however, Katie called the unit the following morning to ensure that the visitation plan was communicated and occurred without delay. The outstanding and compassionate care provided to this patient and her husband by Katie meets the definition of multiple caring factors.

—Heather Davis, MSN, RN, PCCN, SCRN, Advanced Practice Specialist

- What specifically did Katie do that corresponds with RCC? How do you know?

- Did the health system (or context) support the practice of RCC, and if so, how?

- What caring behaviors did Katie display? Should she have done anything different?

- How did this nurse align her performance with the health system's mission?

REFERENCES

Ahmad, N., Ellins, J., Krelle, H., & Lawrie, M. (2014). *Person-centred care: From ideas to action*. Health Foundation.

American Academy of Pediatrics Committee on Hospital Care. (2003). Family-centered care and the pediatrician's role. *Pediatrics*, 12, 691–697. https://doi.org/10.1542/peds.112.3.691

American Association of Colleges of Nursing. (2021). The essentials: Core competencies for professional nursing education. Washington, DC: Author. Available at: https://www.aacnnursing.org/Portals/42/AcademicNursing/pdf/Essentials-2021.pdf

American Geriatrics Society. (2016). Expert panel on person-centered care person-centered care: A definition and essential elements. *Journal of the American Geriatrics Society*, 64(1), 15–18. https://doi.org/10.1111/jgs.13866.

American Nurses Association. (2015). *Code of ethics for nurses, with interpretive statements*. Nursebooks.org

Antonelli, R. C., McAllister, J. W., & Popp, J. (2009). *Making care coordination a critical component of the pediatric health system: A multidisciplinary framework*. The Commonwealth Fund.

Balint, E. (1969). The possibilities of patient-centered medicine. *Journal of the Royal College General Practitioners, 17*(82), 269–276.

Brummel, S. K., Butler, D., Frieder, M., et al. (2016). Person-centered care: A definition and essential elements. *Journal of the American Geriatrics Society, 64*(1), 15–18. https://doi.org/10.1111/jgs.13866

Chandra, S., Mohammadnezhad, M., & Ward, P. (2018). Trust and communication in a doctor–patient relationship: A literature review. *Journal of Healthcare Communities, 3*(3), 36.

Eklund, J. H., Holmström, I. K., Kumlin, T., Kaminsky, E., Skoglund, K., Höglander, J., Sundler, A. J., Condén, E., & Meranius, M. S. (2019). "Same same or Different?" A review of reviews of person-centered and patient-centered care. *Patient Education and Counseling, 102*(1), 3–11. https://doi.org/10.1016/j.pec.2018.08.029

Ekman, I., et al. (2011). Person-centered care—Ready for prime time. *European Journal of Cardiovascular Nursing, 10*, 248–251. https://doi.org/10.1016/j.ejcnurse.2011.06.008

Epstein, R. M., & Street, R. L. (2011). The value and values of patient-centered care. *Annals of Family Medicine, 9*(2), 100–103. https://doi.org/10.1370/afm.1239

Epstein, R. M., Fiscella, K., Lesser, C. S., & Stange, K. C. (2010). Why the nation needs a policy push on patient-centered health care. *Health Affairs, 29*(8), 1489–1495. https://doi.org/10.1377/hlthaff.2009.0888

Fawcett, J. (1984). The metaparadigm of nursing: Present status and future refinements. *The Journal of Nursing Scholarship, 16*, 3, 84–87.

Fazio, S., Pace, D., Flinner, J., & Kallmyer, B. (2018). The fundamentals of person-centered care for individuals with dementia. *The Gerontologist, 58*(suppl 1), S10–S19. https://doi.org/10.1093/geront/gnx122

Gerteis, M. (1993). Coordinating care and integrating services. In M. Gerteis, S. Edgman-Levitan, J. Daley, & T. L. Delbanco (Eds.), *Through the patient's eyes: Understanding and promoting patient-centered care* (pp. 45–71). Jossey-Bass.

Goldfarb, M. J., Bibas, L., Bartlett, V., Jones, H., & Khan, N. (2017). Outcomes of patient and family-centered care interventions in the ICU: A systematic review and meta-analysis. *Critical Care Medicine, 45*(10), 1751–1761. https://doi.org/10.1097/CCM.0000000000002624

Goldstein, E., Farquhar, M., Crofton, C., et al. (2005). Measuring hospital care from the patient's perspective: An overview of the CAHPS hospital survey development process. *Health Services Research, 40*, 1977–1995.

Groom, L. L., Brody, A. A., & Squires, A. P. (2021). Defining telepresence as experienced in telehealth encounters: A dimensional analysis. *Journal of Nursing Scholarship, 53*(6), 709–717.

Guney, S., & Gandhi, R. K. (2022). Leveraging AI to understand care experiences: Insights into communication across racial and ethnic groups. *NEJM Catalyst*. Available at: https://catalyst.nejm.org/doi/full/10.1056/CAT.21.0480

Gusmano, M. K., Maschkem, K. J., & Solomonm, M. Z. (2019). Patient-centered care, Yes; Patients as consumers, No. *Health Affairs, 38*(3), 368–373. https://doi.org/10.1377/hlthaff.2018.05019

Hobbs, J. L. (2009). A dimensional analysis of patient-centered care. *Nursing Research, 58*, 52–62. https://doi.org/10.1097/NNR.0b013c31818c3e79

Hughes, T. M., Merath, K., Chen, Q., et al. (2018). Association of shared decision-making on patient-reported health outcomes and healthcare utilization. *The American Journal of Surgery, 216*(1), 7–12, https://doi.org/10.1016/j.amjsurg.2018.01.011

Institute of Medicine. (2001). *Crossing the quality chasm: A new health system for the 21st century*. Washington, DC: National Academies Press.

Jafarpoor, H., Vasli, P., & Manoochehri, H. (2020). How is family involved in clinical care and decision-making in intensive care units? A qualitative study. *Contemporary Nurse, 56*(3), 215–229. https://doi.org/10.1080/10376178.2020.1801350

Johnson, B. H., & Abraham, M. R. (2012). *Partnering with patients, residents, and families: A resource for leaders of hospitals, ambulatory care settings, and long-term care communities.* Institute for Patient- and Family-Centered Care.

Johnson, B. H. (2000). Family-centered care: Four decades of progress. *Families, Systems, & Health, 18*(2), 137–156. https://doi.org/10.1037/h0091843

Jutterström, L., Hörnsten, Å., Sandström, H., Stenlund, H., & Isaksson, U. (2016). Nurse-led patient-centered self-management support improves HbA1c in patients with type 2 diabetes—A randomized study. *Patient Education and Counseling, 99*(11), 1821–1829. https://doi.org/10.1016/j.pec.2016.06.016

Kaba, R., & Sooriakumaran, P. (2007). The evolution of the doctor–patient relationship. *International Journal of Surgery, 5*(1), 57–65. https://doi.org/10.1016/j.ijsu.2006.01.005

King, B. M., Linette, D., Donohue-Smith, M., & Wolf, Z. R. (2019). Relationship between perceived nurse caring and patient satisfaction in patients in a psychiatric acute care setting. *Journal of Psychosocial Nursing & Mental Health Services, 57*(7), 29–38. https://doi.org/10.3928/02793695-20190225-01

Kuo, D. Z., Houtrow, A. J., Arango, P., et al. (2012). Family-centered care: Current applications and future directions in pediatric health care. *Maternal and Child Health Journal, 16*(2), 297–305. https://doi.org/10.1007/s10995-011-0751-7

Labrague, L. J., De los Santos, J. A. A., Tsaras, K., et al. (2020). The association of nurse caring behaviors on missed nursing care, adverse patient events and perceived quality of care: A cross-sectional study. *Journal of Nursing Management, 28*, 2257–2265. https://doi.org/10.1111/jonm.12894

Lee, K. H., Lee, J. Y., & Kim, B. (2020). Person-centered care in persons living with dementia: A systematic review and meta-analysis. *The Gerontologist, 62*(4), e253–e264. https://doi.org/10.1093/geront/gnaa207

Lewin, S., Skea, Z., Entwistle, V. A., Zwarenstein, M., & Dick, J. (2001). Interventions for providers to promote a patient-centered approach in clinical consultations (Review). *The Cochrane Collaboration, 3*, 1–63. https://doi.org/10.1002/14651858CD003267

Lipkin, M., Quill, T. E., & Napodano, R. J. (1984). The medical interview: A core curriculum for residencies in internal medicine. *Annals of Internal Medicine, 100*(2), 277–284. https://doi.org/10.7326/0003-4819-100-2-277

Maycut, C. & Wild, C. (2019). Relational comportment: Embodying caring as a contemplative journey. *International Journal for Human Caring, 23*(4), 295–301. http://dx.doi.org/10.20467/1091-5710.23.4.29

Mead, N., & Bower, P. (2000). The evolution of the doctor–patient relationship. *International Journal of Surgery, 5*(1), 57–65. https://doi.org/10.1016/j.ijsu.2006.01.005

Mezey, M., Kobayashi, M., Grossman, S., Firpo, A., Fulmer, T., & Mitty, E. (2004). Nurses improving care to health system elders (NICHE): Implementation of best practice models. *Journal of Nursing Administration, 34*(10), 451–457. https://doi.org/10.1097/00005110-200410000-00005

Mitchell, P. (2008). Patient-centered care—A new focus on a time-honored concept. *Nursing Outlook, 56*(5), 197–198. https://doi.org/10.1016/j.outlook.2008.08.001

Morgan, S., & Yoder, L. H. (2012). A concept analysis of person-centered care. *Journal of Holistic Nursing Practice, 30*(1), 6–15. https://doi.org/10.1177/0898010111412189

National Committee for Quality Assurance. (n.d.). Patient-centered medical home (PCMH) recognition. http://www.ncqa.org/programs/recognition/practices/patient-centered-medical-home-pcmh

Naylor, M. D., Brooten, D., Campbell, R., et al. (1999). Comprehensive discharge planning and home follow-up of hospitalized elders: A random clinical trial. *Journal of the American Medical Association, 281*(7), 613–620. https://doi.org/10.1001/jama.281.7.613

NEJM Catalyst. (2017). What is patient-centered care? Available at: https://catalyst.nejm.org/doi/full/10.1056/CAT.17.0559

Patient Protection and Affordable Care Act, Pub. L. No. 111-148, 124 Stat. 119. (2010). http://www.gpo.gov/fdsys/pkg/PLAW-111publ148/pdf/PLAW-111publ148.pdf

Patient-Centered Outcomes Research Institute. (2021). Available at: https://www.pcori .org/

Price, R. A., Elliott, M. N., Cleary, P. D., et al (2015). Should health care providers be accountable for patients' care experiences? *Journal of General Internal Medicine, 30*(2), 253–256. https://doi.org/10.1007/s11606-014-3111-7

Radwin, L. E. (2003). Cancer patients' demographic characteristics and ratings of patient-centered nursing care. *Journal of Nursing Scholarship, 35*(4), 365–370. https:// doi.org/10.1111/j.1547-5069.2003.00365.x

Reinhart, R. J. (2018). In the news: Americans' satisfaction with their healthcare. Gallup. Available at: https://news.galup.com/poll/226607/news-americans-satisfaction -healthcare.aspx

Reynolds, A. (2009). Patient-centered care. *Radiologic Technology, 81*(2), 133–147.

Schall, M., Sevin, C., & Wasson, J. H. (2009). Making high-quality patient-centered care a reality. *Journal of Ambulatory Care Management, 32*(1), 3–7. https://doi.org/10.1097/01 .JAC.0000343118.23091.8a

Sepucha, K. R., Atlas, S. J., Chang, Y., et al. (2018). Informed, patient-centered decisions associated with better health outcomes in orthopedics: Prospective cohort study. *Medical Decision Making, 38*(8), 1018–1026. https://doi.org/10.1177/0272989X18801308

Shaller, D. (2007). Patient-centered care: What does it take? *The Commonwealth Fund.* http://www.commonwealthfund.org/usr_doc/Shaller_patient-centeredcarewhat-doesittake_1067.pdf

Sidani, S., & Fox, M. (2014). Patient-centered care: Clarification of its specific elements to facilitate interprofessional care. *Journal of Interprofessional Care, 28*(2), 134–141. https:// doi.org/10.3109/13561820.2013.862519

Sinaiko, A. D., Szumigalski, K., Eastman, D., & Chien, A. T. (2019). *Delivery of patient centered care in the U.S. health care system: What is standing it its way?* Available at: https://www.academyhealth.org/sites/default/files/deliverypatientcenteredcare_ august2019.pdf

Sinclair, S., Kondejewski, J., Jaggi, P., et al (2021). What works for whom in compassion training programs offered to practicing healthcare providers: A realist review. *BMC Medical Education, 21*, 455. https://doi.org/10.1186/s12909-021-02863-w

Smith, K. A., Bishop, F. L., Dambha-Miller, H., et al. (2020). Improving empathy in healthcare consultations—A secondary analysis of interventions. *Journal of General Internal Medicine, 35*, 3007–3014. https://doi.org/10.1007/s11606-020-05994-w

Stewart, M., Brown, J. B., Weston, W. W., & Freeman, T. R. (2003). *Patient-centered medicine: Transforming the clinical method* (2nd ed.). Radcliffe Medical Press.

Stollenwerk, D., Kennedy, L. B., Hughes, L. S., & O'Connor, M. (2019). A systematic approach to understanding and implementing patient-centered care. *Family Medicine, 51*(2), 173–178.

Volland, J. (2020). What patients want providers to know about "Medical History" NRC health. Available at: https://nrchealth.com/what-patients-want-providers-to-know -about-medical-history/

Wagner, E. H. (1998). Chronic disease management: What will it take to improve practice? *Effective Clinical Practice, 1*(1), 2–4. https://ecp.-acponline.org/augsep98/cdm .pdf

Wasson, J. H., & Baker, N. J. (2009). Balanced measures for patient-centered care. *Journal of Ambulatory Care Management, 32*(1), 44–55. https://doi.org/10.1097/01 .JAC.0000343123.53585.51

Weissman, J. S., Millenson, M. L., & Haring, R. S. (2017). Patient-centered care: Turning the rhetoric into reality. *The American Journal of Managed Care, 23*(1), e31–e32.

Youssef, A., Wiljer, D., Mylopoulos, M., et al. (2020). "Caring About Me": A pilot framework to understand patient-centered care experience in integrated care—A qualitative study, *BMJ Open*, *10*, e034970. https://doi.org/10.1136/bmjopen-2019-034970

Zhao, J., Gao, S., Wang, J., et al. (2016). Differentiation between two healthcare concepts: Person-centered and patient-centered care. *International Journal of Nursing Sciences*, *3*, 398–402.

CHAPTER 6

Relational Capacity

"We all have ability. The difference is how we use it."

—Charlotte Whitten

CHAPTER OBJECTIVES:

1. Describe the term, relational capacity
2. Contrast individual and collective relational capacities
3. Evaluate organizational relational capacity as a meaningful asset in health systems

THE MEANING OF RELATIONAL CAPACITY

Relational capacity in simple terms refers to the individual and collective ability to relate (in the work environment). More specifically, the term, relational capacity, as it is used here was influenced by the work of Seligman et al., known as the father of positive psychology (2005). In this way of thinking, the focus is placed not what undermines individuals, but rather on what contributes to happy, productive, and healthy individuals such that they can positively contribute, enjoy their work life, and realize their full potential (Seligman et al., 2005). During the last 15 to 20 years, positive psychological approaches have been applied to the workplace (Luthans et al., 2015, 2016; Luthans & Avolio, 2007), offering organizations an alternative, but intentionally positive perspective from which to meet their objectives. Such an overriding ethos provides the basis for individuals, groups of individuals (e.g., healthcare teams), departments, or entire organizations to continuously engage people in high-quality connections. Relational capacity is increasingly seen as a needed strength in individual health professionals as well as in health systems. Collective relational capacity is especially crucial to attain health systems' visions, to complete missions, to implement lasting change, and ultimately, to self-advance.

The development of healthy, creative relationships is a dynamic social process that is by nature self-advancing. People tend to relate to and engage with those who are amiable and who share useful information that is other-focused. Furthermore, relational capacity involves trust and responses that are

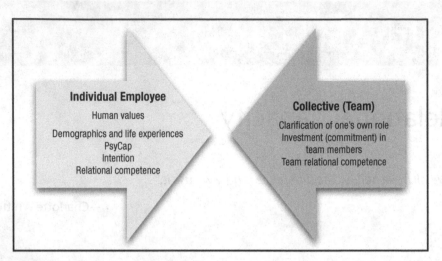

FIGURE 6.1 Organizational relational capacity.

interesting and appealing versus those that are flat or off-putting. Relationship capacity can be thought of on an individual, team or department level, and organizational levels (Figure 6.1).

INDIVIDUAL RELATIONAL CAPACITY

Obviously, relational capacity varies by individual on a continuum from those who are overwhelmed by or simply cannot connect to others and those who are actively engaged in high-quality relationships. In nursing, modes of being with (or caring for) another were well explained by Haldorsdottir (1991) as extending from lifegiving or biogenic (caring) relationships on the one hand to life-destroying or biocidic relationships on the other (uncaring). Sandwiched between these two extremes are the categories of life sustaining (bioactive), life neutral (biopassive), and life restraining (biostatic).

At the extreme biocidic end of the spectrum, relationships between patients and nurses were described as depersonalized, distressful, cold, and characterized as robbing joy from patients. At the other biogenic extreme, relationships between patients and nurses were affirming, protective, warm, and growth producing. It is these life-giving (positive) relationships that were described as professional, creating the ideal conditions for healing or goal attainment. Thus, the ability of nursing and health systems to positively relate is crucial for the well-being of patients and families as well as employees and customers.

To effectively (positively) relate in organizations, one must consider both the individual as well as collective teams. Individual characteristics such as personal values, life experiences, demographics; positive psychological characteristics (psychological capital [PsyCap]) (Luthans et al., 2007); the intention to relate; and the competencies required to relate (in a caring manner) comprise the components that contribute to relational capacity.

Certainly, one's values or belief systems impact the ability to relate. Schwartz's (1994, 2006, 2011, 2012) theory of basic human values suggests that one's dormant or unexpressed values and beliefs guide behavior. More specifically, one's values are abstract and tend to be tied to emotions, not objective facts; thus they are difficult to pinpoint, vary among individuals, and are not necessarily tied to reality. Values provide a motivational aspect as they frequently are attached to an individual's desired goals. As such, values guide our evaluations of people, behaviors, and events and are ordered in importance. In essence, values serve as guiding principles that direct one's behavior (Schwartz, 2012); in this case, engaging relationally.

Schwartz has defined 10 universal values that guide people's behavior and contends that they overlap and compete with each other (see Table 6.1). For example, the power to achieve (pursuit of self-interests) may conflict with the benevolence value (concern for the welfare and interests of others) at a point in time, impacting behaviors or attitudes tied to high-quality relationships.

Typically, people's demographics and life circumstances or experiences shape the priority attached to their values. For example, a person's age or generation and their education and family structure will influence to a large extent their view of the world, ultimately affecting potential behaviors. According to Schwartz & Bardi (1997), changing life experiences influence an individual to upgrade the importance attributed to values they can readily attain and downgrade the importance of those whose pursuit is blocked. However, this relationship changes when considering the power and security values; when they are easily attained, their importance drops. For example, people who suffer economic hardship and social upheaval attribute more importance to the values of power and security than those who live in relative comfort and safety (Inglehart, 1997).

In summary, people's age, education, gender, and other characteristics largely determine the life circumstances to which they are exposed. These include their family dynamics, socialization and learning experiences; the social roles they play; the culture they are born into; the expectations and sanctions they encounter; and the abilities they develop. Thus, differences in background

TABLE 6.1 Schwartz's Motivational Human Values

Universalism
Benevolence
Conformity
Security
Power
Stimulation
Achievement
Self-direction
Tradition
Hedonism

Source: Adapted from Schwartz, S. H. (1994). Are there universal aspects in the structure and contents of human values? *Journal of Social Issues, 50*, 33. https://doi.org/10.1111/j.1540–4560.1994.tb01196.x

characteristics represent differences in the life circumstances that ultimately influence the value placed on various priorities (Schwartz, 2011).

The psychological state of individuals, particularly those who exhibit the positive characteristics of hope, resilience, optimism, and self-efficacy, termed PsyCAP, was first labeled as an important construct by Luthans & Youssef (2004). In their important contributions to human strengths in the workplace, Luthans et al. defined PsyCap as "a core psychological factor of positivity in general, and the investment/development of 'who you are'" (Luthans et al., 2005, p. 253). As a state-like resource, high levels of PsyCap have been found to positively influence well-being, health outcomes, such as lower body mass index (BMI) and cholesterol levels and satisfaction with one's relationships (Lorenz et al., 2016). The four characteristics of PsyCap are considered resources or strengths that can be developed both individually and collectively, positively impacting performance in organizations (Luthans, 2005; Luthans & Youssef, 2007; Luthans & Youssef-Morgan, 2017).

The characteristic of *optimism* refers to positive acknowledgment of one's immediate and future successes. The characteristic of *resiliency* is defined as "when beset by problems and adversity, sustaining and bouncing back and even beyond (resilience) to attain success" (Luthans et al., 2007, p. 3). The concept of *hope* is derived from the work of Snyder (2000), who reported that hope is a multidimensional construct composed of both an individual's determination to set and maintain effort toward goals (described as *willpower* or *agency*) and that individual's ability to discern alternative courses of action to attain those goals (described as *way power* or *pathways thinking*). Finally, as defined by the well-known research psychologist, Bandura (1997), *self-efficacy* refers to people's convictions about their own capacity to successfully execute a course of action that leads to a desired outcome. Bandura has argued that if adequate levels of ability and motivation exist, self-efficacy will impact an individual's decision to perform a specific task and their level of persistence in performing that task despite problems, disconfirming evidence, and even adversity. Weak efficacy beliefs can contribute to behavior avoidance and anxiety, whereas strong efficacy beliefs can promote behavior initiation and persistence. This is especially crucial when considering the caring behaviors.

If individuals perceive their own capacity for caring to be limited, performance of the caring behaviors in clinical situations may be inadequate and may even influence avoidance of situations requiring interaction. Thus, it behooves nursing educators to ensure caring competency upon graduation!

The concepts of self-efficacy, optimism, hope, and resiliency have been incorporated into a theoretical definition of the construct, relational capital (PsyCap), and when combined have a synergistic effect. Specifically, researchers have found that PsyCap is a core construct that predicts performance and satisfaction better than any of the individual strengths that make it up (Luthans et al., 2005; Luthans et al., 2008; Luthans et al., 2010). Using a valid and reliable measure, the Psychological Capital Questionnaire (PCQ; Luthans et al., 2007), PsyCap can be reasonably measured and used in organizations for training/counseling programs. PsyCap can now be measured using a short form (PCQ-12; Avey et al., 2011) that has the advantage of decreased burden and applicability across cultures. As an individual resource, PsyCap can change over time and be developed through training interventions. Importantly, overall PsyCap is correlated with satisfaction and investment in relationships (Luthans & Youssef-Morgan, 2017).

In organizations, PsyCap has been shown to positively influence employee performance (self-rated, supervisor-rated, and objective), desirable employee attitudes and citizenship behaviors, and longitudinal well-being. Likewise, PsyCap has been inversely related to turnover intentions, work stress, and anxiety (Luthans & Youssef-Morgan, 2017). These findings are important for health-care work environments where renewed importance for employee well-being is taking hold. However, conceptualizing PsyCap at a team-based or collective level is still evolving. It is reasonable to suggest, however, that more optimistic employees working together may positively influence organizational relationships. Ultimately, PsyCap remains a strong component of relationship capacity that, together with other individual strengths, can be leveraged in organizations.

Intention refers to purposeful actions performed to achieve immediate outcomes and future goals. Husserl (1980) identified intention as a phenomenological trait that characterizes a mental state or experience as being "directed toward something." Intention in its simplest form was defined more precisely as a thinking–feeling response that motivates action (Anscombe, 1957/1963). Dossey & Keegan (2009) defined intention as "the conscious determination to do a specific thing or to act in a specific manner; the mental state of being committed to, planning to, or trying to perform an action" (p. 21). According to Anscombe, the basic building blocks of intention are an identified reason to act, the desire to act, and consideration for the feasibility of acting, all of which converge to form an intention (or choice) to achieve attainable and beneficial goals.

BOX 6.1: Thus, the intention to relate (or connect) is a combination of an individual's awareness of a reason to act, the resulting desire it influences, the feasibility of an identified set of actions, and finally the choice to act. This combination of factors is a process of thinking and feeling that is subjective in nature and results in a conscious (fully aware) choice to relate.

When used in reference to nursing practice, the term, intention, is found primarily in holistic theoretical frameworks and in theories focused on caring (Sofhauser, 2016). Here, intention refers to "being with" patients without attachment to outcomes, that is, working with patients and families in the moment with limited regard to what needs to be accomplished in the future.

Intention is behaviorally oriented and is different than the term, *intentionality*. Intentionality refers to a state of being or one's whole frame of reference at a point in time. It signifies a deep or a grounding dimension that sets the stage for *how* one directs their thoughts. Acting with intention (relational intention) is enhanced when one is fully aware, purposeful, and centered (see Figure 6.1). Associated behaviors become more authentic, even reverent. Relational intention is apparent when behavior is positively directed toward the other using the caring behaviors to initiate, cultivate, and sustain relationships. One's competence, on the other hand, infers ability or expertise.

In general, the term *competence* refers to one's knowledge, skills, and attitudes; *relational* competence, therefore, refers to an individual's knowledge, skills, and attitudes for relating interpersonally, including helping to engender trust, safety, and dignity in recipients. This ability to comprehend, move toward another, to develop mutuality, staying open, even enjoying the experience, is a necessary component of relational capacity. According to Carpenter et al. (1983), relational competence consists of five dimensions that predispose individuals to *initiate* relationships and five dimensions that help *enhance* or *maintain* those relationships over time. Initiation skills are assertiveness, dominance (the desire and ability to be in charge of one's own situation and to engage), and independence and belief in one's ability to relate (Carpenter, 1993). Shyness and social anxiety were seen as factors that were detrimental to initiating relationships. Maintenance factors were intimacy (tendency toward helping and support), ability to trust, interpersonal sensitivity, altruism, and perspective taking (ability to see all sides of an issue). These factors are aligned with the caring behaviors or processes described in Chapter 3 and are often at least superficially dealt with as part of health professional curricula. Proficiency in their use is essential if relational competence is to flourish. Nurses, in particular, are known for the maintenance factors, but assertiveness, dominance, and beliefs about one's abilities to relate are not necessarily discussed, learned, or evaluated.

Communication is also considered a fundamental dimension of relational competence. In fact, the majority of activities in health systems involve communication, often among individuals who are not well known to each other. Effective communication begins with caring about the way a message is delivered and caring about the people whom you engage in dialogue (Hertz, 2015). Using simple explanations, personal stories, humor, and authentic presence conveys such caring. In particular, registered nurses, as the most often observed and consistent health professionals in most clinical settings, must have the ability to communicate effectively. Particular forms of communication, such as discussing bad news, dialoguing with other health professionals, communicating during conflict, conversing about spiritual concerns, talking with patients/families from different cultures, public speaking, and actively listening amid the busy workflow associated with healthcare delivery are challenging activities for nurses and often it is easier to avoid them. Yet, professional nurses are educated to communicate effectively with emphasis placed on skills such as questioning, reframing, clarifying, using open-ended questions, demonstrating cultural sensitivity, and specialized techniques for communicating with those who cannot actively interact (such as those who are comatose, psychologically impaired, or under the influence of medications). Using these skills in everyday practice builds trust and teamwork, strengthening relational competence.

COLLECTIVE RELATIONAL CAPACITY (TEAM CARING)

The healthcare needs of today's public demand specialized skills requiring groups of health professionals working together in the best interests of patients and families. For example, patients with diabetes often have problems with chronic obesity, heart disease, and frequently need assistance with behavioral changes (American Diabetes Association, n.d.). The comprehensive care of patients with diabetes, therefore, is often best met through teams of dietitians, nurses, endocrinologists, cardiologists, primary care physicians, psychology professionals, and others who work together to help patients meet their health goals. Regular interaction among these professionals is not enough; rather, "effective healthcare teams share common goals, understand each other's roles, demonstrate respect for each other, use clear communication, resolve conflict effectively, and are flexible (Grumbach & Bodenheimer, 2004, p. 1246). Although a qualitative study with a sample size of 36, Wei et al. (2020) found that the underlying facilitator of effective collaboration among healthcare teams was a culture of caring, for example, groups of health professionals who related in a caring, collaborative manner (team caring). This characteristic contributed to health organizations and positive patient outcomes (see Chapter 4).

However, situating a discipline such as nursing *within* the interprofessional team with respect to daily processes of care requires clarification of one's own role as a member of that interprofessional team. This enables nurses to appreciate their unique contribution as well as those of the other team members. In fact, as interprofessional practice evolves toward the norm in health systems, nurses should be able to demonstrate the significance of their unique perspective and skill sets for different patient populations. Just as relationships with patients and families take time, so do relationships with team members. Investing in team members in terms of committing to ongoing interactions that reach the levels of connection and knowing (Duffy, 2003) is key.

Nurses, however, have documented problems relating to *each other* with known instances of intimidating and disruptive behaviors (DB) (Monteau, 2017). DB, such as bullying, lateral violence, physical aggression, incivility, verbal abuse, and refusing to communicate have been linked to problems in nursing recruitment, turnover, and retention. However, study findings suggest that the consequences of DB go far beyond nurses' job satisfaction and morale and affect the health of the work environment, including interprofessional collaboration, which may well, in turn, have a negative impact on clinical outcomes, including safety. In fact, DBs are linked to increased frequency of adverse medical events and medical errors, decreased patient safety, lower quality of care, and higher patient mortality, in addition to organizational outcomes such as cost, staff turnover, and job dissatisfaction (Rehder et al., 2020).

Inadequate professional collaboration among healthcare professionals may cause much distress to patients and their families, who often want consistent information and a sense of certainty about their diagnosis and treatment alternatives. In addition, relational difficulties among clinicians may impede the recruitment of patients to clinical trials, cause confusion about courses of action, and create a loss of confidence in the team's ability to meet patient needs.

Consider the following:

Kelly is a recent baccalaureate graduate who is working her first job on the orthopedic floor of a general community hospital. One of her patients, Mrs. Powers, a 58-year-old White female, is experiencing newly developed shortness of breath postop day 2 after a total knee replacement. Kelly becomes concerned and calls the orthopedic surgeon to report Mrs. Powers' status change. She becomes nervous on the phone and cannot deliver a clear, concise report. The physician becomes irritated and asks for detailed information (lab results, lung sounds) that Kelly cannot produce. He finally tells her to call him back "when she can do her job thoroughly and has her information straight."

Kelly, visibly shaken by this encounter, approaches an experienced nurse, Joan, to ask for help. Kelly is inexperienced in assessments and the possible complications of knee surgery and feels dispirited after the phone conversation with the physician. Joan, who is busy with her own patients, does not appreciate the meaning of this experience for Kelly and dismisses her concerns saying, "You will have to wait — I am up to my eyeballs with this patient." Under her breath, she says, "I don't get these new grads—you'd think that after 4 years, they could listen to a few lung sounds, check lab results, and call a physician. I am so sick of doing their job for them."

Kelly walks away and does her own assessment, this time listening for lung sounds and checking the chart for lab results. Nothing seems amiss. Mrs. Powers' shortness of breath is abating, and Kelly attributes the whole episode to her own lack of experience. She calls the physician back and reports that everything seems okay now.

Two hours later, Mrs. Powers' shortness of breath has returned but is worse than earlier, and she needs to sit straight up in bed to catch her breath. She looks sweaty and a little off color as well. Kelly calls another senior nurse (Mary) who comes into the room, takes down the patient's bedclothes and examines both legs. The one unaffected by the surgery is swollen and slightly reddened. Mary assesses Mrs. Powers' lungs and applies oxygen, all the while explaining to Kelly what she is doing. Simultaneously, she reassures Mrs. Powers, who is getting visibly upset. Convinced that the patient is stable for the immediate future, Mary takes Kelly outside the room and explains what is going on, why she has done what she did, and then coaches Kelly on what to say and how to convey her concerns (organize her thoughts) during the subsequent phone call to the physician. She allows Kelly to "teach back" her report and stays with her during the phone call. This conversation goes a little smoother, and the physician orders some blood work and a CT scan and assures Kelly she will be there soon. After the call, Mary reviews the entire experience with Kelly, offering further advice on complete assessments and complications after orthopedic surgery.

This case is typical, particularly during summer months, when new nurses take their first positions after graduation. Can you characterize the type of behaviors used by Joan, the experienced nurse, and by the physician in the beginning of the case? How do you think they contributed to Kelly's sense of efficacy as a nurse or her desire to remain employed on that unit? How did they contribute to the patient's sense of safety or confidence in her recovery? The second nurse, Mary, was also busy, but understood the importance of this "teaching moment" and used her caring knowledge, skills, and attitudes to relate professionally to Kelly, the patient, and the physician, all the while keeping her focus on "what's best for the patient." She role-modeled certain behaviors, relayed information, reassured the patient, and allowed Kelly to ask questions and practice her reporting skills—Mary understood her unique role as an experienced nurse on this team. She also invested in Kelly by supporting her during the conversation and making time for her.

Or reflect on this account in which a senior nurse was "floated" to help on another unit, a typical anxiety-provoking situation in nursing:

It is customary in this health system for nurses working on the inpatient hospice unit to provide support and expertise with subcutaneous access ports in patients who are housed on other units. On the day shift in such an organization, the hospice unit was called to provide a routine flush for an access port in a patient on a medical–surgical unit. An experienced hospice nurse went to the unit in another building. Upon arrival, she introduced herself to the unit secretary, told her why she was there, and asked her to find the charge nurse so she could find out who the patient was and where supplies and equipment were kept. The charge nurse responded that she was busy with another patient, and the hospice nurse would have to wait about 10 minutes. Fifteen minutes later, the charge nurse was still not available, leaving the hospice nurse unaware of the patient or where to find the supplies for the procedure. Finally, when the charge nurse became available, she said it was the patient in bed 79B, leaving the hospice nurse to fetch the supplies—an uncomfortable situation since she did not know the unit. She went about collecting the necessary equipment rather haphazardly, performed the flush as requested, documented it, and told the secretary she had finished. The whole episode took longer than an hour.

Two weeks later, she was asked to perform the same procedure; however, this time when she arrived on the unit, a licensed practical nurse (LPN) greeted her, took her to see the patient, and helped collect the needed supplies; she then stayed and assisted. It was an easy and efficient experience that lasted 20 minutes.

For an expert nurse providing services in an unknown unit, the first incident was unpleasant and inefficient; in the second incident, the LPN collaborated with the hospice nurse, contributing to an efficient and pleasant work experience. The LPN used her relationship skills to affirm the hospice nurse, facilitating a calm experience and an efficient procedure. It is no wonder that many nurses don't like to "float"!

In addition to understanding one's role and working hard to generate quality relationships on an interprofessional team, a third aspect of collective relational competence is the teams' shared relational competence. Earlier in this chapter, relational competence was described in terms of initiation and maintenance of relationships. The senior nurse, Mary, in the previous example, exuded relational competence. She was assertive yet caring, dominant (understood and exercised her leadership role in this situation), and confident (viewed herself as able). Mary also understood the work or had a strong knowledge base in the care of postop orthopedic patients and communicated well, imparting information, supporting the new nurse, and soliciting feedback. Thus, effective relational capacity in health teams consists of clarification of one's individual role as a contributing member of a team, investment in each team member, and collective relational competence.

BOX 6.2: Relational competence is the glue that holds a health team together and ensures its success in meeting patient and team member needs. It helps ease friction during conflict, calm difficult personalities, persuades, softens the sadness of disappointing moments, and, most importantly, guarantees that the team's work is focused on the patient and family.

Interprofessional teams can function for a short while without relational capacity, but eventually they will break down and unknowingly distress team members and potentially place patients in jeopardy. Individual health professionals depend on their larger and multidisciplined work group for support in handling the hard relational work that is central to healthcare. In such teams, members trust each other, hold productive mini-meetings (called *rounds* in healthcare), have fun together, feel safe and acknowledged—overall, they use collective relational capacity to get the work done. The more an interprofessional work group is conscious of itself as a collective that serves important functions in supporting the individual work of its members, the more successful that group will be in its overall role of meeting the health needs of patients and families, and, by default, health systems.

ORGANIZATIONAL RELATIONAL CAPACITY

In health systems, relational capacity is a meaningful asset that is based on developing, cultivating, and sustaining high-quality individual and collective relationships. It can be further described to include external organizations or work groups that influence or impact the business of healthcare, including customers, suppliers, employees, accrediting organizations, governments (including international), partners, other stakeholders, and, sometimes, even competitors. Health systems with higher levels of relational capacity often have wide networks of relationships with others who impact healthcare and healthy ties with all of its key stakeholders. This relational strength, if nurtured and allowed to emerge, is naturally self-advancing, directly impacting performance.

In health systems, it is relationships that drive the work. Relationships that health professionals develop with their peers, their bosses, their patients, families, and even the organization, all impact the quality and costs of services provided. Relationships are commonplace in health services and often are so implicit that they go unnoticed. For example, despite the fact that health professionals spend the majority of their time "relating," this is not routinely acknowledged, studied, or attended to. At the core of health systems, however, are the specific ways individuals are tied to and interact with one another and the organization itself. In fact, Gittell (2009) states that "shared goals and mutual respect form the basis for collected coordinated action" (p. 14). Such relationships uniquely characterize and provide a framework for organizational work.

The essence of organizational relating is more than just getting along with people and attaining goals; it is about realizing that we are not alone in this work and that, together, people create, grow, and develop, and are productive workers. This relationship factor is almost a hidden asset for it is not readily seen, but it sure goes a long way toward healthy performance. For example, employees' level of engagement, willingness to go above and beyond, and relational competence with patients and families are not easy to observe but directly impact patients' experiences (a reimbursable outcome), other employees' satisfaction with work, and the bottom line.

Consider this scenario:

I was skeptical when we began treating patients with electroconvulsive therapy (ECT); I even asked my manager if ECT really works. She shrugged with a "maybe" or "I hope so." But then she went on to say, "I've seen remarkable changes in patients' demeanor and affect and give credit to ECT for the improvements. As I got more involved with the ECT program and expansion, I'm inspired by its success rate." This is an example of how some nurses felt about ECT when it was first introduced to provide comprehensive care in their community. Many nurses were uncomfortable with the treatment or doubted the process, were unaware of current ECT evidence, and there were longstanding cultural barriers and stigmas associated with the treatment. Nevertheless, in San Diego County, UC San Diego Health System and Kaiser Permanente were two of the few hospitals that offered ECT as a treatment option for depression in Southern California. As more space and workforce was required to meet the needs of the county, these two hospitals joined forces to provide collaborative care to patients.

Over time, using team-based education and ongoing collaboration and learning together, ECT is now perceived well among the nursing staff. In fact, when asked about the team he works with and his perception of their attitudes toward ECT, one of the psychiatrists says the best way to describe it is "gratifying." He has seen nurses' response to the procedure go from hesitant to reassuring. He is very proud when nurses are seen comforting patients and advocating for the therapy, with the conviction that they will soon feel better. The psychiatrist compares this situation to a pebble in a pond, where each person is able to walk away and share his or her positive experience with ECT with others, often decreasing the stigma attached to it.

Team members at UCSD Health can now attest to the incredible impact of ECT as some of their patients enter treatment catatonic and unable to communicate and then "return" to talking, smiling, and participating in the world around them. Any stigma surrounding ECT as a treatment option for depression is rarely displayed at this system. Rather, the team's support for patients and families, collaboration, education, human respect, and individualized care has been an incredible journey for all involved.

In summary, the two organizations have learned from each other and grown together to ensure best practice with the support of psychiatric departments, doctors, anesthesia providers, and nurses. This long-lasting relationship answers a call from the community looking for ECT as an answer to their chronic depression that has otherwise been left unanswered.

Now, after some time co-relating in this program, nurses are advocates for patients and the treatment and encourage student nurses to participate. As one nurse stated, "I have seen patients transition from a catatonic state to one in which they will have an engaged conversation with you. I like to demonstrate the patient's experience with ECT to everyone who is interested." As a result, nursing students often will shadow the staff during the procedure and are always grateful for the opportunity.

—Lindsay C. Holt, PhD, RN, CPAN

It is obvious that the relationships between the two health systems, their leaders, and clinicians drove this work. Being open, learning together, ensuring that the procedures were undertaken with the utmost human respect, inclusion of family, and patient preference was paramount. Often, the choice to try ECT takes time, but nurses at this system supported patients as they made the decision to pursue treatment, advocating for them throughout the process; and their leaders ensured that learning opportunities were available throughout.

Building organizational relational capacity is a major responsibility of the leaders of health systems. Typically, health systems' leaders are judged based on quality, safety, and system (financial) outcomes, the assumption being that this is good for patients and the system. Yet, the quality of relationships in an organization may be a key driver of organizational metrics. As leaders, then, it is vital to notice the quality of relationships and what is contributing to and benefitting from them. Leaders who spend time with their staff, share common interests, ask them how they are doing, what they are working on, and have a sense of humor have a good chance of gaining a level of respect that will form the basis for future relationships. Valuing relationships with coworkers is also important as a source of ongoing learning. Although we are all busy, allocating time to nurture relationships is an essential aspect of leadership.

To assess the relational capacity within a health system, the leader could start by asking questions. For example, leaders might ask:

- Does the system invest time and effort in selecting employees with the right relational competences?
- Do the socialization practices (onboarding, continuing education, unit level interactions) in the system reflect the relational values and culture of the organization? Are these practices well thought out? Or are they considered a waste of time?
- What type of orientation and mentoring is available to new employees?
- Do leaders focus on relationships as their primary work activity?
- Are leaders of meetings in an organization capable of engaging members? Do the members rely on each other to get the work done?
- Are there systems in place to help employees (all employees) deal with work–family dynamics?
- Does the system honor individuals' and teams' needs for reflection and conscious awareness?
- What meaningful rewards are in place to recognize high-quality relationships?

BOX 6.3: After all, leadership is a dynamic *process* encompassing self-awareness, practicing one's values and beliefs, applying meaningful motivations, developing and using a supportive team, and living an integrated life. In essence, leadership is a way of being versus just doing a job. Thus, for those who teach leadership in health systems, helping students learn how to enable relational capacity is paramount.

Likewise, health educators have a responsibility to teach and help students learn the importance of relationships to healthcare practice. Particularly in online courses, maintaining and nurturing high-quality faculty–student relationships is key. Educating in this way requires faculty members who are comfortable and relationally competent themselves and who understand the benefits of such learning. Frankel et al. (2011) proposed three areas necessary for faculty development. Although directed toward medical education, these ideas are important for all health professionals, especially in light of the high dependency and teamwork required in modern-day health services. The three areas for faculty development are mindful practice, formation (ethical development), and communication skills. Future recommendations for faculty development include (a) making relationship-centered care a central competency in all healthcare interactions, (b) developing a national curriculum framework with input from patients, (c) requiring performance metrics for professional development, (d) partnering with national healthcare organizations to disseminate the curriculum framework, and (e) preserving face-to-face educational methods for delivering key elements of the curriculum.

BOX 6.4: Although it may be painful for health educators to acknowledge that time-honored approaches to learning and curricula need major revision, articulating the relational outcomes we most desire and asking which methods will best help us to achieve them are important first steps in reconstructing educational programs that will produce graduates with individual and collective relational capacity.

As organizational relational capacity also includes relationships with external partners, it is significant that health systems in recent years have placed an increased focus on academic–service partnerships. For example, many schools of nursing are now formally partnering with clinical sites for teaching and research, improving care, and instilling principles of lifelong learning (Jones et al., 2021). Conceptually, such partnerships entail sharing power and resources, and some empirical evidence is available related to their success. For example, some have evaluated academic–practice partnerships to build alliances, fulfill health needs of communities, and advance the professional nursing workforce (Karikari-Martin et al., 2021; Gilliss et al., 2021). The strength of the relationships among the partners has been key to their success.

Building organization relational capacity is enabled by the individual and collective relational capacity of employees. Nurses, in particular, have a unique opportunity to make a profound difference in patient and system outcomes based on the highly relational characteristics of their discipline. The time is now to use our collective relational capacity to enhance the health of patients, health systems, and ourselves.

SUMMARY

Relational capacity, a resource necessary for quality caring at the individual, collective, and organizational levels, is explored. Human values, life experiences, intentions, PsyCap, and relational competence are described as important elements of individual relational capacity. Team or collective relational capacity in which groups of health professionals working together in the best interests of patients and families is also discussed. Case studies illuminate the importance of relational capacity on patient and employee outcomes. Finally, organizational relational capacity is highlighted as an often unobserved system asset that positively impacts performance. Examples for leadership and education are used.

CALL TO ACTION

Relational capacity is an individual and collective trait and an organizational strength that impacts self-advancement. Relational capacity is everyone's responsibility. **Assess** your own relational capacity—include your underlying values, PsyCap, caring intention, and relational competence. Shared relational capacity among health teams contributes to organizational relational capacity. **Build** relationships, particularly those with yourself, with patients and families, with other health professionals, and with the health system.

REFLECTIVE QUESTIONS/APPLICATIONS

For Professional Nurses in Clinical Practice:

- Discuss the interprofessional practice among nurses on your unit. Is it of high quality? Why or why not?
- Is there an expectation that relational capacity is necessary for RN work at your institution? If so, how is it evaluated?
- Reflect on your own individual relational capacity using the components presented in this chapter. Where do you stand? What do you need to do to improve it?
- What patient outcomes do you think might be enhanced with greater relational capacity?
- Which experienced nurse would you have been in the case study, Joan or Mary? Why?
- Take a minute and think back to a team that you absolutely loved being a part of. Did that have anything to do with the relational capacity of the team? How did you contribute to that team's relational capacity?

For Professional Nurses in Educational Practice:

- What specific curricular revisions have you developed that address individual, collective (team), and organizational relational capacity competencies? How do you evaluate it? What teaching/learning strategies do you use to help undergraduate and graduate students learn how to relate?

- Reflect on the need for relational capacity among teams of health professionals. How does your educational program facilitate graduates' competencies to work effectively in teams?

- What can you do to select, develop, and mentor students to enhance their individual relational capacity? Specifically, how can they best learn how to listen, be optimistic, develop hope, communicate, understand their unique contribution to healthcare, and *do* the ongoing personal work necessary to build relational capacity?

- How might you suggest incorporating relational capacity building into your online courses?

- Provide some suggestions for exposing students' values and belief systems that would provide them some insight into their behavior.

For Professional Nurses in Leadership Practice:

- What is the state of relational capacity at your organization? How do you know?

- How do you specifically hold yourself accountable to build relational capacity at work?

- Reflect on the hiring process in place at your institution. Does it include assessment of individuals' relational capacity? What would it take to revise this?

- How is collective (team) relational capacity monitored and measured at your institution? What could you do to enhance this process?

- How do you facilitate the individual relational capacity of health professionals under your supervision? What specific activities (orientation, mentoring, career development, etc.) support this?

- Does your leadership team understand the importance of relational capacity at all levels as it relates to the bottom line? If not, how will you facilitate their development?

- Create a plan for dramatically altering the selection, orientation, socialization process, and ongoing career development of employees to enhance organization relational capacity. Who should be involved? What methodology would be used? How long will it take? What implications for RN practice would occur? How would you ensure that the plan is enacted as developed? How would you evaluate its implementation?

PRACTICE ANALYSIS

Bill, a 60-year-old male with pancreatic cancer, has been hospitalized for almost 2 weeks and is in the intensive care unit for the past 5 days. His physical deterioration and suffering have created anguish in his wife and in the health-care team. The attending physician discussed with the wife the likelihood of her husband having a cardiac and/or respiratory arrest, described the actions the team would take for a full resuscitation as well as the varying levels of resuscitation approved by the treatment setting, which included a do-not-resuscitate option, and asked her to express her preferences regarding resuscitation. The wife initially chose the do-not-resuscitate status for her husband and completed all of the official paperwork to implement that decision. During the next 12 hours, the wife actively solicited from nursing and medical staff their definitions of do-not-resuscitate. She then contacted the attending physician to rescind her decision, choosing instead to have a full resuscitation order in place. She explained her decision change as, "When I saw that the nurses and doctors did not all define resuscitation in the same way, I decided that I would not leave that in their hands. I am my husband's wife and will be to the end." This new decision was enacted and over the next 4 days, the patient showed clear signs of dying. His wife stayed with him in the intensive care unit and witnessed the changes in her husband's physical appearance. She began commenting on those changes and on her husband's obvious suffering. Within 2 hours of his death, the wife told the nurse that she did not want her husband to be resuscitated. This information was immediately conveyed to the physician who, once again, changed the order in the electronic health record.

- What individual and collective (team) relational capacity was exhibited in this case?

- What was the state of organizational relational capacity in this unit? How might the nurse leader in this unit evaluate and improve organizational relationship capacity?

- What could have been done differently by the health professionals in this situation?

REFERENCES

American Diabetes Association. (n.d.). Living with diabetes. http://www.diabetes.org/living-with-diabetes

Anscombe, G. E. M. (1957/1963). *Intention*. Harvard University Press.

Avey, J., Reichard, R. J., Luthans, F., & Mhatre, K. H. (2011). Meta-analysis of the impact of positive psychological capital on employee attitudes, behaviors, and performance. *Human Resource Development Quarterly*, 22(2), 127–152. https://doi.org/10.1002/hrdq.20070

Bandura, A. (1997). *Self-efficacy: The exercise of control*. Freeman.

Carpenter, B. N. (1993). Relational competence. In D. Perlman & W. H. Jones (Eds.), *Advances in personal relationships, a research manual* (Vol. 4., pp. 1–28). Jessica Kingsley.

Carpenter, B. N., Hansson, R. O., Rountree, R., & Jones, W. H. (1983). Relational competence and adjustment in diabetic patients. *Journal of Social and Clinical Psychology, 1*(4), 359–369. https://doi.org/10.1521/jscp.1983.1.4.359

Dossey, B., & Keegan, L. (2009). *Holistic nursing: A handbook for practice* (p. 21). Jones & Bartlett.

Duffy, J. (2003). Caring relationships and evidence-based practice: Can they co-exist? *International Journal for Human Caring, 7*(3), 45–50.

Frankel, R. M., Eddin-Folensbee, F., & Inui, T. S. (2011). Crossing the patient-centered divide: Transforming health care quality through enhanced faculty development. *Academic Medicine, 86*(4), 445–452. https://doi.org/10.1097/ACM.0b013e31820e7e6e

Gilliss, C. L., Poe, T., Hogan, T. H., Intinarelli, G., & Harper, D. C. (2021). Academic/clinical nursing integration in academic health systems. *Nursing Outlook, 69*(2), 234–242.

Gittell, J. H. (2009). *High performance healthcare: Using the power of relationships to achieve quality, efficiency and resilience.* McGraw-Hill.

Grumbach, K., & Bodenheimer, T. (2004). Can health care teams improve primary care practice? *Journal of the American Medical Association, 291*, 1246–1251. https://doi.org/10.1001/jama.291.10.1246

Haldorsdottir, S. (1991). Five basic modes of being with another. In D. Gaut & M. Leininger (Eds.), *Caring: The compassionate healer* (pp. 37–49). The National League for Nursing.

Hertz, H. (2015). *Effective communication requires caring, explaining, listening, and living the role.* https://www.nist.gov/baldrige/effective-communication-requires-caring-explaining-listening-and-living-role

Husserl, E. (1980). Ideas pertaining to a pure phenomenology and to a phenomenological philosophy: Second book: Studies in the phenomenology of constitution. Kluwer Academic.

Inglehart, R. (1997). *Modernization and postmodernization: Cultural, economic, and political change in 43 societies.* Princeton University Press. (LEHMAN-SOCIAL WORK RESERVES HM101 .I554 1997).

Jones, K., Burnett, G., Sztuba, L., & Hannon, R. (2021). Academic practice partnerships: A review of a statewide population health nursing leadership initiative. *Public Health Nursing, 38,* 64–76. https://doi.org/10.1111/phn.12833

Karikari-Martin, P., Zapata, D., Hesgrove, B., Murray, C. B., & Kauffman, K. (2021). Academic–Service partnerships: Increasing the advanced nurse workforce. *Journal of Nursing Education, 60*(4), 190–195.

Lorenz, T., Beer, C., Pütz, J., & Heinitz, K. (2016). Measuring psychological capital: Construction and validation of the compound PsyCap scale (CPC-12). *PLoS One, 11*(4), e0152892. https://doi.org/10.1371/journal.pone.0152892

Luthans, F. (2005). *Organizational behaviour* (10th ed.). McGraw-Hill International Edition.

Luthans, F., Avey, J. B., Avolio, B. J., & Peterson, S. J. (2010). The development and resulting performance impact of positive psychological capital. *Human Resource Development Quarterly, 21,* 41–67. https://doi.org/10.1002/hrdq.20034

Luthans, F., Avolio, B., Walumbwa, F., & Li, W. (2005). The psychological capital of Chinese workers: Exploring the relationship with performance. *Management and Organization Review, 1,* 247–269. https://doi.org/10.1111/j.1740-8784.2005.00011.x

Luthans, F., Avolio, B. J., Avey, J. B., & Norman, S. M. (2007). Positive psychological capital: Measurement and relationship with performance and satisfaction. *Personality and Psychology, 60,* 541–572.

Luthans, F., Norman, S. M., Avolio, B. J., & Avey, J. B. (2008). The mediating role of psychological capital in the supportive organizational climate–employee performance relationship. *Journal of Organizational Behavior, 29,* 219–238. https://doi.org/10.1002/job.507

Luthans, F., & Youssef, C. M. (2004). Human, social, and now positive psychological capital management. *Organizational Dynamics, 33*, 143–160. https://doi.org/10.1016/j.orgdyn.2004.01.003

Luthans, F., & Youssef, C. M. (2007). Emerging positive organizational behavior. *Journal of Management, 33*(3), 321–349. https://doi.org/10.1177/0149206307300814

Luthans, F., Youssef, C. M., & Avolio, B. J. (2007). *Psychological capital.* Oxford University Press.

Luthans, F., Youssef, C. M., & Avolio, B. J. (2015). *Psychological capital and beyond.* Oxford University Press.

Luthans, F., & Youssef-Morgan, C. M. (2017). Psychological capital: An evidence-based positive approach. *Annual Review of Organizational Psychology and Organizational Behavior, 4*, 339–366. https://doi.org/10.1146/annurev-orgpsych-032516-113324

Monteau, M. (2017). Eliminating intimidating and disruptive behavior. *The American Journal of Nursing, 117*(4), 13. https://doi.org/10.1097/01.NAJ.0000515212.62097.57

Rehder, K. J., Adair, K. C., Hadley, A., et al. (2020). Associations between a new disruptive behaviors scale and teamwork, patient safety, work-life balance, burnout, and depression. *Joint Commission Journal of Quality and Safety, 46*(1), 18–26. https://doi.org/10.1016/j.jcjq.2019.09.004

Schwartz, S. H. (1994). Are there universal aspects in the structure and contents of human values? *Journal of Social Issues, 50*, 19–45. https://doi.org/10.1111/j.1540-4560.1994.tb01196.x

Schwartz, S. H. (2006). Basic human values: An overview. http://segr-did2.fmag.unict.it/Allegati/convegno%207-8-10-05/Schwartzpaper.pdf

Schwartz, S. H. (2011). Studying values: Personal adventure, future directions. *Journal of Cross-Cultural Psychology, 42*(2), 307–319. https://doi.org/10.1177/0022022110396925

Schwartz, S. H. (2012). An overview of the Schwartz theory of basic values. *Online Readings in Psychology and Culture, 2*(1). https://doi.org/10.9707/2307-0919.1116

Schwartz, S. H., & Bardi, A. (1997). Influences of adaptation to communist rule on value priorities in Eastern Europe. *Political Psychology, 18*, 385–410. https://doi.org/10.1111/0162-895X.00062

Seligman, M. E. P., Steen, T. A., Park, N., & Peterson, C. (2005). Positive psychology progress: Empirical validation of interventions. *American Psychologist, 60*, 410–421.

Snyder, C. R. (2000). *Handbook of hope: Theory, measures, and applications.* Academic Press.

Sofhauser, C. (2016). Intention in nursing practice. *Nursing Science Quarterly, 29*(1), 31–34.

Wei, H., Corbett, R. W., Ray, J., & Wei, T. L. (2020). A culture of caring: The essence of healthcare interprofessional collaboration. *Journal of Interprofessional Care, 34*(3), 324–331. https://doi.org/10.1080/13561820.2019.1641476

CHAPTER 7

Feeling "Cared For"

"They may forget your name but they will never forget how you made them feel."

—Maya Angelou

CHAPTER OBJECTIVES:

1. Describe the consequences of "feeling cared for."
2. Evaluate how nurses actualize "feeling cared for."
3. Distinguish among the measurement, improvement, and research associated with "feeling cared for."

THE POSITIVE EMOTION OF "FEELING CARED FOR"

Feeling "cared for" is a positive emotion that develops over time through connected and caring relationships. In Heidegger (1962), the philosopher described "feeling cared for" as a universal phenomenon involving meaningful closeness with others. In a later phenomenological nursing study, Bunkers (2004) found the meaning of "feeling cared for" among 10 poor women to be "contentment with intimate affiliations arising with salutary endeavors while honoring uniqueness amid adversity" (p. 63). An important finding in Bunker's research was that "feeling cared for" emerged as a separate phenomenon from the caring process itself. It included acknowledgment of the unique individual who has the freedom to choose connection as well as separation. This is consistent with the Quality-Caring Model© (QCM), which views "feeling cared for" as a consequence of (separate from) the caring process.

BOX 7.1: Repeated connections between patients and health professionals that are of a caring nature foster this optimistic human emotion of "feeling cared for." For example, nurses, through their intimate repetitive interactions with patients and families, create connections that value and affirm the other. This transformative process facilitates "feeling cared for," energizing patients and families to relax, disclose, participate, learn, and activate healthy responses.

"Feeling cared for" is a reflection of the significance or value of a person that is essential to well-being (Flett, 2018). It enables one to feel noticed, important, and needed – ultimately, that they matter. Most human beings desire this positive emotion as it protects against stress and suffering, invigorates, promotes resilience, and increases caring for others. During illness, patients and families often experience some degree of suffering–this very personal experience was witnessed during the COVID-19 pandemic when patients were often physically separated from family members during hospitalization. However, physical, emotional, and even spiritual suffering occurs frequently during illness, prompting nurses to intervene. Helping patients "feeling cared for" by addressing their suffering, making sense of the situation, and supporting their needs for healing enables the motivation, inspiration, and encouragement patients need for self-advancement or progress. Thus, "feeling cared for" not only enables human significance, but it engenders confidence, feeling understood or being known, appreciated, inspired, connected, hopeful, secure, and ultimately a renewed sense of wholeness.

Yet hospitalization often places individuals at risk for non-caring relationships, often resulting in anxiety, isolation, prolonged recovery, and sometimes pain or discomfort unrelated to disease. For example, individuals who are made to feel invisible, without a voice, not taken seriously, or treated impersonally during their healthcare experience often articulate feeling anxious, sometimes fearful, disconnected, and frequently vulnerable or unsafe (Kenward et al., 2017).

In fact, these negative emotions have been tied to increased heart rate and blood pressure, increased cortisol levels, and may alter the immune system (Adler, 2002). In a systematic review of healthcare neglect in three countries, Reader & Gillespie (2013) found feelings of not being cared for in hospitalized patients; and in particular, caring neglect was described as "being rude, not responding to patient complaints of pain, purposefully delaying help for patients, intentionally ignoring patients, avoiding contact with patients, preferring to socialise with colleagues rather than treat patients, and prioritising some patients over other others due to liking them more" (p. 8). Furthermore, there were wide discrepancies in patient perceptions of not feeling cared for compared to nurses' perceptions, which resulted in physical and emotional harm. Such harms are incongruent with the current definition of nursing as a caring discipline (American Nurses Association [ANA], 2021) and are counter to current ethical and quality standards!

Consider the following case:

Anna was postop a lobectomy for adenocarcinoma of the left lung. She completed her 6-month CT scan and was hoping for a negative result. Instead, the result she obtained via the electronic health record showed two additional nodules in the left middle lobe. Having witnessed her father's death from lung cancer and knowing her own history, she was fearful and called her surgeon to discuss the results. Although the office staff indicated he would call her, he did not return her call for two days. On the third day in the early evening, the surgeon called and asked Anna, "What is the problem?" When Anna explained that she would like more information about her CT scan results, the surgeon replied, "Yes, there are two nodules. Many people have lung nodules. If there was anything to be worried about, I would have notified you. If all my patients called me about every little thing, I would never be able to get my work done, including your surgery." Anna was left feeling worthless, exasperated, a burden, and belittled. She resolved not to see this surgeon again.

How does this conversation alleviate Anna's anxiety or the ethical responsibility of a health professional to treat this patient as a whole person who was worthy of respect? How did the surgeon's answer "enable" Anna's future discussions with physicians?

Feeling cared for is a positive reaction that has been associated with improved social connectedness and some physiological alterations. In fact, studies have shown that positive emotions were significantly connected to health, and in some cases, actually protected against and slowed the progression of cardiovascular disease (Thong et al., 2017; Kansky & Diener, 2017). Other studies have shown correlations between positive emotions and psychological health and team performance (Waters et al., 2021). In a qualitative study, stroke patients reported on how caring behaviors promoted "feeling cared for" during hospitalization. Phrases such as, "I was not left out of the loop; they checked on me frequently, the feelings of apprehension and/or fear eased up a bit, and I started to sense, 'I am in good hands and should not worry,' and finally, my children asked questions, and they took the time to explain what was going on." These expressions of "feeling cared for" were reflective of the caring behaviors: attentive reassurance, attending to basic human needs, and affiliation needs (Salinas et al., 2020).

BOX 7.2: Feeling "cared for" by health professionals provides patients with the energy or drive to continue treatment or make behavioral changes, interact, learn, and maybe even follow through; in other words, it may be tied to one's ability to engage, progress, or advance. It seems to buffer stress, promote resilience, relieve the burden of expectations, lessen some uncertainty, and increase confidence and comfort. This reaction is a necessary antecedent to future interactions and more terminal outcomes. Thus, it is imperative that nurses appreciate their role in motivating this important intermediate outcome.

Because of the continuous and highly emotional involvement with patients and other health professionals, demanding patient situations, required competencies, fluctuating workflow, and stressful system-related issues, "feeling cared for" from the perspective of the health professional is significant to healthy work environments. Closely allied with the term, mattering, the sense of the difference one makes in the work environment, can be thought of as an indicator of organizational health and employee success (Reece et al., 2021). In fact, when employees feel cared for, the meaning of their work may deepen, and creative work involvement may be enhanced (Stephens & Carmeli, 2017). Yet, allowing oneself to "feel cared for" is often difficult for some health professionals. As experts in caring, nurses know how to care for others but find it strange to receive such regard. At one Quality-Caring© organization, the notion of team caring was formalized in a 45-minute group meeting that regularly convened once a week to process the week's work. A few rules were established, such as only positive or affirming words could be used, everyone was to be heard, and members were to actively listen. This group time allowed members to recognize the collective work of the group, solve emergent problems, celebrate successes, work on affirming projects, receive caring from each other, and share resources to face the challenges of the upcoming week. Unknowingly, the consequences of this group process resulted in collective "feeling cared for," strengthening individual members and allowing them to better see their possibilities. Another interesting result was the gradual re-evaluation of individual members concerning their unique strengths and contribution to the work.

BOX 7.3: There is a reciprocal nature to caring. When one truly cares for others, the carer also benefits (and when caring is withheld, the opposite happens). Thus, "feeling cared for" is enhanced when caring is extended to others. As a health professional charged with the safety of vulnerable individuals, it is the nurse's role to extend caring first.

THE UNIQUE ROLE OF THE NURSE

Feeling cared for is a significant and differentiating nursing-sensitive intermediate outcome that can be observed and measured. Thus, it could be considered a "marker" of quality nursing care. As a result of caring relationship–centered professional encounters, patients develop this positive emotion that connotes "I matter; I am viewed as capable; I am appreciated for who I am; I am safe." The importance that patients attribute to feeling recognized as worthy and capable individuals with the potential for decision making is the essence of "feeling cared for" and influences their future interactions, intermediate health outcomes, and ultimately self-advancement (see Figure 7.1). However, power differences can sometimes thwart this process.

Typically, in healthcare situations, authority gradients (or hierarchies of power) exist that place patients and families in dependent relationships (with respect to clinicians), with well-meaning health professionals assuming the power during healthcare interactions (see Figure 7.2). Authority gradients have been frequently described in healthcare safety situations where various workers, with differences in status, perceive power or authority pressures that result in failure to relay important information or failure to act (Cosby & Croskerry, 2004).

Consider the following case:
A new graduate nurse is working on a busy pulmonary acute care unit. She notices that one of her patients with asthma is more dyspneic and a little tachycardic. The new graduate nurse knows she should communicate this to the physician, but he has a reputation for getting agitated when interrupted. So, she decides to communicate it to the charge nurse, but when approached, the charge nurse, who is very

busy, appears annoyed. Because of her lack of confidence and the perceived lack of caring by those in power, the new graduate decides to wait. Unfortunately, the patient worsens and has a near-respiratory arrest, requiring intubation, mechanical ventilation, and a visit to the ICU.

What could have been done differently in this situation? Who could have attended to this new graduate's need for feeling cared for?

Authority gradients often create unintended barriers that, in high-risk environments, may lead to errors and even sentinel events. Thus, preventing or neutralizing them as soon as recognized is essential. Likewise, when well-meaning

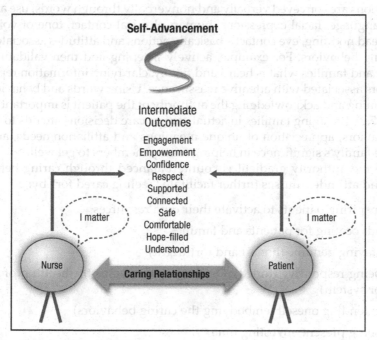

FIGURE 7.1 Consequences of "feeling cared for."

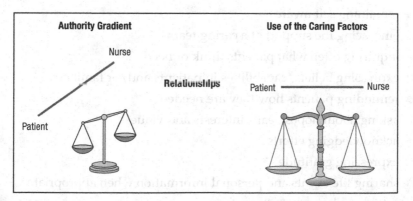

FIGURE 7.2 Nature of relationships between patients and nurses.

health professionals exert authority over or are perceived by patients to be the ones with power, the result may be situations in which patients are afraid to speak up, impeding communication and the transfer of important information (and in some cases, the occurrence of error). This lopsided and somewhat conditional patient–health professional relationship does not honor the shared partnership that should exist between patients and health professionals, but rather, creates an imbalance of power that many times is experienced as degradation, sometimes damaging to present and future interactions.

Nurses who are experts in the caring behaviors, however, routinely use them to convey mutuality and reciprocity in relationships (see Figure 7.1), thereby equalizing authority between patients and health professionals (see Figure 7.2). Such actions are conveyed verbally and nonverbally through words, use and timing of language, facial expressions, human physical contact, tone of voice, distance, head nodding, eye contact – basically actions and attitudes associated with the caring behaviors. For example, actively listening and then validating with patients and families what is heard and finally, clarifying information represents behaviors associated with attentive reassurance. Using words and behaviors that are affirming and acknowledging the authority of the patient is important (Tables 7.1 and 7.2). Engaging families in actual care or care decisions attends to the caring behaviors, appreciation of unique meanings and affiliation needs, and conveys the family's significance in helping family members to get well.

Once the authority gradient is counterbalanced through caring behaviors, skills, and attitudes, nurses further facilitate "feeling cared for" by:

- inspiring patients to activate their own resources
- advocating for patients and families
- staying genuine (honest and forthright)
- being responsive (tuned in to the patient versus the health professional or system)
- extending oneself (embodying the caring behaviors)
- being present; investing time
- displaying technical competence and demonstrating compassion
- remaining self-aware
- embracing the support of a caring team
- inquiring often what patients think or need
- expressing beliefs/capabilities in patients and/or families
- reminding patients how they are needed
- asking about hopes, fears, interests and values
- acknowledging efforts
- expressing gratitude
- sharing life events and personal information when appropriate
- setting and expecting boundaries

TABLE 7.1 Differences in Verbal Messages Based on Authority

Health Professional Is the Authority	Patient Is the Authority
Time to do your dressing.	Hello, Mr. Smith. I am checking up on you as I said I would. Is it okay with you if I change your dressing now?
I have so many patients today, I couldn't get here any sooner.	Hi, Mrs. Mallon. You've been on my mind for the past 30 minutes. Is this a good time to discuss your medication?
Hi honey, you seem to be doing fine today.	Hello, Mrs. Lanoue. It's nice to see you today.
Your meds have not come up yet.	Jane, there has been a delay in the delivery of your medications from the pharmacy. What can I do to make you comfortable while we wait a few more minutes?
I know how you feel but I have been busy with three other patients and another nurse called in sick.	You sound really angry about this.
That won't work on this unit.	Mr. Horn, I like your idea!
I know how to do this!	How do you do it, Mrs. Kelly?
Calm down, they will take you as soon as they can. They are busy down there.	Mr. Gannon, your test was scheduled for 10 a.m. but they just notified me that it will be delayed. They said they could take you about 1 p.m. I will make sure you get a lunch tray as soon as you get back.

TABLE 7.2 Nonverbal Messages That Convey Caring

Maintain eye contact
Smile
Sit comfortably and not too far away
Face the patient, always
Pay attention while someone is dialoguing with you, don't do any other activity
Do not allow interruptions, such as phone calls, unless it is an emergency
Excuse and explain yourself *if* it is an emergency and you have to leave
Be enthusiastic and energetic
Allow patients to talk without interruption
Listen for cues to underlying feelings
Dress professionally
Use soft, gentle touch
Use relaxed body posture, even leaning in
Acknowledge patients' words, nod head, say "yes"

Professional nurses manifest caring and the resultant positive emotion of "feeling cared for" as they assist healthcare consumers and other health professionals in preventing or healing health problems. Giving and receiving another's attention, respect, support, and protection while assisting in human and affiliation needs builds relationships versus tearing them down. Listening to one's personal and professional wisdom and learning how to grow despite negative emotions and events enables others to accept and *"feel* cared for." In doing so, nurses benefit as well, feeling as if they matter; are more secure in their role; more caring to self, coworkers, and families; calmer and more centered; connected to the values inherent in professional nursing; and part of a larger whole (see Figure 7.1).

MEASURING "FEELING CARED FOR"

Evaluation and demonstration of the influence of caring processes (or caring behaviors) on specific health outcomes reveals the value of caring relationships not only to the nursing profession, but also to the patients, their families, health systems, and policy makers. Both qualitative and quantitative approaches can assist in assessing "feeling cared for." For example, patient interviews and focus groups are often used to gather data from patients. Using such techniques, interview guides that ask specific questions about feeling cared for could provide useful data for decision making or to improve practice. Quantitative data are useful to assess and improve practice as well as to provide evidence for decision making. They are also used in research to generate connections among variables, test caring interventions, and validate and refine theory. Because the phenomenon of "feeling cared for" has been conceptualized and defined, it *is* measurable, albeit with recommendations.

Measurement, a fundamental aspect of quantitative analysis, is generally understood as a process by which attributes or dimensions of a phenomenon are assigned a value (to eliminate guessing or uncertainty). "Feeling cared for" can be measured in terms of its degree, its observed current state, improvements over time, what it is associated with, how it compares among groups, and patients' opinions of it. Using a systematic method of collecting data (to ensure accurate and consistent application) and employing focused instruments is implicit in measurement. Measuring phenomena is commonly associated with some error – either in the instrument itself, how the data were collected, or in the characteristics of the sample. Reducing this error is a major goal of high-quality instruments. Understanding how an instrument was developed is important because it has implications for its accuracy, application in practice, and interpretation of results.

BOX 7.4: Although many have attempted to measure caring (Sitzman & Watson, 2019), the human emotion of "feeling cared for" as a consequence of caring actions assumes that the patient is the authority for care received and the resultant unit of analysis. Although many tools are available to measure caring, there are fewer that measure this phenomenon *from the patient's point of view*, explicitly reveal the conceptual definition of caring that guided item development, are valid and reliable, are low in burden, and were tested in diverse populations with large sample sizes.

Thus, there is much confusion about what and how to measure "feeling cared for." For further information on measurement and methods of assessment, see Gray & Grove (2022). This text provides a good overview of quantifying variables, including reducing measurement error and ensuring accurate, reliable, and sensitive assessment. In the context of this brief background regarding measurement and assessment of "feeling cared for," the importance of choosing appropriate instruments with the most credibility is stressed.

First, recognizing the definition or conceptual framework from which the items in an instrument were generated is paramount. The emotion of "feeling cared for" in a recipient is a consequence of health professionals' caring actions and suggests a preconceived notion of what caring means and an assessment of its outcomes from the patient's point of view. In the QCM, the meaning of caring is derived from the caring behaviors, which were developed from multiple theories (see Chapter 2), and the measurement of "feeling cared for" is recommended to be generated from the patient's point of view. It is likewise important to understand the context in which an instrument was developed to better assess its usefulness in a particular setting. For example, the patient population, setting, age group of respondents, emotional states of respondents, and severity of illness all have a bearing on the results. Therefore, if an instrument was developed in acute care, administering the same instrument in a community setting would not necessarily yield the same results, unless it was later tested in that population.

Next, the clarity of items, including the degree of readability, is important. If an item was meant to measure mutual problem solving, for example (a caring behavior), but the way it was worded connoted trust, the answers would not be valid. In addition, if the items on a caring instrument were worded in language that was difficult to understand, the respondents may not accurately be able to answer it. How an instrument is administered impacts its results – for example, potential biases of the data collector, burden to the patient (e.g., how long it took), consistency of administration, and interrater reliability (multiple data collectors using the same approach) all affect how an instrument performs. Burden to the patient and the evaluation team is also important as they may affect accuracy of responses and availability of results. Obviously, validity (accuracy) and reliability (consistency) of instruments are a major concern, and these properties should be explicitly made known to potential users (see Table 7.3 for a list of criteria from which to judge caring instruments).

In the aforementioned Sitzman & Watson (2019) text, several caring instruments are presented in a matrix format for ease of locating. Some measure the importance of caring behaviors, others measure caring from the patients' point of view; in certain populations, others measure caring from the nurses' point of view, some measure caring in nursing students, and still others measure caring among peers and within families or groups. Furthermore, information on the theoretical basis and psychometric properties was added. Thus, although the measurement of caring is evolving, moving towards construct validity remains a goal (Coates, 2019).

One instrument that has moved in that direction is the Caring Assessment Tool (CAT)© (Duffy et al., 2014). The CAT is a 27-item instrument designed to capture patients' perceptions of feeling cared for by nurses (Duffy et al., 2014). Using a sample of 1,111 adult patients in 12 U.S. hospitals located in four geographically distinct regions of the United States, an exploratory factor analysis

TABLE 7.3 Criteria for Choosing Caring Instruments

Criteria	Questions for Consideration
Conceptual framework	On whose theory or conceptual base were the items developed?
Purpose	What was the original purpose of the instrument?
Context	In what patient population or setting has the instrument been tested and used?
Perspective	From whose viewpoint is the tool seeking information – patients, families, students, or nurses?
Clarity	Are the items understandable? Are the directions easy?
Administration	How is the questionnaire administered - paper and pencil, electronically, over the internet? What is the time required for completion? How is scoring accomplished?
Psychometrics	Is the tool valid and reliable? How was this established? Was it established in a similar population? Are the forms of validity and reliability consistent with your purpose?
Burden	How easy is it for patients to complete?

identifying a single factor, provided an acceptable fit (73% of variance explained; comparative fit index = .989). Furthermore, high internal consistency (coefficient alpha = .97) remained after item reduction to 27. The resultant 27-item instrument is easy to understand and is shorter, reducing patient and administrative burden, ideal for use in busy health settings. It has been used extensively in studies of patient–nurse interactions as an indicator of "feeling cared for," perceived nurse caring behaviors, and patient-centered care. The CAT has been tested electronically (Duffy et al., 2012) and is available in English, Spanish, and Japanese (see example items in Figure 7.3). It offers a means of measuring "feeling cared for" by nurses from the patient's point of view, is theoretically derived, has been evaluated in multiple studies, and is accurate, reliable, easy to administer, and low in burden, allowing for regular assessment in the real-world environment.

An adaptation of the CAT developed to measure nurses' "feelings of being cared for" by their managers has also been evaluated. The CAT–administrative version supports the idea that nurse managers have an important role in fostering an environment where caring relationships between patients and nurses can flourish (Cara et al., 2011). This is especially significant in post-pandemic healthcare systems where caring work environments are growing in importance. Based on the QCM, Wolverton et al. (2018) used a cross-sectional design with a convenience sample of 703 clinical nurses from five hospitals in the Midwestern, Mid-Atlantic, and Southern Regions of the United States to evaluate the CAT-Administration version (CAT-adm)©. Findings revealed a one-factor solution, similar to that observed with the CAT (see above). After item reduction, the 25-item CAT-adm questionnaire with a Cronbach's alpha of .98 was developed. As caring patient–nurse relationships flourish in environments where leaders create and sustain caring cultures, the measurement and continual improvement of nurse manager caring behaviors is essential to advancing excellence. In fact, this revised instrument was used in a correlational design to examine the relationship between staff nurses' perceptions of nurse manager caring behaviors

Since I have been a patient here, the nurses					
Are responsive to my family	NEVER 1	RARELY 2	OCCASIONALLY 3	FREQUENTLY 4	ALWAYS 5
Pay attention to me when I am talking	NEVER 1	RARELY 2	OCCASIONALLY 3	FREQUENTLY 4	ALWAYS 5
Support me with my beliefs	NEVER 1	RARELY 2	OCCASIONALLY 3	FREQUENTLY 4	ALWAYS 5
Respect me	NEVER 1	RARELY 2	OCCASIONALLY 3	FREQUENTLY 4	ALWAYS 5
Help me feel less worried	NEVER 1	RARELY 2	OCCASIONALLY 3	FREQUENTLY 4	ALWAYS 5

FIGURE 7.3 Sample items on the Caring Assessment Tool (CAT).

and acute-care patient experience scores (Kostich et al., 2021). Although limited by sample size (67 participants from 17 departments in one large academic medical center in the Midwest), findings indicated a moderately positive relationship between the staff nurses' perceptions of the nurse manager's caring behaviors and the patients' overall hospital rating of patient experience ($r = .497; p < .043$). This correlation represents nurse managers' caring presence, attentiveness, and availability to the clinical nurses in this sample. Furthermore, nurses' feelings of "being cared for" by nurse managers was greater when managers were somewhat more visible ($r = .375; p < .002$). Thus, the CAT-adm provides hospital administrators, nurse managers, and researchers with a measure suitable for practice improvement using a psychometrically sound and less burdensome instrument to collect data. Some examples of its use for ongoing quality assessment are listed below:

- Periodic internal evaluation to assess nurse manager caring behaviors with findings used to structure ongoing leadership development.
- Evaluation of improvement in nurse manager caring behaviors based on pre–post assessment of educational interventions targeted to department-level leaders.
- As a performance indicator used during nurse leader evaluations.
- As a supplement in the evaluation of healthy work environments.

As an increasing number of institutions realize the energizing value of caring cultures, the CAT-adm will be further employed. It is important to note that both the CAT and the CAT-adm studies used multisite samples and showed a one-factor solution. Obviously, further studies are needed to confirm these findings in the ongoing effort to achieve construct validation.

To conclude, a growing knowledge base regarding the measurement of caring is emerging; however, there continue to be issues related to adequacy of sample sizes and designs, the conceptual base of available instruments, adequate psychometrics, and the perspective of the evaluator. With regard to the latter factor, the recipient of caring (usually the patient) is the most direct source of "feeling cared for" in clinical situations. This perspective is always the most advantageous because the perceptions of caring of patients and nurses have been known to differ (Thomas et al., 2019). Similarly, when measuring caring among nursing students, families or caregivers, or nurses themselves, it is important to collect the data directly from those being "cared for."

IMPROVING "FEELING CARED FOR"

While *measuring* "feeling cared for" refers to quantifying the concept, *improving* "feeling cared for" refers to using evidence to make judgments about the phenomenon and then revising practice accordingly. Evidence about the quality of "feeling cared for" can be derived internally and externally. In fact, patient–RN relationships are often not assessed at all or are conducted by proxy through questionnaires conducted after hospitalization. However, regularly evaluating and using evidence to improve "feeling cared for" is the first step in its improvement. Internally, health professionals' reflections on practice, narratives from patients and families, qualitative and quantitative techniques with regular use of valid and reliable questionnaires generate data from which to make revisions in practice. Externally, multisite data (such as those generated through regional and national collaboratives) can establish benchmarks from which to improve practice. Research using larger samples and robust designs provide evidence needed for actionable practice changes.

Internal to health systems, health professionals engage patients and families in caring relationships, but patients themselves (the recipients) are generally the best authority for evaluating the relationship. Thus, efforts to measure and improve "feeling cared for" should include their voice. Generally, improvement requires a process designed to help reach conclusions about clinicians' practice or health systems' attainment of certain objectives or behaviors. Measurement is inherent in performance or practice improvement because it often provides the basis for performance reviews, continuation or revisions of programs, and improvements in services. Data are collected, both ongoing (formative) or at the conclusion (summative) of an initiative and are used to make informed decisions.

Because "feeling cared for" is theorized to result from caring professional practice, the caring behaviors provide practical guidance on "how to care" (see Chapter 3 for some examples). In the context of a caring relationship, the health professional uses instrumental and relational values, knowledge, and skills to meet specific health outcomes. The knowledge, skills, and behaviors tied to caring relationships vary among health professionals, patients, and settings and fluctuate further by system characteristics. Thus, to ensure that patients and families as well as health professionals themselves "feel cared for," an ongoing process of evaluation, analysis of data, reflection on data, and practice revisions are needed. Unfortunately, well-designed relational improvement programs are often overlooked or not conducted because of the perceived complexity of the process, including the collection of data while simultaneously caring for patients. Healthcare professionals, in particular, seem to rely on patients' comments or their own passion and feelings to conclude that their practice is meeting patient needs. However, without proper evaluation and improvement, the value or usefulness of caring relationships cannot be known.

An evaluation model provides a framework to guide this process. In the context of caring professional practice, the QCM provides an overarching framework from which to guide quality improvement efforts. Using this model, structural components of professional practice include characteristics of the participants and the system. In this case, patients, providers, or organizational demographic data provide important information that may impact the processes or outcomes of practice and should be captured. For example, patients who are severely ill or have multiple comorbidities may influence how professional nurses use the caring behaviors and what outcomes can be realistically attained. Moreover, nurses with certain credentials (i.e., education, certifications) may provide care that varies from their peers, which could impact the results. Organizations that use specific staffing models or that provide more educational opportunities for professional nurses may inadvertently impact the processes and outcomes of care. Taking these factors into consideration during improvement processes allows one to modify the resulting data, lending credibility to the outcomes.

Evaluating the process of caring (use of the caring behaviors) by assessing "feeling cared for" provides evidence related to *how* professional practice is working. This assessment is useful when staff and patient opinions about care vary, to engage in evidence-based discussions about recommendations for improvement, or to make adjustments or decisions about continuation of certain practices. In the acute care environment, it is especially important to capture these perceptions as close to real time as possible to be able to knowledgably change practice to benefit individual patients and families. Regularly assessing caring processes allows clinicians and administrators to monitor improvements in nursing practice, to link caring processes with nursing-sensitive outcome measures, to study ways that structural indicators such as staffing patterns or nurse credentials affect caring processes, and to examine trends over time.

RESEARCHING "FEELING CARED FOR"

To extend the understanding and strengthen the evidence of caring relationships as a significant variable in the healthcare process, much more research must be conducted and disseminated. Continuing to build on the rich foundation of caring science using multiple methods will enrich the knowledge base. Refining existing measures of "feeling cared for" with a particular emphasis on construct validity using the patient's view will allow for more multisite comparisons. Qualitative studies permitting in-depth assessment of "feeling cared for" and its immediate consequences, cultural influences and "feeling cared for," the complexities of caring relationships, how caring capacity develops, and requirements for caring relationships are necessary. Using approaches such as observation, interviews, focus groups, narratives, and other interpretive methods will enrich the science.

Quantitative methods linking "feeling cared for" to specific patient, nurse, and system outcomes will strengthen the evidence regarding the value of caring in clinical practice. Similarly, linking "feeling cared for" to student learning outcomes and administrative caring to healthy work environments for professional nurses will provide the basis for innovation in these settings. Most importantly, developing caring-based interventions for testing in quantitative studies is necessary to provide high levels of evidence for caring-based nursing practice and to validate caring theory.

Caring-based interventions designed to elicit "feeling cared for" in recipients are complicated to design, and the practical implications of funding for such evaluations can be challenging. Nevertheless, caring-based interventions must be tested to better understand how they contribute to overall healthcare outcomes. Choosing a caring-based conceptual framework to support the intervention followed by an application based on prior research and organized to meet the needs of the population under study is paramount. Developing a protocol describing the content, strength, and frequency of the intervention allows for replication. Using probability sampling and longitudinal studies, questions such as, "What is the effect of the intervention on specific outcomes of care?" can be answered. Integrating cost-effectiveness components will add to the understanding of the intervention's worth.

Nationally, the Patient-Centered Outcomes Research Institute (PCORI) (2021), authorized by Congress in 2010, focuses on researching health outcomes of importance to patients. In 2021, the PCORI leadership released the proposed national priorities for health which will be used to establish their research agenda. The priorities and resultant goals include:

1. Increase evidence for existing interventions and emerging innovations in health

   Goal: Strengthen and expand ongoing comparative clinical effectiveness research focused on both existing interventions and emerging innovations to improve healthcare practice, health outcomes, and health equity.

2. Enhance infrastructure to accelerate patient-centered outcomes research

   Goal: Enhance the infrastructure that facilitates patient-centered outcomes research to drive lasting improvements in health and transformation of both the research enterprise and care delivery.

3. Advance the science of dissemination, implementation, and health communication

   Goal: Advance the scientific evidence for and the practice of dissemination, implementation, and health communication to accelerate the effective sharing of comparative clinical effectiveness research results for public understanding and uptake into practice.

4. Achieve health equity

   Goal: Expand stakeholder engagement, research, and dissemination approaches that lead to continued progress toward achieving health equity in the United States.

5. Accelerate progress toward an integrated learning health system

   Goal: Foster actionable, timely, place-based, and transformative improvements in patient-centered experiences, care provision, and ultimately improved health outcomes through collaborative, multisectoral research to support a health system that understands and serves the needs and preferences of individuals.

(PCORI, 2021)

Since 2012, PCORI has funded more than $1.4 billion in research projects, many of which pertain to the patient's inclusion and decision making regarding their care. "Feeling cared for" as a positive consequence of caring professional relationships may fit into one of these new priorities and provide an approach for ongoing studies.

Similarly, the National Institute of Nursing Research (NINR) uses a research lens approach to frame the perspective through which to examine a health challenge. Several are suggested, each of which offers a valuable perspective by which to investigate health-related questions. The NINR Strategic Plan will prioritize research framed through the following five lenses:

- health equity
- social determinants of health
- population and community health
- prevention and health promotion—with a particular emphasis on eliminating health disparities.
- systems and models of care

(National Institute of Nursing Research, 2021)

Caring-based interventions could be designed and framed through these lenses. For example, in school-age children, promoting wellness might be improved through targeted interventions provided in the context of caring relationships with school nurses or counselors, or increasing regular exercise through a caring-based walking group among elderly women living in assisted-living facilities might be evaluated. Studies using social determinants of health to individually reduce symptoms of chronic disease may be examined. Non-pharmacologic interventions, such as increasing access to information on lifestyle modification for those with chronic disease and provided in the context of caring relationships with healthcare professionals are examples of how caring-based interventions might be evaluated using the framing approach identified by NINR. Furthermore, identifying barriers to health equity, correlating "feeling cared for" with reduction of specific symptoms, testing patient-defined models of care, or using qualitative methods to elicit lived experiences or culturally congruent ideas related to prevention and health promotion will meet this mandate.

Likewise, adopting healthy behaviors to improve nurses' well-being in the workforce are gaining acceptance. Caring-based interventions that seek to increase self-caring or studies that identify factors associated with self-caring practices are warranted. How self-caring impacts the quality of work life or well-being, especially over the long term, is increasingly important. Supporting caregivers, especially those caring for patients with chronic disease, with long-term caring-based interventions and demonstration projects that honor the importance of caregivers for the health of loved ones are issues of deep concern for nursing. Research questions such as, "Do caring relationships with health professionals improve self-caring and quality of work life?" or "How well does a caregiver–care recipient caring relationship sustain itself over time?" need answers.

Studying caring end-of-life interventions based on patient preferences would provide evidence of nursing's value in this vulnerable population. In addition, understanding how enhancing communication among health professionals (collective relational capacity) might improve decision making or decrease physical and psychological burden in patients and their families would greatly enhance our knowledge base. Creative technological innovations that incorporate "feeling cared for" among patients, caregivers, and the healthcare team may enhance nursing's value by first evaluating the concept; and second, by applying analyses in ways that enhance clinical outcomes. For example, evaluation of "feeling cared for" in real time (using technological solutions) may help investigators develop interventions that enhance nurses' delivery of person-centered care and subsequently improve patient outcomes. Finally, ongoing and accelerating preparation of nursing scientists who are especially passionate about the value of "feeling cared for" as it relates to these priority areas is important.

Faculty members can also impact the understanding of caring-based pedagogies on student learning. For example, the following questions may advance the knowledge base of nursing education:

- How are caring relationships best learned in simulated teaching environments?
- How is caring competence best evaluated?
- What are the relationships between learning in caring environments and student outcomes?
- What are the best strategies for learning and practicing interprofessionalism?
- How are nurse caring relationships extended during learning transitions?
- What is the best preparation for nurse faculty for teaching caring relational professional practice?

Vital to the discussion of educational research is the preparation of the next generation of scientists. Without role models conducting research in health professions schools, graduate students will not get the chance to participate in advancing the notion of "feeling cared for" and its link to important clinical, learning, or system outcomes. Researchers involved in such research must involve students at all levels, explain their methods and results during class discussions, invite participation in specific projects, demonstrate the consistency between conceptual frameworks and specific research variables, and model the process of conducting research. Examples of this include undergraduate student honors programs, research practicums, joint publications, and faculty–service partnerships in which research is a component.

At the systems level, it is important to know how best to adopt and improve relationship-centered professional encounters such that "feeling cared for" in recipients can be tied to important and reimbursable outcomes (e.g., patient experience, 30-day readmission rates, adverse outcomes). Some examples include:

- Examining the benefits of carefully evaluating clinician–patient relationships in real time and using results to make actionable practice changes.
- Evaluating the impact of caring cultures on health professionals' work satisfaction, resilience, grit, retention and turnover.
- Identifying ways to improve relationship-centered interprofessional teams.
- Understanding how the use of information technology might assist patients and families to provide feedback about their care.
- Identifying ways to re-prioritize relationships in clinical workflow.
- Comparing departments in an organization in terms of how leadership impacts caring relationships.
- Evaluating the benefits of academic–service partnerships for improving "feeling cared for" among recipients.
- Determining the relationships between nurse caring and reimbursable patient outcomes.
- Examining the influence of nurse caring on patient activation.

Finally, using strategies such as interprofessional research teams (team science); applying methods in which data are pooled from multiple sites; and integrating biological, behavioral, and cost-effectiveness strategies will eventually enable us to better understand how health professionals with certain characteristics perform the caring processes, the proper "dose" required for "feeling cared for" in particular patient populations, the most effective ways to learn caring, and the relative worth of caring practices. Dissemination of findings through publications and presentations and their use in the revision of policy will help translate credible results to the bedside and hopefully transform the work environment such that health professionals find added meaning in the work they do. Understanding how "feeling cared for" improves health outcomes and contributes to evolving theory will provide the rationale for new patient-care delivery systems that align caring relationships with valuable assets.

SUMMARY

"Feeling cared for" is a positive emotion that occurs as a distinct consequence of caring relationships and is theorized to influence important intermediate and terminal health outcomes. The importance of "feeling cared for" to health outcomes is reviewed as are the benefits to health professionals themselves. The unique role of the nurse in facilitating "feeling cared for" is reviewed in terms of specific attitudes and behaviors. Measuring "feeling cared for" using well-designed and effectively applied instruments is crucial to evaluating and improving caring practice. The criteria for judging instruments are presented along with a discussion of those important characteristics. The CAT and CAT-adm are presented, and examples are provided of their use in clinical settings with emphasis on the recipient's voice. Research on "feeling cared for" is considered, and emphasis is placed on advancing the science through multiple methods and approaches. National research priorities are reviewed. Building on the existing research and developing caring-based interventions combined with advanced investigational strategies will eventually enable more robust findings and validate evolving theory. Dissemination of results and quickly translating credible findings to practice environments will inspire new possibilities for future learning and practice environments.

CALL TO ACTION

Positive emotions are connected to health. "Feeling cared for" is a positive emotion that positively influences patients' well-being. **Generate** "feeling cared for" in your patients. Evaluating "feeling cared for" and using those results to improve professional practice, linking it to important outcomes, explaining differences among groups and individuals, and accelerating adoption by health systems of relationship-centered professional encounters is the responsibility of health professionals and leaders. **Compare** and then **choose** ways to best measure "feeling cared for" in your setting. Regularly **evaluate** and use the results to improve "feeling cared for." **Brainstorm** potential research questions that could be examined, including how you would **participate**.

REFLECTIVE QUESTIONS/APPLICATIONS

For Professional Nurses in Clinical Practice:

- Discuss your views on whether patients in your organization "feel cared for." Why do you think you have answered this way?
- Is there an expectation that facilitating "feeling cared for" is a necessary component of RN work at your institution? If so, how is it evaluated?
- Reflect on your own individual ability to receive "feeling cared for" by members of the health team. Where do you stand? How could you better accept this positive emotion from others?
- What patient outcomes do you attribute to "feeling cared for?" Why?
- What have you learned about measurement as a result of reading this chapter?
- Appraise one qualitative and one quantitative research study on caring relationships. What are the variables? How are they measured? Are the results credible? Would you adopt the findings in practice? Why or why not?

- How do you participate in research? Take a minute and create a PICO (Population, Intervention, Comparison, and Outcome[s]) question that might advance your understanding of "feeling cared for." What will you do with this question?

For Professional Nurses in Educational Practice:

- What specific curricular activities have you developed to enhance the unique role of the nurse in facilitating "feeling cared for" among patients and families and among the health team? How do you evaluate them?

- Reflect on the need for acceptance of "feeling cared for" among the inter-professional team. How does your educational program facilitate a graduate's capacity to accept positive emotions from their team members?

- What can you do to advance the understanding of measurement among undergraduate and graduate students?

- How would you suggest facilitating team caring during educational programs?

- Provide some suggestions for exposing students to national research priorities and publication/presentation opportunities.

- Identify two or three research priorities from those discussed in this chapter. How can the study of "feeling cared for" contribute to these priorities? Give specific examples.

- Develop a caring-based intervention to facilitate "feeling cared for" among a population of your choice.

- Design a study to examine the impact of a nursing intervention on "feeling cared for" among junior high students with asthma.

For Professional Nurses in Leadership Practice:

- What is the state of "feeling cared for" among patients at your organization? How do you know?

- How do you specifically hold yourself and your staff accountable for "feeling cared for" among patients and families? Should they be?

- Reflect on the performance improvement process in place at your institution. Does it include assessment of "feeling cared for"? Why or why not? What would it take to revise this?

- How do you facilitate research at your organization? What specific research questions are you investigating?

- Does your leadership team understand the importance of "feeling cared for" as it relates to the bottom line? If not, how will you facilitate their development?

- Discuss how you would go about partnering with a health professions school to provide research/quality improvement consultation to your staff, design studies that measure "feeling cared for," and submit proposals to potential funders.

■ Create a plan to dramatically alter the performance improvement process to include the routine evaluation of "feeling cared for" from the patient's point of view. What methodology would be used? How long will it take? What would be the implications for RN practice? How would you ensure that the plan is enacted as developed? How would you evaluate its implementation?

PRACTICE ANALYSIS

Alicia is a 37-year-old female who is admitted to an outpatient surgery center for a breast biopsy. She is observed by a nurse as sitting with her husband in the waiting area rapidly moving her crossed right leg and staring straight ahead. The perioperative nurse approaches her, introduces herself, and brings her into the operating suite in preparation for surgery. The nurse sits down with Alicia, asks her how she would like to be addressed, and begins explaining the procedure. The nurse then stops talking and allows Alicia and her husband to ask questions. Alicia begins by responding that she is scared and asks if her husband can accompany her. The nurse reassures Alicia and affirms that her husband can accompany her to the pre-op area. She then explains how she had the same procedure and relates to Alicia how it went. She stays with Alicia through the procedure and when she is in the recovery area, talks to her husband about Alicia's progress. When Alicia is ready, she explains the discharge instructions and follow-up care. The couple remains anxious about the impending pathology results. The nurse provides them with her phone number should they have any further questions.

■ Do you think Alicia and her husband felt "cared for?" How can you be sure? Would you have felt this way in this scenario?

■ What does the nurse do specifically to help Alicia feel "cared for?" What does she miss?

■ Did the nurse use any of the caring behaviors in her interactions with this couple? If so, what were they?

REFERENCES

Adler, H. M. (2002). The sociophysiology of caring in the doctor–patient relationships. *Journal of General Internal Medicine, 17*(11), 883–890. https://doi.org/10.1046/j.1525 -1497.2002.10640.x

American Nurses Association. (2021). *Nursing: Scope and standards of practice* (4th ed.). Author.

Bunkers, S. S. (2004). The lived experience of feeling cared for: A human becoming perspective. *Nursing Science Quarterly, 17*(1), 63–71. https://doi.org/10.1177/ 0894318403260472

Cara, C. M., Nyberg, J. J., & Brousseau, S. (2011). Fostering the coexistence of caring philosophy and economics in today's health care system. *Nursing Administration Quarterly, 35*(1), 6–14.

Coates, C. (2019). The evolution of measuring caring: Moving toward construct validity. In K. L. Sitzman, & J. Watson, J (Eds.), *Assessing and measuring caring in nursing and health sciences* (3rd ed.). Springer Publishing Company.

Cosby, K., & Croskerry, P. (2004). Profiles in patient safety: Authority gradients in medical error. *Academy of Emergency Medicine, 12*, 1341–1345. https://doi.org/10.1197/j.aem.2004.07.005

Duffy, J., Brewer, B., & Weaver, M. (2014). Revision and psychometric properties of the caring assessment tool. *Clinical Nursing Research, 23*(1), 80–93. https://doi.org/10.1177/1054773810369827

Duffy, J., Kooken, W., Wolverton, C., & Weaver, M. (2012). Evaluating patient-centered care: Feasibility of electronic data collection in hospitalized older adults. *Journal of Nursing Care Quality, 27*(4), 307–315. https://doi.org/10.1097/NCQ.0b013e31825ba9d4

Flett, G. (2018). The psychology of mattering: Understanding the human need to be significant. Academic Press.

Gray, J. R., & Grove, S. K. (2022). *The practice of nursing research: Appraisal, synthesis, and generation of evidence* (9th ed.). Saunders.

Heidegger, M. (1962). *Being and time*. Harper & Row.

Kansky, J., & Diener, E. (2017). Benefits of well-being: Health, social relationships, work, and resilience. *Journal of Positive School Psychology, 1*(2), 129–169. https://journalppw.com/index.php/JPPW/article/view/20

Kenward, L., Whiffin, C., & Spalek, B. (2017). Feeling unsafe in the healthcare setting: Patients' perspectives. *British Journal of Nursing, 26*(3), 143–149. https://doi.org/10.12968/bjon.2017.26.3.143

Kostich, K., Lasiter, S., Duffy, J., & George, V. (2021). The relationship between staff nurses' perceptions of nurse manager caring behaviors and patient experience. *Journal of Nursing Administration, 51*(9), 468–473. https://doi.org/10.1097/NNA.0000000000001047

National Institute of Nursing Research. (2021). NINR research lenses. https://www.ninr.nih.gov/aboutninr/ninr-mission-and-strategic-plan

Patient-Centered Outcomes Research Institute. (2021). Proposed national priorities for health. https://www.pcori.org/sites/default/files/PCORI-Proposed National-Priorities-for-Health-English-June-2021.pdf

Reader, T. W., & Gillespie, A. (2013). Patient neglect in healthcare institutions: A systematic review and conceptual model. *BMC Health Services Research, 13*, 156. https://doi.org/10.1186/1472-6963-13-156

Reece, A., Yaden, D., Kellerman, G., Robichaux, A., Goldstein, R., Schwartz, B., Seligman, M., & Baumeister, R. (2021). Mattering is an indicator of organizational health and employee success. *The Journal of Positive Psychology, 16*(2), 228–248.

Salinas, M., Salinas, N., Duffy, J. R., & Davidson, J. (2020). Do caring behaviors in the quality caring model promote the human emotion of feeling cared for in hospitalized stroke patients and their families? *Applied Nursing Research, 55*, 151299. https://doi.org/10.1016/j.apnr.2020.151299

Sitzman, K. L., & Watson, J. (2019). *Assessing and measuring caring in nursing and health sciences* (3rd ed.). Springer Publishing Company.

Stephens, J., & Carmeli, A (2017). Relational leadership and creativity: The effects of respectful engagement and caring on meaningfulness and creative work involvement. In S. Hemlin, & M. Mumford, (Eds.), *Handbook of research on leadership and creativity* (pp. 273–296). Edward Elgar Publishing.

Thong, I. S., Tan, G., & Jensen, M. P. (2017). The buffering role of positive affect on the association between pain intensity and pain related outcomes. *Scandinavian Journal of Pain, 14*, 91–97. https://doi.org/10.1016/j.sjpain.2016.09.008

Thomas, D., Newcomb, P., & Fusco, P. (2019). Perception of caring among patients and nurses. *Journal of Patient Experience, 6*(3), 194–200. https://doi.org/10.1177/2374373518795713

Waters, L., Algoe, S. B., Dutton, J., Emmons, R., Fredrickson, B. L., Heaphy, E., Moskowitz, J. T., Neff, K., Niemiec, R., Pury, C., & Steger, M. (2021). Positive psychology in a pandemic: Buffering, bolstering, and building mental health. *Journal of Positive Psychology*, *17*(3), 303–323. https://doi.org/10.1080/17439760.2021.1871945

Wolverton, C. L., Lasiter, S., Duffy, J. R., Weaver, M. T., & McDaniel, A. M. (2018). Psychometric testing of the caring assessment tool: Administration (CAT-Adm©). *SAGE Open Medicine*, *6*, 2050312118760739. https://doi.org/10.1177/2050312118760739

CHAPTER 8

Practice Improvement

"For good ideas and true innovation, you need human interaction, conflict, argument, debate."

—Margaret Heffernan

CHAPTER OBJECTIVES:

1. Compare the terms, practice and competence.
2. Describe the phrase "learning from the work" or leaning in practice.
3. Distinguish between the terms, quality improvement and practice improvement.

THE NATURE OF PROFESSIONAL PRACTICE

Most work roles defined as practices highlight the importance of application, engagement, performance, and sometimes, creative processes. However, it is also recognized that higher levels of practice are associated with repeated performance or rehearsals. Review and more in-depth reflection on practice advances a practice even further. It follows that effective nursing professional practice involves repeated exposure and clinical application of knowledge, skills, and attitudes, all influenced by current available evidence. In health systems, clinical practice is supported by education and leadership practices, all unified by knowledge generated externally (from empirical studies or theory) or internally (from performance improvement or reflection on experiences) (see Figure 8.1). Using internal and external evidence, health professionals continuously learn about and adjust their individual practices, lifting the overall profession's contributions. For example, health professionals take in and use data daily (e.g., patient assessments, performance evaluations, administrative and financial documents) and acquire and apply information through procedures, protocols, and policies. They converse, share documents, and record data and information. However, they often do not take the time to reflect on these data (or information) either alone or in groups, limiting the knowledge available that could be used in a meaningful way to improve practice. Additionally, empirically available evidence is often not activated in a timely fashion, further limiting

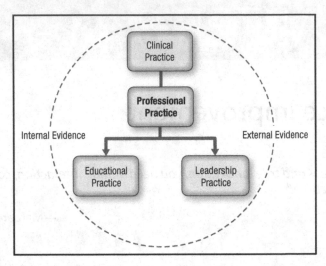

FIGURE 8.1 Professional practice.

practice improvement (Gassas, 2021). However, by examining trends and eval-uating available information, practice revisions can be designed that readily integrate available knowledge into the work and ultimately allow for beneficial adaptations. A preliminary report revealed that employees who participated in such practices found added value, connectedness, and empowerment at work, while positively influencing clinical outcomes (Brennan & Wendt, 2021). Health professionals' connections to patients, families, and each other are powerful opportunities to examine the available evidence, reflect on practice, engage oth-ers, and impact outcomes; however, a certain level of competence is required to adequately engage in ongoing learning about practice.

In the health professions, the term, competence, is used as an expression of expertise (Bathish et al., 2018). Clinical competence is tied to quality patient care, but actually varies by the performer and the context. Benner (2021) defines a competent nurse as one who has a clinical grasp of situations, can predict likely future changes, and resultant patient needs (p. 223). She goes on to define the well-known proficient and expert nurse who performs at increasingly higher levels. Dreyfus & Dreyfus (2008), however, added yet an even higher level of performance, that of mastery, where the expert practitioner performs beyond best practice to include innovative practice when unique situations demand it. Yet, many in the health professions believe that after a certain amount of exposure and repeated performance (or experience), competence is attained, leading to maximal performance (i.e., the traditional apprenticeship approach to health education). In today's world, however, many would argue that clinical performance beyond competence is necessary to meet the accelerated complex demands for expert and innovative practice!

Ericsson et al. (1993) offered a position that maximum performance for individuals in a given domain is not attained automatically with extended experience, but rather is increased as a result of deliberate efforts to improve. In fact, the focus of his framework for expert performance is the result of an extended process of skill acquisition mediated by large, but not excessive, daily amounts of *deliberate* practice. "Deliberate practice is purposeful with the learner engaging in well-defined exercises while receiving guidance, with the end goal of reaching the level of an expert" (Schmidt & Fenner, 2020, p. 396). In this process, receiving feedback on performance is essential to progress with the end goal of mastery (Schmidt & Fenner, 2020). It is important to note that after taking into consideration demographic variables, education, and experience, Bathish et al. (2018) showed that deliberate practice in nursing made the greatest contribution among other variables to competence. No significant relationships were found between years of experience or education and competence. This empirical evidence for the relative impact of deliberate practice on RN competence was consistent with other studies and reinforces the expectation that life-long learning approaches are imperative for nurses to continuously progress toward expert or mastery levels of care. In addition, the Deliberate Practice in Nursing Questionnaire [DPNQ] has been designed to measure deliberate practice in nursing, affording us the opportunity to examine whether nursing professional expertise is at a level that meets the national demands for high-quality healthcare in the increasingly complex healthcare environment of today (Bathish et al., 2016).

At the systems level, the practice of healthcare is complicated, unpredictable, sometimes unfriendly, and often mysterious to patients, families, health professionals, and even top executives. In this complex system (see Chapter 3), new information and knowledge are available each day (some would say each minute). Translating this empirical evidence into clinical practice is a professional obligation that fulfills health professionals' commitment to society, while creating value for health systems; and continuously improving practice is associated with the last concept of the Quality-Caring Model (QCM): Self-advancing health systems. Self-advancing health systems are progressive, dynamic systems that successfully integrate available information into clinical practice through ongoing relational processes, adjusting practice (patterns) as needed at the local level in order to naturally progress or improve. This ongoing relational work is grounded by the caring behaviors, but influenced by the context and the integration of best evidence. Incorporating patients and families as full partners in this ongoing continuous improvement process generates individual and collective practice changes (informed by evidence) allowing for natural self-advancement.

However, tremendous variability in nurses' activation of evidence-based practice (EBP) persists (Melnyk et al., 2018). Moreover, EBP competency scores were not reported to be significantly different between nurses in Magnet® and non-Magnet designated organizations! As a result, the varying EBP competency levels among nurses and systems may lead to poorer health outcomes, increased costs, and disparities in care. This situation may be compromised even further by the pandemic-related nursing shortage, loss of limited clinical sites for nursing students, and lack of resources for EBP in hospitals.

Over the last 20 years, the health system has focused on designing elaborate performance improvement (PI) and decision-support departments; employed numerous consultants; bought sophisticated software programs; engaged in benchmarking; sent employees to expensive training programs; and constructed policies, reports, and data collection mechanisms to foster internal practice improvement. Each of these mechanisms, although inherently beneficial, has been implemented peripherally to clinical practice, as separate or discrete activities whose goal is to improve the system's performance overall. Furthermore, patients and families are frequently not included in healthcare evaluations of the care received, limiting this important contribution to practice improvement. In some organizations, tensions exist between organizational PI departments and those who provide care. This is a critical challenge for busy health professionals who are doing their best to provide safe, quality patient care. To meet national healthcare goals, including the use of best available evidence, it is crucial that we find ways to empower health professionals and patients to rapidly improve the care they offer and receive.

Since expert clinical practice evolves over time and is influenced by supportive practices and the working environment, considerations for ongoing learning are mounting. For example, interactions among employees; imitating efficient clinicians; reflecting together during rounds; sharing tools, care plans, flowcharts and articles; and ongoing translation of evidence must be considered as opportunities for improving practice. Involving and coaching clinical nurses in these activities while providing feedback on knowledge and skills may also advance improvements.

Consider the following:

A caregiver's mental health and well-being are intimately linked with a stroke survivor's health outcomes and quality of life (Sutter-Leve et al., 2021). Unfortunately, nurses in one health system conducted a literature review on the topic and found a systematic review revealing that caregiver support interventions were limited and inconsistent. Left unaddressed, they believed that the burden might have negative consequences for the caregiver and the individuals they care for.

At this Comprehensive Stroke Center, the nurses understood the importance of supportive caregivers. A geographical survey of comparable local health organizations revealed gaps in practice in the organization's current state compared to evidence-based recommendations and community standards of care regarding stroke caregiver support during their transition between hospital and discharge. Given this background, they conducted a practice improvement project addressing caregiver support during transitions of care for stroke survivors and their caregivers after hospital discharge. The population, intervention, control, and outcomes (PICO) question used was: Among stroke survivors and family caregivers discharging from a comprehensive stroke center, will a caregiver preparedness assessment in conjunction with a stroke survivor and caregiver support program, compared to usual care, influence discharge readiness and address gaps in caregiver readiness?

Using recommendations from the literature and clinical practice guidelines published by the American Heart Association and American Stroke Association (Winstein et al., 2016), participants (English and Spanish speaking stroke survivors and their family caregivers) who were admitted to the neuro ICU or PCU were included. A baseline assessment of family caregiver readiness was conducted, then individualized interventions based on their responses were initiated, and a subsequent assessment was conducted upon discharge. In addition to these individualized interventions, an updated family caregiver support pamphlet was distributed to all family caregivers of stroke survivors.

The recruitment process was affected by the recent COVID-19 surge as hospital visitation policies were tightened up and patient census shifted to accommodate the increase in COVID-19 cases in the health system. As a result, some patients who met the criteria for the project did not have any family caregivers at the bedside to engage with, while others were present on an inconsistent basis. Despite this, a 78% participation rate was noted. Using the Preparedness for Caregiving Scale (Abu et al., 2020; Hagedoorn et al., 2020), pre and post assessments were completed. Two months into this pilot project, preliminary statistical analysis illustrated an improvement in family caregiver readiness (p = .0189). Based on this information, it is evident that the proposed intervention has established some benefit for family caregiver support. Providing a tailored approach for person-centered care of stroke survivors and their families by identifying their unmet needs allowed for RN time and resources to be focused on areas of most importance to the family caregiver and the patient.

—Abby Edilloran, BSN, RN, SCRN

This kind of problem in clinical care was noticed, investigated, and followed up in a purposive manner with attention to current evidence. How was it that this group of nurses in the midst of a pandemic were motivated enough to see this project through? They were concerned about a potential gap in good practice, came up with a method to evaluate a possible solution (one that is innovative and included the patient/family in the process), designed a practice improvement project that could be evaluated, and helped others in their geographic area as well. Their relational processes of sharing knowledge, person-centered care using several of the caring behaviors, and attention to "what's best for the patient" resulted in collective learning.

BOX 8.1: In health systems, caring relationships among health professionals (relational capacity), together with continuous active engagement in learning, directly influences health professionals' expertise and the quality and rate of self-advancing systems. Using this knowledge is necessary for individual and system self-advancement.

LEARNING IN PRACTICE (OR LEARNING FROM THE WORK)

Learning typically refers to acquiring new knowledge or skills and sometimes developing new world views (values and beliefs). New knowledge is expected to generate new behaviors in an individual; at the group level, it is expected to improve communication and interactions; and at the organizational level, it is associated with changes in vision, structure, policies, and new products or services/programs. However, learning is usually characterized as an isolated event—such as taking a course, obtaining a certification, or completing a continuing education program. As such, it often occurs *before* one does the work and is fragmented from it, sometimes not connected at all. Such learning, although important, does not honor the important relationship between the new knowledge gained and its translation into clinical practice. However, the term *continuous learning* is anticipated to generate a deeper and more purposeful learning that is aimed at ongoing development, change, or improvement (most notably at the department or organizational level). Continuous learning (i.e., lifelong learning) is a learning outcome of most health professional programs. Thus, individual health professionals who engage in continuous learning and who work in organizations that facilitate *learning from the work*, a method desperately needed at this time in history, are better equipped to rapidly translate new knowledge into clinical practice.

Learning in the workplace or real-world learning emphasizes continual learning by doing the work *after* graduation from a professional program. This type of contextual learning attempts to bridge the education—practice gap in a sociocultural clinical setting. It uses informal discussions (such as during rounds), reflection on experiences, internal clinical performance data, and external empirical evidence to determine gaps and connections to best practices. Such an approach involves interaction among various professionals within the work environment, feedback received through exchanging and sharing of information, and resultant changes in knowledge or the generation of ideas designed to improve processes or outcomes of care. It is a relational form of learning that gradually emerges from collective dialogue and work-related activities. As such, it is often unique and unpredictable; however, it enables employees and organizations to adapt their strategies and action plans in the course of doing work, to achieve increased knowledge, better performance, and even certain organizational goals. Such an environment is characterized by curious employees who feel safe enough to "wonder out loud" and who use problems, disruptions, and confusion at work in a positive way to fashion new strategies or approaches to practice. Leaders in such systems foster learning as a priority and encourage dialogue and the testing of new ideas. Learning from the work in this manner transforms the nature of the work environment from passive performance of routine tasks to a dynamic actionable practice that is perfected in context and over time. Learning and improving practice in this manner often occurs without even realizing it. Infusing learning into the everyday workflow is pragmatic and adds meaning, creates connections, and ultimately, facilitates the design of contemporary and novel approaches to practice. Taking this approach requires high-quality relationships and team member interactivity as key interventions to enable health professionals to make the best use of opportunities to improve practice (Parboosingh et al., 2011). For example, rounding together or discussing case examples aligns current practice with professional standards and new information, which can trigger group learning and resulting behavioral changes. Working on a project generated from a pattern first noticed during bedside handoffs is pertinent to the local situation and engenders practice changes that have meaning. Learning in the workplace frames continuous learning from a bottom up versus a top down approach and in so doing facilitates advancement.

On a larger scale, such activity mushrooms from a single department to the entire organization. The term *organizational learning* was originally coined by Senge (1990) in the *Fifth Discipline* and later became focused as a professional discipline through the Organizational Learning Center (OLC) at Massachusetts Institute of Technology. Later, the organization formed the Society for Organizational Learning (SOL). More recently, the continued gap between data and action provided the impetus for the term, learning health systems who "continuously, routinely, and efficiently study and improve themselves (Friedman et al., 2016, p. 1).

LEARNING HEALTH SYSTEMS

The U.S. Agency for Healthcare Research and Quality (AHRQ) defines a learning health system (LHS) as a health system in which internal data and experience are systematically integrated with external evidence and that knowledge is put into practice. As a result, patients get higher quality, safer, more efficient care, and healthcare delivery organizations become better places to work (AHRQ, 2019).

Focusing more on the here and now is a fundamental change in a system that has been emphasizing, collecting, and disseminating outcomes data after the fact for nearly two decades. The adoption of a *learning* health system that incorporates health professionals' lifelong learning, real-time information, including patient perspectives and measures of patient-centeredness, external evidence, performance transparency, and leaders who build supportive infrastructures for learning are recommendations from the report "Best Care at Lower Costs: The Path to Continuously Learning Health Care in America" (Institute of Medicine [IOM], 2012). Today, LHSs are urgently needed, particularly systems that promote collaboration among other health systems, community-based organizations, and government agencies to enable evidenced-based responses to health emergencies (Romanelli et al., 2021). Combining data from the EHR with external evidence, the patient's voice, and a supportive infrastructure that promotes collaborative review and reflection, interpretation of data, and performance transparency generates a continuous learning cycle of data-driven practice improvement that fuels real-time informed responses. Such learning from the work enables rapid, iterative, and expert practice changes that are informed by evidence while also allowing for more collaboration and meaning in the workplace.

Learning from the work on individual work units (departments or microsystems [Côté et al., 2020] where various health professionals work together on a regular basis) capitalizes on the context and shared relational purpose to foster knowledge and practice improvement/innovation. Furthermore, it uses situation-specific language and understanding of the unique patient population to advance practice. Finally, focusing on care processes as they are being delivered and revising them in real time demands integrating data access and collection into everyday workflow, using specialized software for rapid analysis, and reflecting on the results.

Reflection involves dialogue and deep thinking about practice and is a way for health professionals to judge the implications of the data, to generate ideas for change, and to take action on those ideas. Called *sensemaking* by Kitzmiller et al. (2010), "sensemaking is a social process of searching for answers and meaning that drives the actions people take" (p. 96). The COVID-19 pandemic in particular with its accelerated levels of uncertainty, presented a unique opportunity for deeper understanding or sensemaking under extreme circumstances (Christianson & Barton, 2020).

BOX 8.2: Making and valuing the time to regularly reflect on care processes (this is not an ad hoc process) and using the time to deeply think about and question former behaviors and their relationships to the underlying professional practice helps employees make wiser choices in the future. A facilitator can help a group stay connected to clinical practice and find ways to practically apply new knowledge (Harvey & Lynch, 2017). This approach builds learning into the workflow, helps systems learn from mistakes, ensures internal knowledge complements external knowledge, and can generate real impact.

Similar to health system learning, a learning health network is an action-oriented group that uses the same continuous learning cycle with a larger group of health systems and/or universities usually organized around specific populations to leverage data, share new knowledge, and generate quick, standardized solutions or practice improvements. It includes robust collaboration between patients and families, clinicians, and researchers who work together to accelerate practice solutions. Such networks can expand the location where care is delivered to include community-based and hospital-based practice. They can also easily address the social determinants of health in populations; promote connections among many clinicians, particularly those in remote areas; and adapt the PI process for community use. For example, Burman et al. (2021) described two learning networks using the Extension for Community Healthcare Outcomes (ECHO) model (Arora et al., 2017). This learning network model combines technology (video conferencing), case analysis, training, and continuous evaluation to determine effectiveness. The examples highlighted in the article focus on nursing practice and results provided support that the ECHO model can be applied to professional development. In nursing, this model focused on key nursing responsibilities, but learning networks can also be useful in situations such as disasters and pandemics to share knowledge and problem-solve practice solutions (especially in rural areas) quickly.

BOX 8.3: Learning health systems and networks share a common passion—improving practice—and rely on data, regular interaction among members, and reflection to accomplish their goals.

THE VALUE OF PRACTICE IMPROVEMENT

Practice improvement involves health professionals using best evidence (both PI and research), clinical information (e.g., from the EHR), and collaborative review and reflection to design actionable practice changes that continuously improve patient health outcomes, the patient experience, health system efficiency, and the work experience of healthcare professionals (Hosain et al., 2020). It includes the capacity to give and receive clinical and scientific information on behalf of good patient care, to integrate information and technology into the workflow, to balance inquiry and action wisely in daily caregiving, to work interdependently with team members through caring relationships, to reflect on practice, engage patients and families, to use measurement and data to revise patient care, implementation of practice changes, and evaluation (see Table 8.1).

Although they have similar meanings, practice improvement represents more of a culture or a way of being that is close to the clinical work and integrated within it. Quality improvement, on the other hand, is often seen as a series of separate projects that are conducted by individuals not necessarily working directly in clinical care. As such, practice improvement encourages all clinicians to exercise their curiosity, engage, and use data. It views learning from the work as a priority and is inclusive to both clinicians and patients/families. Table 8.2 highlights differences in traditional versus contemporary practice improvement.

Implementation is a phase of practice improvement that is often undervalued in health systems; consequently, limited attention is paid to its success. However, it is a key phase in the successful translation of evidence into practice that often is plagued by real-world challenges and barriers. Thus, a multitude of implementation theories and strategies have been developed over the last 10 years to facilitate such changes (Grol & Wensing, 2020). The COVID 19 pandemic, however, has accelerated the need for the use of routinely collected data that are applied in real time to create practice-based changes (Wensing et al., 2020). This quick action-oriented approach is dependent on teams of interdependently working health professionals working "in relationship" to examine evidence, reflect on current practice, and rapidly re-create practices that meet the real world needs of patients and families. Such practice is challenging, requiring effective communication, leadership support including resources, and feedback in the form of outcomes of the practice change.

TABLE 8.1 Components of Practice Improvement

Leverage technology to give and receive evidence—both internal and external
Integrate evidence into the workflow
Balance inquiry and action wisely; work engagement
Work interdependently "in relationship"
Reflection on practice
Engage patients and families
Use measurement and data to design new practice approaches
Implementation of practice changes
Evaluate for impact and sustainability

TABLE 8.2 Differences Between Traditional and Contemporary Practice Improvement

	Traditional Practice Improvement	Contemporary Practice Improvement
Label(s)	QI/PI	Practice improvement/continuous learning
Drivers	Corporate needs assessments	Local patient/clinical needs
Emphasis	Discipline specific; focused on externally derived outcomes	Context specific, practice based (department); focused on daily processes of care
Knowledge acquisition	Centralized, structured approach with predictable outcomes	Decentralized, small work groups learning through relating in everyday practice
Involved individuals	QI professionals, leadership/management	All employees, health professionals, leaders
Role of leadership	Problem identification, policy development, and implementation	Communicates the priority of learning from the work and resultant practice improvement; encourages inquiry, dialogue, and the evaluation of new ideas; attends to process; fosters safety culture
Role of patients/ families	Minimal participation	Direct and active patient involvement
Training	QI personnel; leadership	Continuous learning individually and collectively; multiple avenues for training exist; regular feedback on performance
Value added	Improvement occurs in batches	Practice improvement is ongoing and embedded in the work; facilitates the use of evidence and the design of contemporary and innovative approaches; adds meaning to the work

PI, performance improvement; QI, quality improvement.

Evaluating practice changes in the context of a fluctuating health system requires speedy feedback on the quality of patient services, employee wellness, and system efficiencies. Thus, the impact of practice changes on key indicators is needed information that is best directed back to those clinicians who are implementing the practice changes. Such feedback fuels motivation and enables sustainment of changes or their continuation over time, by valuing clinicians' contributions as owners of the process. Sustainment of practice changes is a more dynamic indicator of success that reflects the everchanging needs of patients and the development of new evidence, that fits within the QCM's major concept of self-advancing systems.

Although traditional research, EBP, and various quality improvement strategies have been shown to improve safety and quality, health professionals, their relationships, and the challenges of their work are readily visible and provide rich ground for learning *if only they would notice their practice and turn it into opportunities for learning*. Embedding learning in the work by fostering caring relationships among team members who *tune in* to work-related observations, sensations, and available objective data may provide added value to health systems by connecting the dots between everyday clinical practice, health outcomes, and employee work experience. For example, using the expertise of team members to meet the needs of patients (and involving them in the process), solving clinical problems *before* they become catastrophes (receiving immediate answers from expert team members), and increasing individual health professionals' knowledge and performance through sharing collective knowledge, all add meaning to the work, honor patient preferences, and may improve patient outcomes (or at least reduce adverse outcomes). The importance of including patients in the process of practice improvement (mutual problem-solving) cannot be overstated. Patients' unique perspectives (which may be surprisingly different from health professionals) provide a reasonable stance from which to evaluate the care received in terms of whether their needs and preferences were met or not. A recent study showed that patient and stakeholder engagement provided important feedback that was used to optimize the intervention and study processes (Sauers-Ford, 2021).

BOX 8.4: Practice improvement is important to patients and families not only because they expect safe, quality care but also because it may increase their sense of autonomy and participation in health decisions. As patients engage in mutual problem solving (one of the caring behaviors—see Chapter 3), motivation for future interactions with health professionals is energized. Furthermore, the process of engaging with health professionals may in itself translate to healthy behaviors and meet the conditions for individual self-advancement—learning, growing, changing, taking risks, progressing, coping, and integrating (self-caring).

From the health professional's perspective, learning from the work uplifts clinical practice from routine, mundane, repetitive activities to meaningful, knowledge-based work. Knowledge-based practice or EBP is essential to safe, high-quality patient outcomes. Such practice eliminates confusion and ambiguity regarding interventions and may also act to diffuse conflicting situations. Learning from the work may enhance health professionals' self-confidence and feelings of accomplishment necessary for self-advancement, a form of self-caring.

Although these are significant examples of the value of contemporary practice improvement, greater potential value lies in members' *use* of new knowledge to try out an approach (innovation value) or change their ways of doing business (change practice) as a result. The value may also be realized when a measurable positive impact occurs within the work team or the organization as a result of a changed practice—for example, practice variation and resultant costs may decrease or patient experiences may improve. Value is further added when routine practice improvement is aligned with the academic pursuits of the team members, enhancing efficiency, and rewarding individual team members (e.g., using group learning in course-related assignments, disseminating group learning through external publications and presentations). When the interactions of the learning team influence the participants (and the organization) to reexamine the definition of success, value is added. Finally, when learning from the work becomes integrated into the workflow, and practice is continuously improved from the inside out, patients and families receive beneficial, more up-to-date care that reflects health systems' primary missions, linking purpose to everyday clinical work.

SUMMARY

The dynamic nature of professional practice allows for the use of evolving clinical data, empirical evidence, and health team relational creativity to design innovative practice changes that improve patient, employee, and system outcomes. However, optimal practice improvement is facilitated by master performers (in this case, clinicians) who *deliberately practice*, consistent with the principles of lifelong learning, and professional expectations. Key to such deliberate practice is the relational processes used by health professionals in daily clinical care that enable learning from the work. Real world learning or learning from the work is a form of lifelong learning that facilitates meaningful experiences that enrich both patient and health professionals. At the system level, learning in this manner combines clinical data with empirical evidence, patients' perspectives, health professionals' reflection, and creativity to generate new knowledge that is almost impossible to efficiently acquire otherwise. Using that knowledge, health teams who work together *learn in practice* and take action to drive practice improvement. Such learning assists health professionals to make sense of their actions, to question their ways of doing business, and to use each other's expertise to continually improve. The value added by learning health systems who integrate learning into everyday workflow, meets the needs of patients and families and health professionals themselves, while fostering health system self-advancement.

CALL TO ACTION

Improving professional practice is a complex and relational process. Learning from work and the practice changes it elicits depends on caring-based teams of health professionals who actively combine real-world data with empirical evidence to design new ways of providing care. **Learn** from your professional colleagues by paying attention to practice, sharing your own expertise, engaging patients, and relating in a caring manner to continuously improve.

REFLECTIVE QUESTIONS/APPLICATIONS

For Professional Nurses in Clinical Practice:

- Describe how practice is improved in your organization. Why do you think you have answered this way? Are patients included? What is the role of the clinical nurse?

- Is there an expectation that practice improvement is a necessary component of RN work at your institution? If so, how is it done? How is it evaluated?
- Reflect on your own individual ability to learn from practice. How do you do it? What do you do with the knowledge and skills you acquire? How could you better integrate this into the workflow?
- What positive outcomes in health professionals do you attribute to the process of "learning from the work"? Why? What positive outcomes in patients do you attribute to this process? Why?
- What have you learned about practice improvement as a result of reading this chapter?
- Evaluate the quality improvement process at your institution. What is specified in the overall plan? What is the role of individual health professionals?
- Is your health system a "learning health system? Why or why not? How do you know? What could be different?

For Professional Nurses in Educational Practice:

- How does *learning* occur in your work? How does this differ between programs or departments?
- Reflect on the need for lifelong learning as a competency in your program. How does the curriculum facilitate this competency? How do you evaluate it?
- What can you do to advance the understanding of practice improvement among undergraduate students and graduate students?
- How might you suggest facilitating *learning from the work* during your educational programs?
- Provide some suggestions for exposing students to learning health systems.
- As a health professions educator, discuss how you use reflection as a strategy for lifelong learning. Suggest three possible educational research questions involving reflection on practice. Be specific.
- Develop an intervention aimed at practice improvement among your professional discipline. How could you make it interprofessional?

For Professional Nurses in Leadership Practice:

- What is the state of practice improvement at your organization? How do you know?
- How do you specifically hold yourself and your peers accountable for providing the infrastructure necessary for learning from the work among health professionals?
- Reflect on the performance improvement process in place at your institution. Does it take advantage of team relationships and principles of

learning health systems? Why or why not? What would it take to revise this?

■ How do you facilitate practice improvement at your organization? What specific methods are used?

■ Does your leadership team understand the value of integrating learning into clinical workflow? If not, how will you facilitate their development?

■ What characteristics of learning health systems are apparent in your organization? What domain are they organized around? Who are the leaders and members? How is their work incorporated into the overall performance improvement structure at the organization?

PRACTICE ANALYSIS

The executive team of a large regional health system expressed its frustration at once again needing to open previously closed clinical beds because of increasing patient needs. In years past, members had completed the painful work of closing these beds, modifying staffing, and associated expenses. After this painstaking process, they had at least felt a sense of accomplishment at having made hard but necessary decisions.

However, since the COVID-19 pandemic started, the team has faced multiple decision points related to "rightsizing" and finally decided to limit this vicious cycle by taking steps to shift their focus from a short-term crisis resolution approach to a more long-term solution using a learning health system approach. Facing obvious and painful failures in trying to solve recurring needs for patient beds, members recognized how little they really understood about their needs for hospital beds and decided to focus on better understanding it. They made a commitment to develop a deeper and shared understanding of what drives the need, the types of beds required, and how they were calculated, and to proactively and consistently manage them. They dialogued about the key variables or criteria that would indicate their success.

The team then identified that the emergency department morning report, the daily observation unit huddle, and health department projections might offer opportunities for reflections on needs. Because data from these forums were already available, they provided a relatively quick and easy way for team members to get the data, dialogue about what was driving the needs, provide the basis for suggestions and innovations, and gradually evolve into some tangible learning on the issue. This subtle shift to using already established information to "learn" from their practice was enlightening.

To start with, team members shared their beliefs and understanding regarding what contributed to the system's bed requirements. Thereafter, they deliberately turned these statements into hypotheses to test with each member considering what they were involved in or what data they had that would serve as the basis for learning. For example, the director of the observation unit was curious whether his assumptions about the relationship between patients' activity tolerance and next-day admissions would hold up. The director of the ICU had questions about whether previous cuts in patients' beds might have actually resulted in less availability for patients with respiratory deficits to be admitted on medical units. Initially, they simply added brief reviews of admitting trends (such as the prior 3 days of admissions) to their discussions and included staffing patterns with projected hires, transfers, and resignations to the weekly executive reports. Over time, through several iterations, they began to see new patterns and investigated such dynamics as the relationship between patient acuity in the ED, staffing requirements, and admission status. In daily safety meetings, they reflected on these findings and how they adjusted requirements and then described different approaches that they had tried to increase beds and associated staffing in certain areas. (At one meeting, the director of medicine reported about asking his team what they would do if stable ventilated patients were admitted for the next 6 months. The creative responses that he received inspired some of his peers to try the same experiment.)

At each iteration, the group saw that the combined results of their different approaches to learning about re-opening hospital beds became the topic on which they reflected. With the benefit of their peer-to-peer relationships, team members teased out unspoken assumptions, lessons learned, and so on. They began to question the actions they had chosen in the past and realized that they needed more powerful and timely patient requirements and staffing projections. They acknowledged how delays in feedback—in the form of unanticipated patient needs—affected their ability to proactively manage the situation. These sessions inevitably led to new questions and novel ideas.

- What specific approaches did the team use to "learn" about patient needs? How are they different from or the same as traditional performance improvement approaches?

- What about the team's interaction did you notice that was new or novel? How might this work lead to even more practice improvement?

REFERENCES

Abu, M., Arafat, R., & Ayahrul, S. (2020). The readiness of family in treating post-stroke patients at home: A literature review. *Enfermería Clínica*, 30, 293–296. https://doi.org/10.1016/j.enfcli.2019.07.106

Agency for Healthcare Research and Quality. (2019). About learning health systems. Agency for Healthcare Research and Quality. https://www.ahrq.gov/learning-health-systems/about.html

Arora, S., Kalishman, S. G., Thornton, K. A., et al. (2017). Project ECHO: A telementoring network model for continuing professional development. *The Journal of Continuing Education in the Health Professions*, 37(4), 239–244. https://doi.org/10.1097/CEH.0000000000000172

Bathish, M., Aebersold, M., Fogg, L., & Potempa, K. (2016). Development of an instrument to measure deliberate practice in professional nurses. *Applied Nursing Research*, 29, 47–52. https://doi.org/10.1016/j.apnr.2015.04.009

Bathish, M., Wilson, C., & Potempa, K. (2018). Deliberate practice and nurse competence. *Applied Nursing Research*, 40, 106–109. https://doi.org./10.1016/j.apnr.2018.01.002

Benner, P. (2021). Novice to mastery: Situated thinking action and wisdom. In E. S. Mangiante, J. Peno, & J. Northrup (Eds.), *Teaching and learning for adult skill acquisition: Applying the Dreyfus and Dreyfus model in different fields* (pp. 215–236). Information Age Publishing.

Brennan, D., & Wendt, L. (2021). Increasing quality and patient outcomes with staff engagement and shared governance. *OJIN: The Online Journal of Issues in Nursing, 26*(2). https://doi.org/10.3912/OJIN.Vol26No02PPT23

Burman, M. E., McGee, N., Proctor, J. L., et al. (2021). ECHO: A model for professional development in nursing through learning networks. *The Journal of Continuing Education in Nursing, 52*(4), 198–204. https://doi.org/10.3928/00220124-20210315-09

Christianson, M. K., & Barton, M. A. (2020). Sensemaking in the time of COVID-19. *Journal of Management Studise, 549*(2), 572–576.

Côté, A., Beogo, I., Abasse, K. S., Laberge, M., Dogba, M. J., & Dallaire, C. (2020). The clinical microsystems approach: Does it really work? A systematic review of organizational theories of health care practices. *Journal of the American Pharmacists Association, 60*(6), e388–e410. https://doi.org/10.1016/j.japh.2020.06.013

Dreyfus, H., & Dreyfus, S. (2008). Beyond expertise: Some preliminary thoughts on mastery. In K. Nielsen, S. Brinkmann, C. Elmholdt, L. Tanggaard, P. Musaeus, & G. Kraft (Eds.), *Qualitative stance; essays in honor of Steiner Kvale* (pp. 113–124). Aarhus University Press.

Friedman, C. P., Allee, N. J., Delaney, B. C., et al. (2016). The science of learning health systems: Foundations for a new journal. *Learn Health Syst, 1*(1), e10020. https://doi.org/10.1002/lrh2.10020

Gassas, R. (2021). Sources of the knowledge-practice gap in nursing: Lessons from an integrative review. *Nurse Education Today, 106*, 105095.

Grol, R., & Wensing, M. (2020). Implementation of change in healthcare. In M. Wensing, R. Grol, & J. Grimshaw (Eds.). *Improving patient care* (pp. 1–20). Wiley.

Hagedoorn, E. I., Keers, J. C., Jaarsma, T., van der Schans, C. P., Luttik, M. A., & Paans, W. (2020). The association of collaboration between family caregivers and nurses in the hospital and their preparedness for caregiving at home. *Geriatric Nursing, 41*(4), 373–380. https://doi.org/10.1016/j.gerinurse.2019.02.004

Harvey, G., & Lynch, E. (2017). Enabling continuous quality improvement in practice: The role and contribution of facilitation. *Frontiers in Public Health, 5*, 27. https://doi.org/10.3389/fpubh.2017.00027

Hosain, J., Reis, O., Verrall, T., Baerwald, A., Davis, B., Muller, A., Jacobson, N., & Ramsden, V. R. (2020). Grounded in practice: Integrating practice improvement into daily activities. *Canadian Family Physician, 66*(12), 931–933.

Institute of Medicine. (2012). Best care at lower cost: The path to continuously learning health care in America. http://www.nationalacademies.org/hmd/Reports/2012/Best-Care-at-Lower-Cost-The-Path-to-Continuously-Learning-Health-Care-in-America.aspx

Kitzmiller, R. A., Anderson, R. A., & McDaniel, R. R. (2010). Making sense of health information technology implementation: A qualitative study protocol. *Implementation Science, 5*, 95. https://doi.org/10.1186/1748-5908-5-95

Melnyk, B., Gallagher-Ford, L., Zellefrow, C., et al. (2018). The first U.S. study on nurses' evidence-based practice competencies indicates major deficits that threaten healthcare quality, safety, and patient outcomes. *Worldviews on Evidence-Based Nursing, 15*(1), 16–25. https://doi.org/10.1111/wvn.12269

Parboosingh, I. J., Reed, V. A., Palmer, J. C., & Bernstein, H. H. (2011). Enhancing practice improvement by facilitating practitioner interactivity: New roles for providers. *Journal of Continuing Education in the Health Professions, 31*(2), 122–127. https://doi.org/10.1002/chp.20116

Romanelli, R. J., Azar, K. M., Sudat, S., Hung, D., Frosch, D. L., & Pressman, A. R. (2021). Learning health system in crisis: Lessons from the COVID-19 pandemic. *Mayo Clinic Proceedings: Innovations, Quality & Outcomes, 5*(1), 171.

Sauers-Ford, H., Statile, A. M., Auger, K. A., Wade-Murphy, S., Gold, J. M., Simmons, J. M., & Shah, S. S. (2021). Short-term focused feedback: A model to enhance patient engagement in research and intervention delivery. *Medical Care, 59*(8 suppl 4), S364.

Schmidt, P., & Fenner, D. (2020). Deliberate practice: Applying the expert performance approach to gynecologic surgical training. *Clinical Obstetrics and Gynecology, 63*(2), 295–304. https://doi.org/10.1097/GRF.0000000000000509

Senge, P. (1990). *The fifth discipline*. Doubleday.

Sutter-Leve, R., Passint, E., Ness, D., & Rindflesch, A. (2021). The caregiver experience after stroke in a COVID-19 environment: A qualitative study in inpatient rehabilitation. *Journal of Neurologic Physical Therapy, 45*(1), 14–20. https://doi.org/10.1097/npt.0000000000000336

Wensing, M., Sales, A., Armstrong, R., & Wilson, P. (2020). Implementation science in times of COVID-19. *Implementation Science, 15*(1), 42. https://doi.org/10.1186/s13012-020-01006-x

Winstein, C. J., Stein, J., Arena, R., Bates, B., Cherney, L. R., Cramer, S. C., Deruyter, F., Eng, J. J., Fisher, B., Harvey, R. L., Lang, C. E., MacKay-Lyons, M., Ottenbacher, K. J., Pugh, S., Reeves, M. J., Richards, L. G., Stiers, W., & Zorowitz, R. D. (2016). Guidelines for adult stroke rehabilitation and recovery. *Stroke, 47*(6). https://doi.org/10.1161/str.0000000000000098

CHAPTER 9

Self-Advancing Systems

"The principle of organization is built into nature. Chaos itself is self-organizing. Out of primordial disorder, stars find their orbit; rivers make their way to the sea."

—Steven Pressfield

CHAPTER OBJECTIVES:

1. Explain the meaning of self-advancing systems.
2. Describe the relationship between processes of care and self-advancing systems.
3. Evaluate the unique opportunities available to health professionals for learning from the experiences they encounter with patients and families.
4. Analyze the benefits of prioritizing human persons to health systems.

THE MEANING OF SELF-ADVANCING SYSTEMS

Self-advancing systems is the last concept in the Quality-Caring Model© (QCM), and the words were specifically chosen. In complex adaptive systems, the language of evolution, adaptation, and self-organization is frequently used to signify the combined effects of multiple interacting parts that, over time, co-create new, and sometimes unexpected responses. The number of interactions in complex systems have a dynamic nature with continuing interactions at the lowest levels forming patterns that provide structure to the system. The direction of the new behaviors or practices is not specified. However, people (or knowledgeable agents) who engage (interact) learn to adjust their behaviors on their own through experience and continuous learning (see Chapter 8) and generate new (or adaptive) beneficial behaviors or solutions that create impact or value (Uhl-Bien et al., 2020). Of course, the context and feedback received (the conditions that people work in) are theorized to influence this adaptive process; thus, adaptive behaviors are not always beneficial. In healthcare, however, the notion that caring relationships are positive influencers that inspire forward movement or progress has informed the label attached to the remaining concept in the model.

The word *advancement* signifies growth, change, development, elevation, improvement, continuance, and expansion. Self-advancing systems are quality systems in that they reflect dynamic, positive progress that enhances the system's performance; and they emerge on their own under the right conditions; thus, they are *self*-advancing. Caring relationships (with self, patients, and families, among health professionals, and in communities) are beneficial in terms of providing feedback and activating positive emotions that energize and support individuals,' groups,' and systems' capacities to change, learn, or respond to their fluctuating conditions. Put another way, living systems (including persons, groups, and the organizations in which they work) are active, interact locally, are capable of discovering new possibilities on their own, co-create patterns that inform behaviors, and repeatedly self-organize (promote order) without conscious planning or control. The multiple connections among the individuals (knowledgeable agents) in a complex system are critical, and their relationships provide important feedback that informs a collective new order. There is no hierarchy of command and control in living systems, but the context and feedback received from the many interconnected relationships fuel adaptation. This phenomenon of self-organization is pervasive, but subtle, and often goes unnoticed. If the context and feedback are nourishing, the potential for reorganization is great; if not, that same potential may be limited. In healthcare, for example, positive feedback may result in greater sensitivity to ongoing conditions, perhaps escalating preventive interventions, resulting in unique, unanticipated but valuable outcomes.

In clinical environments, humans and their social interactions are distinctively self-determining, knowledgeable, and full of promise (assumptions of the QCM). Thus, it is reasonable to expect that through ongoing interactions and feedback over time and within a caring (i.e., *nourishing*) context, new patterns (habits, conduct, behaviors, methods, approaches, and practices) that emerge are optimistically oriented and arise without the need for outside control. Organizations, as living systems similar to individuals, have a natural tendency to arrange themselves, if the ongoing interactions are nurtured (cared for). In this way, new patterns or changes in function or behaviors of employees emerge on their own as forward movement; thus, they are self-advancing. Acknowledging and even exploiting this characteristic in individuals and organizations, instead of reducing it, is the key to quality or excellence.

BOX 9.1: Advancement, therefore, is a natural phenomenon that begins as a local process and is a *product of that process*, not external manipulation. Thus, the use of the word *self* in the term self-advancing systems is fitting.

Self-advancing systems are not linear but have highs and lows and emerge gradually over time and are influenced by context. Through multiple interactions between and among individuals and the environment, interdependencies develop, creating small local differences or changes that can grow exponentially *if cultivated*. These small but positive behaviors may enhance the lives of patients and families, health professionals, and systems at the local level and ultimately lead to larger scale advancement. Furthermore, new forms of behavior and resulting changes cannot be predicted as they occur over time as a result of uncontrollable and numerous connections—drastically changing how we think about progress (or results and outcomes).

For example, the continued focus on quality outcomes several weeks (or months) after care has been delivered is often too far removed from the ongoing interactions of those delivering the care and is not able to keep up with the unpredictable complexity in the system and its context. Because of this phenomenon, improvements in care are often sluggish or weak and frequently do not even endure. Rather, if the focus of a clinical problem or clinical situation is shifted quickly and locally (at the clinical microsystem level) to the *process* of care before it has a chance to spread, it can be very adaptive. That is, if the process of care includes multiple agents (individuals) in the system learning about a problem, drawing from a repertoire of ideas or actions, freely dialoguing about them, and then are permitted to enact them in a context that is supportive and encouraging, new ways of clinical practice are more likely to emerge. See Chapter 8 on practice improvement. Moreover, if a robust frame of reference (e.g., a professional practice model) grounds the practice, individuals can extract concepts from that foundation to modify their ideas and actions, better aligning them with the overall purpose of the discipline or health system.

In health systems, professionals are autonomous individuals with unique knowledge and sets of skills that complement each other. Through ongoing interactions and feedback, their individual expertise becomes integrated in the overall care of patients and families. Successful self-advancing systems use knowledge and anticipation of events to modify their actions (or functions) and prepare for changes. Those that are grounded in strongly held or evidence-based principles are better able to withstand periods of instability or disruptions in the work.

BOX 9.2: Thus, well-balanced groups of health professionals who are grounded in a shared purpose and who continually interact and learn from each other (in caring relationships) can self-advance (themselves, their patients, and health systems) without compromising their individual functionality.

Most self-advancement doesn't happen quickly—rather, it is incremental and best accomplished through simple processes involving interactions operating locally. Interestingly, individual health professionals often are energized and empowered as a result! For example, simple changes in how a handoff is performed, or ways in which patient mobility is enhanced, or how continuous education is delivered in hospitals can lead to large-scale improvements. An example of this is a hospital associated with a larger health system in a diverse area of New York City. Knowing that pressure ulcers were a problem on a unit, the nurses on their own developed a skin care cart (with supplies and equipment) and set up a protocol of accountability for use by all the nurses in the unit. A written communication system was established for use by all RNs on the unit and within a few weeks, skin breakdown was reduced by 50%, and staff members' engagement improved. Although the unit intended to improve incidences of skin breakdown, they did not anticipate the improved staff engagement and pride experienced by the nursing staff. Shortly thereafter, other units started imitating the idea.

On the other hand, in uncertain or chaotic situations (such as the COVID-19 pandemic), individuals and systems are incentivized to rapidly innovate or adapt to accommodate hectic and disorderly circumstances. In the case of COVID-19, the rapid adaptation to telehealth, online learning, outpatient management, point of care diagnostics, new treatments, and limited resources was profound. Many of these advances have remained.

Without dissemination of their ultimate effects, however, changing practices in nursing (or other health professions) often go unnoticed, without tangible evidence of their outcomes. Good ideas can also be impractical, too expensive, or not acceptable (too difficult to implement) to patients or staff. However, through small pilot studies or demonstration projects, practical ways of determining the feasibility of suggested improvements can be established. This approach is performed at the local level (unit), and its evaluation should assess local *and* system variables; thus it represents a shared method that preserves the original idea(s) generated at the local level (and credits them accordingly). The objective is to generate systems capable of adaptation, change, and even novelty by focusing on relevant smaller processes that take place primarily in their natural environment, enabling the system to adapt to real-world situations or events, despite the differences in individuals, the environment, and their interactions over time.

Consider the following:

A nursing chief nurse executive (CNE) is concerned about nurse staffing and turnover rates and their resultant effects on the Consumer Assessment of Healthcare Providers and Systems (HCAHPS®; Goldstein et al., 2005) survey scores. In fact, he has been pestered by the hospital COO to decrease the use of travel nurses who are costing the system thousands of dollars and raise the patient experience scores! He decides that a different staffing model where RNs will practice to the top of their license will be required to meet the requirements for care in his organization. After discussing this with his leadership team, he becomes aware of the preparatory work that will be required in terms of RN education, hiring of assistive personnel, discussions with the medical team, and he begins to wonder just how long this process will take.

At a recent teleconference he attended, a particular presenter discussed how she was able to recruit multiple new RNs to work in a team model using a popular healthcare consultant's approach. To expedite RN recruitment and the new staffing model, he hires the consultant to do the same work at his institution. Over several months (and several thousand dollars), the numbers of RNs hired were minimal, and the staffing model had not yet started. To make matters worse, the travel nurses were still employed, and patient experience scores had not budged!

Was the use of a single consultant too rigid in that particular context or limiting to the process? Could the CNE have used a more innovative approach? What if the nursing staff were presented with the problem and expected to find solutions themselves? Even better, what if the nursing staff already knew about the issue and used group reflections and dialogue to design a revised staffing model themselves? Better yet, what if they included patients in the process?

The first approach is predictable, orderly, and keeps the CNE in control. The second is flexible, messy, and uncontrolled. Will it work? The only way to know is to implement the staff's recommendation and find out. After all, in the near future, when patients are truly in control of their care, health professional—designed approaches may be obsolete anyway!

Despite the interest in advancement and innovation in health systems, diffusion of alternative approaches has been slow. Just like clinical work, it tends to be task oriented (discrete little parts), driven by cost containment, with little discussion about the many interdependent relationships that characterize its complexity. The dominant paradigm is still the sum-of-the-parts mentality in which a health system is viewed as a combination of multiple parts. The problem with such an approach is that health system leaders and some professionals have a tendency to think that if, for example, central line infections or falls have been reduced, the job has been done and the larger concept of safety has been reached. Rather, quality or excellence is an *umbrella* term that is really about continuous forward movement. It consists of multiple dimensions—safety, reliability, accuracy, costs, the overall experience, impact, value and so on. In complex health systems, superior system outcomes (advancement) are not final solutions but part of a systematic, continuous learning process that leads to alternative decisions about practice by the clinicians and patients themselves. This is a much different approach from the mechanistic quality improvement paradigm of specialized personnel measuring and analyzing specified outcomes and reporting them back to department heads.

BOX 9.3: The notion of groups of interdependent, creative health professionals interacting and finding ways to improve practice *on their own* runs counter to traditional organizational thinking that emphasizes the ability of systems to be engineered toward predefined goals within a framework of incentives and punishments.

Self-advancing systems naturally evolve as everyone (including patients and families) shares in the *process* of interaction at the local clinical level, engaging with the work and learning from it, to adjust their behaviors. The challenge for leadership in this time of rapid change is to expect, encourage, and nurture multiple interactions among health professionals through ongoing collaboration, dialoguing, networking, reflecting, and collective learning about patient care such that it becomes enculturated, enabling new solutions—and then to trust and get out of the way!

PROCESS, PROCESS, PROCESS

It's relatively easy to advance (deliver safe, high-quality and valuable care) when resources are plentiful or there is little competition. However today's environment is atypical, demanding alternative strategies for progression. In companies with sustained high reliability (a feature of self-advancing systems), clinical practice is acknowledged as complex and error-prone. Such companies view errors and near misses as opportunities to improve versus finite outcomes, value frontline opinions and recommendations for improvement, and prioritize training and flexibility to minimize failures (Veazie et al., 2022). As such, they emphasize a systems approach and prioritize frontline staff as experts in the decision-making and problem-solving process. Evidence is now emerging that frontline healthcare staff are highly attuned to macro and microsystem problems and are thus uniquely qualified to address small operational failures, thereby reducing errors and near misses in clinical practice settings (Stevens et al., 2017). As an example, the sudden and unanticipated pandemic created an environment that was and continues to be dynamically ambiguous, with unexplained new work roles and routines, disrupted interactions, inadequate resources, and frequent melancholy requiring ongoing risk assessment. We have rarely seen a time when health professionals needed the skills to rapidly identify potential safety concerns, quickly learn how a novel virus produces and spreads symptoms, which treatments work and which do not, and to negotiate the confusing guidance (a.k.a. sensemaking; see Chapter 8). In this environment, health professionals were rapidly driven to interpret and collectively shape their responses to patient and family everchanging needs. This is the *real* work of health systems—noticing cues, a focus on safety, thoughtful interactions among health professionals related to clinical care, accurate and timely communication, followed by informed behaviors. It is clear that self-advancing in today's environment requires knowledgeable *processes* of care.

These processes of care are best found in local clinical units (or departments) and involve attention to the big-picture—person-centered, comprehensive, interdependent, and dynamic ways of thinking and acting. The more task-focused work of yesterday that centered on health professionals or health systems—as opposed to patients and families—was a more linear way of thinking and acting. In nursing, dynamic processes of care translate to holistic, interpersonal, connected, and complete nursing care that is evidence based and provided collaboratively with other health professionals (well-coordinated). Such care is always person-centered with caring relationships as the foundation. It encompasses assessment, ongoing monitoring and surveillance, attention to hygiene (one's own and the patient's), mobility, breathing and circulation, nutritional intake and elimination (including the measurement of intake and output), sleep and rest, planning for transitions, attending to the emotional aspects of illness, education, simple interventions that yield high impact, such as repositioning, anticipating and relieving discomfort, teaching, ambulating or range-of-motion activities, routine spot checking, and regular handwashing.

BOX 9.4: These simple but fundamental nursing acts are essential for optimal comfort, skin integrity, reasonable functional status, positive patient experiences, reductions in hospital or emergency department readmissions, and longer-term independence in the community, all high-impact and *reimbursable* outcomes!

Integrated with basic or fundamental healthcare processes, evidence-based clinical practice guidelines provide health professionals with recommendations for practice that positively influence outcomes. However, how guidelines (which are formulated for the average patient) are implemented for individual patients requires team consideration and patient input. To be useful, guidelines should be well referenced, evaluated regularly, and revised often based on research and sharing of lessons learned. Most importantly, dialog and collaborative decision making among health professionals and patients regarding the use of guidelines in particular situations and the impact of their use have an effect on important outcomes.

Yet, variation in the implementation of evidence-based guidelines are well-known (Devine et al., 2022). The specific steps in a guideline are designed to foster accurate and timely health outcomes. Accountability for processes of care has been fostered through The Joint Commission's use of evidence-based process measures, also referred to as accountability measures (The Joint Commission, 2022). These measures emphasize performance in specific patient populations by allowing for identification of root causes of error or failure.

Attention to clinical processes has many advantages over constantly measuring outcomes of care. However, aspects of clinical processes used for observation should be based on evidence of their contribution to clinical outcomes. For example, are hospitalized older adults assessed for the pneumonia vaccine? Are clinicians regularly monitoring respiratory rates on acute medical units? Are all inpatients assessed for falls on admission? Are nurses rounding regularly? Do nurses respond promptly to signs of deterioration (such as decreasing levels of consciousness or decreased blood pressure)? Such processes of care are linked empirically to specific health outcomes.

Measuring important processes of care (those that are known to influence outcomes) enforces the notion that basic, routine clinical care represents opportunities for improvement. It may prompt more widespread improvement by shifting specific repetitive actions to those that improve overall performance of a department. Along those lines, the message of improvement versus failure (something bad) allows for specifics on where to improve.

After years of focusing on adverse outcomes and medical errors as indicators of quality, many health systems and health professionals still rely on monitoring predominately quality outcomes after care has been delivered. The perpetual attention to measuring adverse outcomes has unintentionally taken us away from the fundamental *processes* of good patient care (such a simple idea, but counterintuitive to modern-day thinking). The big difference between a process-focused health system (or health professional) and an outcome-focused one is that during patient care, the outcome-focused health professional's attention is devoted to concerns about what outcomes will result. With this in mind, the health professional may question whether she or he is doing the intervention correctly, worry that she or he is taking too long, what other health professionals might think, or how the boss will evaluate them. Each of these outcome-focused thoughts interferes with the care ultimately provided! Concerns about the outcome distract one from being present and aware of the uniqueness of the patient and his or her health situation; they may also cause one to doubt the self and take away from the capacity to perform optimally. Health professionals and health systems who take this outcomes stance create outcomes-focused organizations. Over time, outcomes-focused organizations lose focus on the *processes* of good patient care. It is imperative that we concentrate closely and attentively on the *processes* of healthcare.

BOX 9.5: The *processes* of care are really all that we can control in the constantly changing internal and external environment. Focusing on the process—the fundamental practice of good patient care—and trusting that we can perform it well increases the chances of advancement. Clinical practice that is caring, comprehensive, and accurately and reliably delivered will naturally generate positive outcomes that benefit patients and families, health professionals, and health systems.

THE MEANING OF SELF-ADVANCEMENT FOR PATIENTS AND FAMILIES

Each individual patient has a unique experience with various health professionals and health systems along the healthcare continuum ranging from primary care to episodic acute care, restorative care to long-term, or even palliative or hospice care. However, the services provided in fragmented chunks are usually geographically placed and linked to specific disease states. Each of these disease states has associated outcome indicators (e.g., survival, HbA1c levels, O_2 levels, intervention success rates, etc.), and care is usually delivered in the clinician's office requiring multiple visits. The clinician addresses theirr area of expertise without much thought to the overall events the patient undergoes or the multiple interactions occurring within the larger health system. This leads to unpredictable, changing, conflicting, and sometimes dissatisfying healthcare experiences.

Although this example is several years old, consider its underlying theme:
On the day before I get ill, I am an autonomous, capable citizen. I can fill out my tax returns. I can apply my craft. I can make terrific Italian meatballs. I can counsel my adult daughter on how to handle her son's new fears at school. I can finish the Saturday New York Times crossword puzzle. I can binge on three episodes of Game of Thrones while answering 50 emails at the same time.

And then I show up at the healthcare's dinner party, and healthcare strips me. It silences me; it dresses me in a sheet; it takes away my work; it takes away my pleasures, my family; it tells me exactly what to do. "Take a breath, hold your breath." What if, instead, healthcare asked me what I can do and thanked me for doing it? What if, instead, healthcare asked me if I would like to sit or stand ... if I would like to speak or remain quiet? What if healthcare asked me for instructions, not doctor's orders, but people's orders?

(Berwick, 2016)

Experiences of care refer to patients' perspectives on the responsiveness of health providers to their specific needs and include the manner in which care is provided (Institute for Healthcare Improvement [IHI], 2009). Patients' perspectives of their healthcare experiences are essential to providing clinicians with information on how care processes affect responses to illness and are considered a unique and independent dimension of quality. When validly and reliably measured, experiences of care have been linked to specific quality and business outcomes such as allegiance to a health system, fewer complaints, 30-day readmissions, and pain control (Carter et al., 2018; Kleinpell et al., 2019; Quigley et al., 2021). Moreover, in a systematic review that examined evidence from 55 studies, a consistent positive association was reported between patient experience, patient safety, and clinical effectiveness for a wide range of disease areas, settings, outcome measures, and study designs (Doyle et al., 2013).

Using the national HCAHPS Survey (Goldstein et al., 2005), standardized, publicly reported data about patients' experiences of care are collected that allow for meaningful comparison of hospitals and serve as a basis for reimbursement. Prior to the pandemic, patient experience trends remained stagnant; but an overall decline in patients' perception of their care occurred across all healthcare settings as COVID-19 altered visitation practices (Silvera et al., 2021). As policy makers continue to promote value-based payment, it is critical that health professionals attend to patients' unique needs, responding with the caring behaviors, including affiliation needs and allowance for mutual decision making.

Take the case of patients who are receiving care for chronic conditions and are facing life-limiting alternatives. Often, they live in the community but require regular visits to healthcare providers or clinics (e.g., dialysis patients), or they may live in long-term care facilities away from families and friends. They may require help with activities of daily living, might even be depressed, and may take multiple medications that have untoward side effects, may suffer from pain and/or discomfort, and must rely on others. Episodically, such patients may be hospitalized and then return back to the community. In addition to treating the illness, dealing with the emotional aspects of the illness, receiving encouragement and positive reinforcement to modify behaviors (e.g., ambulate, eat well), receiving adequate pain control, obtaining suggestions for diminishing the side effects of multiple medications, achieving a sense of control, or even how to get dressed in the morning are necessary!

In an ideal world, such persons might be able to consistently receive these services in the convenience of their own communities. And, it is highly likely that such processes of care would better provide patients with the caring relationships they need to feel more comfortable, in control, understood, and to be able to detect early warning signs of illness exacerbations *before* there is a need for hospitalization. Such caring processes influence intermediate and longer-term outcomes, such as quality of life and hospital readmissions. In essence, the patient eventually becomes self-caring (able to listen, take responsibility for, repair, and affirm oneself). Isn't this the essence of self-advancement?

THE MEANING OF SELF-ADVANCEMENT FOR HEALTH PROFESSIONALS

Health professionals work in various environments and disciplines; endure demanding jobs with little opportunity for continuing education; work with personnel who may lack commitment or just do not follow through; deal with multiple sources of conflict; sometimes practice in environments that do not recognize or value employee's contributions; or experience periodic burnout, boredom, and even disillusionment. Recently, a secondary data analysis conducted via a web-based survey reported that 41% of healthcare workers (most were nurses) had moral injury scores of 36 or higher (range 10–100; Nelson et al., 2022). Most importantly, although the study had limitations particularly related to the convenience sample and design, findings pointed to breaches of trust with healthcare systems and their leadership. Issues such as inadequate communication, failure to ensure relational support needs were met, prioritizing business operations, inadequate provision of resources, not being present and visible, and lack of palliative care support were expressed by the respondents.

In spite of the discouraging work conditions reported in this paper, registered nurses continue to play a remarkable role in the ongoing delivery of care, healing, and advancement of healthcare. They continue to be the most ethical and trustworthy of professionals (Saad, 2020), are intentional in their willingness to serve, are prepared, and many bravely put their lives on the line during the initial phase of the COVID-19 pandemic. The spotlight placed on nursing working conditions during COVID-19 has generated several positive initiatives that present opportunities for growth, energy, creativity, an enhanced worldview, improved career opportunities, and even personal and professional fun. For example, in addition to increased emphasis on employee wellness, many healthcare professionals have seen recent salary increases, different scheduling options, and even additional benefits. More reliance on technology, particularly artificial intelligence (AI) and telehealth, will provide additional opportunities for growth among health professionals.

BOX 9.6: Working in the health professions allows one to meet and learn from talented patients, families, and co-workers who encourage and support growth. It also provides an identity that is valued in society, opening doors that might otherwise be closed. Most importantly, working in the health professions offers many opportunities to make a difference in the lives of others and in so doing learn about one's own life, *provided we stay awake and apply what we learn from our work on ourselves.*

Health professionals also have daily opportunities for lifelong development through interactions with patients, families, and co-workers, yet many remain unaware of this remarkable resource! On a daily basis, health professionals encounter patient situations that cause them great fear, such as pain, a new cancer diagnosis, chronic disease, loss of function, or death. Over time, such situations can lead to feelings of numbness or even paralysis as they try to protect themselves from the suffering they see every day. Cassel (1982) described suffering as "the state of severe distress associated with events that threaten the intactness or wholeness of the person" (p. 639). Cassel (1992) further adds that "suffering is a consequence of personhood—bodies do not suffer, persons do" (1992, p. 3). Thus, suffering is a human experience that affects all beings, including health professionals. With their special knowledge and skills, health professionals have unique opportunities to consider and learn from the suffering experiences of their patients and families.

Ponder this example:

As a new RN in an academic west-coast hospital, I started on the 12-hour night shift of a busy medical-surgical overflow floor. Through my inexperience, I relied heavily on my interactions with patients. One night I felt drawn to patient JB who had suffered a stroke and was unresponsive. The off-going nurse had told me during report of his grieving wife, who was trying to come to terms with this major life change.

JB was easy to care for, requiring turning, suctioning, and medications occasionally. His flaccid left side gave me no resistance as I took vital signs. I talked to him as I worked. I reminded JB of where he was, what happened to him, and what I'd heard of his wife and family. I always told him what I was doing, when I finished, and when I would be back to check on him. I told him to rest and allow nature to begin healing his brain so he could return to his wife.

As the week progressed his condition deteriorated. A decision was made by JB's family not to resuscitate him should he die. Each night I would continue talking to him while I worked. He remained seemingly inattentive to my care and by the end of the week, JB was no better than when I first saw him. His physician team was taking a non-aggressive approach, spoke daily with his wife, and by the end of the week, it was reported to me that a decision was being awaited from JB's distraught wife about whether to place a feeding tube and transfer him to a skilled facility or not.

I continued to talk to JB each night about what I knew had happened during the day, not knowing if his wife talked to him or spoke to him when she visited. I told him that his CT scan showed increased swelling in his brain and what that meant. As I suctioned him around 5 a.m., I noted JB had lost his gag reflex in response to the suction catheter and that his face seemed slacker. My other assessments and his vital signs were unchanged. As I stood there looking at him, my eye caught a small white glimmer of light that slid down the opposite side of JB's bed and disappeared into the ceiling. I remember thinking that maybe I was more exhausted than I thought, or maybe I had gotten a little too involved with JB. I stood there a few minutes; nothing else occurred.

During my report, I told JB's new nurse of his condition. The nurse went in to see him and when she came out, she told me that JB passed. I went in to see him feeling that maybe he made his own decision. I wondered if I had helped him process his situation, and his passing was his attempt to help his wife with her weighted decision.

On my way home, I believed I had witnessed an extraordinary event that is open to interpretation. I often think of JB, and how I was able to interpret and validate for him what had happened to his health, and perhaps offer him a small part in the last scenario of his life.

—Genesis Bojorquez, PhD, RN, NE-BC, PCCN

What difference do you think this young nurse made in the short life of this patient or his family? What do you think JB's experience taught the nurse about her own life or human suffering? Do you wonder if she paid attention?

Health professionals also encounter situations that cause them great joy—the birth of a healthy baby, the ability of a formerly bedridden individual to walk,

TABLE 9.1 Intermediate Outcomes Associated with the Process of Caring for Others Among Health Professionals

Caring Behaviors	Associated Intermediate Outcomes
Mutual problem-solving	Feeling enabled, empowered, equal, sense of pride
Human respect	Feeling valued, worthy, dignified
Attentive reassurance	Feeling noticed, strengthened, comforted, hopeful
Encouraging manner	Feeling supported, sustained
Appreciation of unique meanings	Feeling understood, validated
Healing environment	Feeling safe, secure, protected
Attending to basic human needs	Feeling healthy, energized
Attending to affiliation needs	Feeling connected, a part of, attached, integral

a pain-ridden patient who is now comfortable, or a surgical patient who is able to re-join the workforce. Thus, health professionals bear witness to incredible anguish and sorrow, but also are presented with many gifts. The process of caring with and for others honors the sacred nature of humans and offers us unique opportunities to see reality, direct our attention toward the human experience of illness (and its associated joys and suffering), and move toward possibilities that have been in front of us all along; for example, learning how to cope in difficult life experiences or periods of uncertainty. Caring relationships with oneself, patients and families, other health professionals, and communities provide the medium for feeling cared for, and for health professionals, this becomes apparent when they are fully engaged in the work, practice organizational citizenship and authentic collaboration, and are open to possibilities (see Table 9.1).

BOX 9.7: Being open to the significance of clinical practice to our own advancement, rather that rushing through the work, shifts our worldview toward the more optimistic aspects of clinical practice. In turn, health professionals find that their work has meaning that transcends income, status, flexible scheduling, and an identity that provides clarity and affirmation. Healthcare is, above all, a series of relationships with ourselves, patients and families, each other, and the larger communities we serve. Actively looking for those positive, upbeat, favorable aspects of our work generates hopeful expectations that nourish our humanity.

A perfect example of noticing an opportunity for personal growth occurred to this author many years ago as a young nurse who had not yet fully confronted death.

After being "pulled" off the critical care unit and "floated" to an oncology unit, I was assigned a 58-year-old woman with breast cancer. She had metastasis to the bone and was in severe pain every time she moved or changed her position. She was alert and oriented, receiving intravenous chemo, and had terrible sores in her mouth. In all, she was suffering tremendously and close to death. She had two grown daughters about my age who were quite fearful of their mother's prognosis and in their anxiety could not stay long in the room—they could often be found pacing in the hall. Witnessing this scenario was hard for me as I had never dealt with death in this manner (my critically ill patients were usually unconscious, and I hadn't yet experienced death in my personal life). I was anxious and didn't know how to interact well with the patient or the family. Somehow, the patient sensed this (could it be that she had children about my age?) and called me over to her bed and asked me to sit down on it. Uncomfortably, I did as I was asked, and the woman took my hand, looked right at me, and began to tell me how she had led a wonderful life (she recounted several stories), that she knew she was dying, and that she was okay with it! She did not seem to be in pain as she told me her story and after she was finished, I was in tears. She was smiling. This beautiful lady taught me the powerful lesson that the process of patient care is rich with life lessons that are to be honored and that even those patients and families who are the most distressed (or suffering) can strengthen our souls, provided we engage with them in the process!

According to Steger (2017), meaningful work "speaks to people's subjective experience that their jobs, work, or careers are purposeful and significant, that their work is harmoniously and energetically synergistic with the meaning and purpose in their broader lives, and that they are enabled and empowered to benefit the greater good through their work" (p. 60). However, a literature review of 71 studies on meaningful work found no consensus in the definitions, and 28 different measurement scales. It was, however, viewed as a positive concept that was associated with higher levels of engagement, job satisfaction, motivation, commitment, well-being, and performance, as well as lower levels of absence and turnover (Bailey et al., 2019). Thus, although the concept of meaningful work is not fully clarified and more research is warranted, the notion that an overall sense of purpose and significance derived from work is consistent with the larger meaning of health professionals' lives and is a crucial matter for health professionals.

Most health professionals are passionate about helping people and making a difference in their lives; furthermore, most like their chosen work (personal conversations), but sometimes get caught up in the negative cultures of some health systems. The constant pressure for efficient throughput, accomplishing endless tasks, and witnessing daily suffering while simultaneously dealing with inadequate resources, inefficient electronic health records, and unhealthy work environments creates conditions in which health professionals do not readily see the importance of their work or who cannot/do not slow down enough to really feel the benefits of their work. Furthermore, many health professionals work endless shifts (often back-to-back) or work two or more jobs, sometimes increasing their own stress.

Although there is no magic formula for *using what we learn from our work to enhance its subjective significance*, slowing down a little to listen, to notice, to feel, and to appreciate how those meaningful moments encountered in clinical practice enrich our lives is crucial. After all, we are also human. Finding meaning by authentically relating to patients and families and other health professionals through the process of clinical practice facilitates feeling cared for *in ourselves* and can lead to some highly significant consequences, such as increased work commitment and engagement, enhanced personal health, self-efficacy, hope, and empowerment (see Table 9.1). The nature of clinical practice is complex and often exhausting; however, it seems as if the more health professionals "roll up their sleeves," linger a little, stay embedded in the important work they do, and pay attention to the *process* of clinical work, the more meaning that work provides. In turn, the impact of that work on health professionals shifts them towards self-advancement.

Reflect on this...

Many young nurses have been socialized for the merit badges that will eventually get them to the coveted ICU or Labor and Delivery (L & D) departments. In many ways, nursing education and nurse residency programs emphasize "getting experience in Med-Surg" as an important step up on the career ladder, rather than an opportunity for personal and professional growth. In fact, after about 6 months to 1 year on the job, many new graduates are already thinking about the next job or the next degree. Few spend time thinking about what makes nursing meaningful, how their experiences increase self-knowledge, or the larger purpose they have in relation to performance improvement, clinical decision-making, interprofessional collaboration, health equity, or community engagement. However, nursing is so much more...

Multiple opportunities exist in the healthcare work environment to connect, to learn, to recognize one's purpose, to know oneself, to better understand how nursing itself generates meaning in one's life. However, the acute care work environment offers few forums for discussing or engaging in such topics.

What would happen if...

— *regular forums existed during nurse residency programs to reflect on pivotal growth opportunities of nursing work?*

— *group reflection was a regular weekly occurrence in hospital departments facilitated by nurses themselves?*

— *opportunities for belonging were consistently extended?*

— *struggles and/or suffering were openly acknowledged and reflected on in an effort to make sense of them or to learn how they altered one's view or practice?*

— *expressive writing was available electronically for health professionals to record their clinical stories and make them available to others?*

One wonders how many newer nurses might figure out "what makes nursing worth doing, whatever the setting?" Or see how doing nursing work creates quality connections that increases one's sense of belonging? Or how making sense of clinical experiences, including suffering, increases one's own personal growth? Or how many nurses might "feel cared for?" Finally, one speculates how many nurses might be able to find their potential for "embodying the caring behaviors?"

THE MEANING OF SELF-ADVANCEMENT FOR HEALTH SYSTEMS

As discussed earlier in this chapter, many health systems today are preoccupied with measuring outcomes or their failure to achieve high-level outcomes, continuing to collect outcomes data primarily *after care has been delivered.* Ignoring the ongoing contextual factors that characterize the environment, and most importantly, failing to really examine, simplify, and solve the *processes* of care yield little success. Yet processes of care are theoretically and empirically linked to important health outcomes (Brooks-Carthon et al., 2016; Donabedian, 1966; Linetzky et al., 2017; Song et al., 2016). Most health systems characterized this way, however, offer various reasons for their inattention to the obvious; for example, the complexity of the work, poor reimbursement (and not enough resources), the younger workforce, an so on, and do not see the potential near-misses, accidents waiting to happen, or poor processes that might impact their outcomes. Curry et al. (2011) suggest that the daily experience of patients reflects the well-being of a health system.

At this point in time, this author would add that the daily experiences of a health system's workforce also reflects the well-being of that system. Realistically, patients' and employees' daily experiences depend on the organization's norms, including its policies, procedures or unwritten rules. The patient experience below illustrates this point:

> As the husband of a university professor who recently "encountered" the health system, I was horrified by the lack of attention to the basic human needs for information, compassion, and problem solving. Here is our story:
>
> I am a software analyst, father of a little girl with a learning disability and another teen-aged son, and was married to a wonderful woman named Laura who is 48. She was a music professor at a prestigious university in Pennsylvania. She started having lower abdominal pain and intermittent nausea in May 2020, which then progressed to her back. She went to her physician multiple times and was told it was stress or muscle tension. The physician prescribed pain meds and muscle relaxants. Then, finally, in August, she was hospitalized for continued pain and multiple tests. While in the hospital, she called me and said, "They told me I have tumors in my ovaries and abdomen and are sending in an oncologist." By the time I got there, the oncologist had visited and gone, not fully explaining to my wife what her diagnosis, treatment plan, or prognosis was. She was anxious, confused, and needed answers. I asked the nurses what was going on, and they said to wait for the oncologist to return.
>
> For 2 days, we waited for the oncologist to come in and explain what he found in my wife. When he did appear, he very systematically suggested that they would treat the pain effectively with medication, and my wife could go home soon. He still didn't explain the diagnosis. I was so exasperated that I asked the nurses to see the complete medical record. They sent me to the administrative suite where I was told it would be a 72-hour wait since they were so backed up with COVID-19 patients. Although my wife continued to be medicated for pain when she asked for it, and the technicians periodically took her blood pressure, no health professional routinely checked in on her or helped us solve our lack-of-information problem.
>
> I continued to ask for information and as our primary physician did not have privileges at this hospital, I asked if the oncologist could at least call him and discuss the case. I also asked for a second opinion and a transfer because I did not like the

care my wife was receiving—it was matter of fact and procedure based. When we were transferred, my wife's transfer summary was incomplete, which meant the new facility could not provide care for several hours as they tried to coordinate the completion of missing data with the former system.. They couldn't provide pain relief or even food during this time. I had to go down to the cafeteria and get my wife a little something so she could eat.

Finally, they came up with the completed transfer summary, read it, and then let me read my wife's medical record.. It was full of information that would have helped my wife and I receive her poor prognosis better. I sat there astounded that it took 4 days to learn that my beautiful wife had inoperable ovarian cancer with metastasis throughout the abdomen and that no one apparently cared that our lives were almost instantaneously turned upside down. No business would operate this way. Why does the healthcare system get away with such poor service? How can health professionals practice this way?

It is now February 2022 and 2 months since Laura died; our children's lives have been so horribly affected, and our home will never be the same. Her last days were peaceful and pain-free (thanks to hospice), but she had several months of repeated hospitalizations. Her encounters with the health system were substandard at best— poor communication, lack of compassion, inattention to basic hygiene, little information or participation in decisions was offered, leadership was unavailable and, most disturbingly, the clinicians did not seem to care. The Accountable Care Act cannot fix these problems—they are fundamental aspects of the work that are usually not dealt with in the face of other seemingly important issues. I am so frustrated...

Clinical processes such as ensuring the delivery of person-centered care would have made this experience bearable; however, numerous health systems fail to appreciate that simple, relationship-centered attitudes and actions used in clinical care (collective relational capacity), and concurrent ongoing practice improvement may, in fact, help them naturally self-advance.

For example, in high-performing nursing homes, a person-centered approach—one where both residents and employees are at the center—was found to be essential for quality outcomes and maintenance (Asante et al., 2021). Furthermore, over a decade ago, Boehmer (2009) suggested that a common denominator of high performing health systems was that they lived their core values. The same holds true today. Health systems can generate sustained value by prioritizing the human person (patient, family, or employee) through relational caring processes that are expressed in daily work, allowing patients, families, and employees to "feel cared for." Attending to sustaining these conditions provides the relational energy for self-advancement (Figure 9.1).

Relational aspects of professional practice that impact performance at the organizational level have been theorized and well documented by Gittell and her colleagues (Bolton et al., 2021; Gittell et al., 2020; Siddique et al., 2019). Labeled *relational coordination*, Gittell suggests that the interdependent nature of interactions among health professionals is optimized when healthcare teams share purpose and knowledge and exhibit mutual respect that together maximize effective coordination of work. At the organizational level, relational

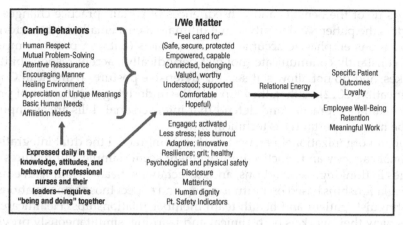

FIGURE 9.1 Prioritizing human persons in health systems.

coordination can be fostered through selective hiring of employees, intervening, measuring and rewarding team performance, resolving cross-disciplinary conflicts proactively, investing in frontline leadership, developing cross-disciplinary care pathways, broadening participation in interdisciplinary patient rounds, and developing shared information systems (Gittell, 2016; Blakeney et al., 2019). The human relational perspective of healthcare, when acknowledged and made explicit as the center of work, includes relationships not only with patients and families but also with other health professionals, oneself, and the communities served.

BOX 9.8: Organizations that attend to the complex interactions in their systems "see" more interconnections in the moment, enable quick adjustments, stay attuned to unfolding relationships longer, are better able to "marry" needs with experience and expertise, and use relationships to solve problems before they spread (or the converse, disseminate solutions to encourage their spread).

Likewise, in self-advancing systems, health professionals (knowledge workers) see their roles as simultaneously practicing and continuously improving the practice. They and their leadership understand that focus on the *process* is key to advancement, and they continuously attend to its accurate performance, rearrangement, revision, and co-creation. The modes of learning about practice are informal, involve relationships, include patients and families, and are sensitive to failures in other organizations (see Chapter 8). For example, errors in other industries provide opportunities for learning about hidden flaws that can be applied to healthcare or assumptions in health systems. Opportunities for practice improvement are often found in routine processes or situations that confront frontline workers versus quality and safety analysts. Frontline workers (those delivering health services, i.e., health professionals) share goals, socialize new members, assign the work, make clinical decisions, create protocols, and learn together. Their focus on the processes of care emphasizes the interdependencies among individuals or departments, better identifies how errors are started, reminds us of the benefits and consequences of certain practice changes, and considers the patient and family as the ultimate focus. Finally, high-performing organizations emphasize accuracy or use of facts (data) in practice improvement, constantly communicate (not just periodically), accept responsibility for mistakes, and do not allow self-serving defensive postures (American Council on Education, 2012). Rather, they tap into the underlying significance of professional healthcare practice and defend that interpersonal skills are as important (maybe more important?) as technical skills.

From an organizational perspective, fully embracing the dual integration of relational capacity and practice improvement seems simple, but requires deep changes in thinking, assumptions, and expectations. Leaders join with employees in relationships based on mutual caring and expect those same relationships to distinguish patient and health team member relationships. Healthcare providers view their work as both clinical and learning, simultaneously providing care while examining ways to improve it. Over time and through experimenting and adapting to practice improvements based on attention to real-time clinical processes, the collective health system begins to accomplish growth naturally while empowering employees and patients alike. The chart in Figure 9.2 serves as a reference point for evaluating self-advancing systems. Starting from the upper left box, health systems where leaders and employees relate well (relational capacity) but do not regularly participate in learning from the work (as described in this book) lack the insight required to engage in practice improvement or are complacent in its importance.

They might also be very focused on measuring performance outcomes or be under-resourced. In the lower left box, both relational capacity and practice improvement are low, indicating that health professionals are very task oriented and prefer the status quo *or* that they do not feel their contributions are recognized. Leadership has little idea about what is going on at the patient level and may perpetuate an overly hierarchical or functional system. Leadership also teeters on trying to please everyone, and in so doing, has strayed from the core aspect of the work. In the lower right box, relational capacity is low while local learning from the work is higher. In this type of organization, practice improvement is seen as important, but departments do not relate well (some withhold

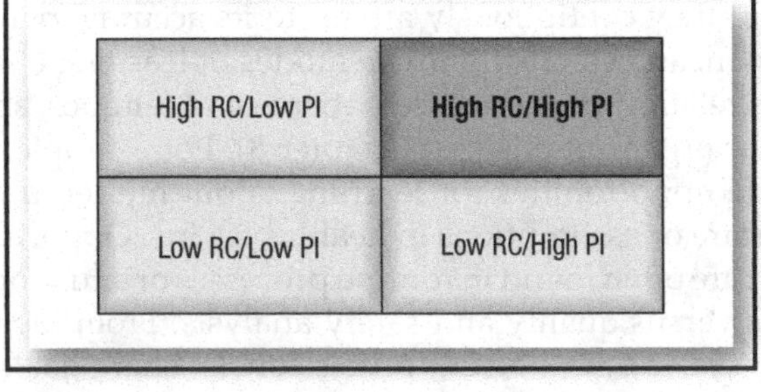

High RC/Low PI	High RC/High PI
Low RC/Low PI	Low RC/High PI

FIGURE 9.2 Reference point for evaluating self-advancing systems.

PI, practice improvement; RC, relational capacity.

information from each other), and there is a lot of competition between people and departments. Employees and some leaders do not feel comfortable outside their own departments, and some continue to advocate for outdated services (sacred cows). Individuals shift blame and deny accountability and view leadership as "in it for themselves." Finally, the upper right box holds the most promise for self-advancement because these systems relate highly (relational capacity) and continuously and regularly learn from the work, improving practice. Clinical practice is always patient centered, based on caring relationships. Characteristics of such systems include:

- a focus on the basics of safe, high-quality, complete and connected patient care
- health professionals and leadership who work together in informal and collegial relationships
- routine encouragement and recognition
- abundant knowledge (learning from the work)
- the patient as *always* part of the decision
- an awareness that outcomes are important, but not all-consuming
- being present but mindful of the future
- holding one another to world-class performance
- small, self-sufficient functional units
- continuous reevaluation
- partnering with stakeholders
- spending time at the bedside

Fully embracing the dual integration of relational capacity and practice improvement, health systems are managing to grow, progress, expand, and without focused attention on outcomes, delivering superior services with high-quality outcomes—that is, they are self-advancing (see Figure 9.3).

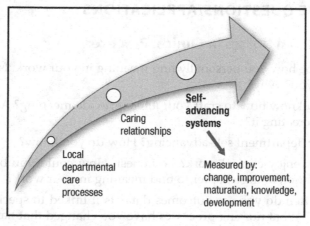

FIGURE 9.3 Self-advancing health systems.

Such advances optimize outcomes, offering value to patients and families, health professionals, and health systems. Caring relationships play a central role and, in fact, energize self-advancing systems. Indeed, such systems are practicing in alignment with their values.

SUMMARY

The last concept in the QCM, self-advancing systems, is introduced and explained in this chapter. It is viewed in a positive light, based on the underlying assumptions about humans and the power of relationships. Focusing on clinical processes as a means of self-advancement is stressed. What self-advancement means to patients and families is described in terms of their unique experiences of care and achievement of self-caring practices. For health professionals, self-advancement is facilitated through genuine caring relationships found in routine clinical practice. The suffering and joys that accompany clinical work can oftentimes provide profound opportunities for generating meaning and ultimately personal growth. Finally, the daily experience of patients and families as well as clinical professionals is characterized as a reflection of a health system's well-being. Relational coordination is explained, and the simultaneous integration of relational capacity and practice improvement is stressed as a means of system advancement.

CALL TO ACTION

Self-advancing health systems effectively use relational capacity and practice improvement to naturally progress, grow, learn, and expand. Embedded in clinical processes, self-advancing systems enhance patient outcomes and expose the meaning of health professionals' work. **Find** the meaning in your work by staying close to the patient and genuinely relating to those with whom you work.

REFLECTIVE QUESTIONS/APPLICATIONS

For Professional Nurses in Clinical Practice:

- Describe how you personally find meaning in your work. Is this important to you? Why?
- Do you know how to craft your job to provide meaning? Are you assertive in creating it?
- Is your department self-advancing? How do you know?
- Do you enjoy clinical work? Be honest. How could you better use the information in this chapter to find meaning in your work?
- How often do you see outcomes data? Is it linked to specific processes of care? What nursing processes have you changed that have positively affected outcomes?

- What have you learned about your own self-advancement as a result of reading this chapter?

- Examine the list of "good, basic, complete nursing care" that is provided in this chapter. Is this occurring on your unit? How often do you assume responsibility for it?

- What is your department's HCAHPS score? What ongoing practice improvements are you involved with that are designed to improve it?

- Nurses report that relating to patients and families holds the most promise for finding meaning in their work. How do you relate to patients and families? Does it help?

For Professional Nurses in Educational Practice:

- How do you teach about progress in health systems? How does this differ in undergraduate and graduate programs?

- Reflect on the need for relational coordination in high-performing organizations. How does this concept translate to the academic enterprise?

- What can you do to help students focus on the importance of good, basic, complete nursing care?

- How might you suggest increasing students' awareness of the meaning and joy associated with clinical work?

- Provide some suggestions for exposing students to the concept of self-advancement.

- As a health professions educator, do any specific potential research questions "pop out" at you as a result of reading this chapter?.

For Professional Nurses in Leadership Practice:

- What is the state of advancement at your organization? How do you know?

- How do you specifically hold yourself and your peers accountable for focusing on the real work of the organization?

- Reflect on the quality improvement process in place at your institution. Does it focus exclusively on outcomes measurement? Are processes of care linked to specific outcomes? Are staff nurses involved in genuine practice improvements? Why or why not? What would it take to revise this?

- How do you facilitate joint relational capacity and practice improvement at your organization?

- Does your leadership team understand the organizational value of the fundamental clinical processes of good, basic, complete nursing care? If not, how will you help them understand?

- In which health systems box of Figure 9.3 does your organization fall? If it is not already in the top right corner, what would it take to move it there?

PRACTICE ANALYSIS

At an academic medical center, pain and functional status of older adults, significant quality outcomes for this population, were observed as problematic. Pain always well controlled was reported by hospitalized older adults as occurring only 58% to 62% of the time (below the national average), and a pain management chart audit ($N = 92$) revealed that regular assessment and nursing knowledge of pain were missing or incorrect 70% of the time. Furthermore, functional decline among older adults was not routinely documented despite the national data that demonstrated the serious nature of this problem as it relates to older adult burden and increased costs. The average length of stay (LOS) for older adults was 5.4 days compared to 3.42 days for all other patients. Finally, only four of the eight domains on the HCAHPS Survey (patient experience of care) reached the 50th percentile for older adults.

In this acute care delivery system, multiple health professionals, organized in separate clinical departments and socialized by discipline, practiced independently. In fact, despite renewed interest in interprofessional collaborative practice (IPCP) education and training, translation of newly acquired behaviors into practice had been slow. Few structures supported it; and after training, health professionals typically reverted to old, traditional modalities of parallel practice. Real IPCP, although known by health professionals to be linked with improved patient outcomes, particularly among hospitalized older adults, was lacking. Health professionals indicated the need to collaborate, but changing long-established clinical workflow was challenging.

A small interprofessional group (two RNs, a clinical pharmacist, an attending physician, and a social worker) began to dialog about the patient population and its needs for improved outcomes. One interested member began to work on an idea of how IPCP could be integrated into the workflow. A model emerged that was person-centered, built upon existing interprofessional education already in existence at the health center, was progressive and comprehensive, and aimed to increase the number of health professionals practicing IPCP (the *process* of patient care). Adopting this approach, the healthcare team would share the common purpose of improving outcomes for older adults and coordinate their work through structured working rounds and expanding the existing nursing performance improvement committee to include all health professionals and interested patients, providing a shared space for dialog about practice improvement. The group committed to try interprofessional rounds with a high degree of participation and use daily structured team checklists and patient input to evaluate and revise their real-time clinical processes. In addition, the re-formed nursing performance improvement committee refocused their work on actionable practice changes that might improve older adults' outcomes. Engaging the team of healthcare providers and patients to examine ways of improving practice was supported by regularly examining patient data looking for patterns, identifying contextual factors and practice patterns that may influence outcomes, and soliciting input from patients. After a couple of informal meetings, the whole group decided to pilot the new approach.

Two clinical units (that admitted most of the older adult population) agreed to implement the IPCP model for 6 months. It was expected that day-to-day activities would be characterized by mutuality, respect, engagement, transparency, accountability, ease, and other like features of cohesive, fully functioning teams, allowing for early recognition of abnormalities, deterrence of errors, more coordinated services, timely responses and anticipation of patient needs, and safe space to raise ideas. During the 6-month time frame, some issues related to leadership during rounds, active participation of members, integrating patients into the membership, and documentation of activities were raised and addressed. Based on the mutual respect and continued engagement of members, however, the innovative team held together and at the end of 6 months, older adult functional decline was reduced by 12%, pain control advanced to greater than 80%, and HCAHPS scores improved slightly.

- What features of high reliability organizations are evident in this case?
- What did the leaders do to support self-advancement in this situation?
- How does this example demonstrate health professionals practicing in alignment with their professional values?

REFERENCES

American Council on Education. (2012). Assuring academic quality in the 21st century: Self-regulation in a new era. A Report of the ACE National Task Force on Institutional Accreditation. http://www.acenet.edu/news-room/Documents/Accreditation-TaskForce-revised-070512.pdf

Asante, B. L., Zúñiga, F., & Favez, L. (2021). Quality of care is what we make of it: A qualitative study of managers' perspectives on quality of care in high-performing nursing homes. *BMC Health Services Research, 21*(1), 1–10.

Bailey, C., Yeoman, R., Madden, A., Thompson, M., & Kerridge, G. (2019). A review of the empirical literature on meaningful work: Progress and research agenda. *Human Resource Development Review, 18*(1), 83–113.

Berwick, D. (2016). *Eight ways to shift the power back to patients*. Twenty-eighth annual National forum on quality improvement in healthcare, concluding address. Institute for HealthCare Improvement. https://www.hhnmag.com/articles/7916-don-berwick-offers-8-ways-to-shift-the-balance-of-power-back-to-patients

Blakeney, A. R., Lavallee, D. C., Baik, D., Pambianco, S., O'Brien, K. D., & Zierler, B. K. (2019). Purposeful interprofessional team intervention improves relational coordination among advanced heart failure care teams. *Journal of Interprofessional Care, 33*(5), 481–489.

Boehmer, R. M. (2009). *Designing care: Aligning the nature and management of health care.* Harvard Business Press.

Bolton, R., Logan, C., & Gittell, J. H. (2021). Revisiting relational coordination: A systematic review. *The Journal of Applied Behavioral Science, 57*(3), 290–322. https://doi.org/10.1177/0021886321991597

Brooks-Carthon, J. M., Lasater, K., Rearden, J., Holland, S., & Sloane, D. M. (2016). Unmet nursing care linked to rehospitalizations among older black AMI patients: A cross-sectional study of US hospitals. *Medical Care, 54*(5), 457–465. https://doi.org/10.1097/MLR.0000000000000519

Carter, J., Ward, C., Wexler, D., & Donelan, K. (2018). The association between patient experience factors and likelihood of 30-day readmission: A prospective cohort study. *BMJ Quality & Safety*, 27(9), 683–690.

Cassel, E. J. (1982). The nature of suffering and the goals of medicine. *New England Journal of Medicine*, 306(11), 639–645. https://doi.org/10.1056/NEJM198203183061104

Cassel, E. J. (1992). The nature of suffering: Physical, psychological, social, and spiritual aspects. In P. L. Stark, & J. P. McGovern (Eds.), *The hidden dimension of illness: Human suffering* (pp. 1–10). National League for—Nursing Press.

Curry, L. A., Spatz, E., Cherlin, E., Thompson, J. W., Berg, D., Ting, H. H., Decker, C., Krumholz, H. M., & Bradley, E. H. (2011). What distinguished top performing hospitals in acute myocardial infarction mortality rates? A qualitative study. *Annals of Internal Medicine*, 154, 384–390. https://doi.org/10.7326/0003-4819-154-6-201103150-00003

Devine, P., O'Kane, M., & Bucholc, M. (2022). Trends, variation, and factors influencing antibiotic prescribing: A longitudinal study in primary care using a multilevel modelling approach. *Antibiotics*, 11(1), 17.

Donabedian, A. (1966). Evaluating the quality of medical care. *Milbank Memorial Fund Quarterly*, 44, 166–206. https://doi.org/10.1111/j.1468-0009.2005.00397.x

Doyle, C., Lennox, L., & Bell, D. (2013). A systematic review of evidence on the links between patient experience and clinical safety and effectiveness. *British Medical Journal Open*, 3(1), e001570. https://doi.org/10.1136/bmjopen-2012-001570

Gittell, J. H. (2016). *Transforming relationships for high performance: The power of relational coordination*. Stanford University Press.

Gittell, J. H., Logan, C., Cronenwett, J., Foster, T. C., Freeman, R., Godfrey, M., & Vidal, D. C. (2020). Impact of relational coordination on staff and patient outcomes in outpatient surgical clinics. *Health Care Management Review*, 45(1), 12–20.

Goldstein, E., Farquhar, M., Crofton, C., Darby, C., & Garfinkel, S. (2005). Measuring hospital care from the patients' perspective: An overview of the CAHPS hospital survey development process. *Health Services Research*, 40(6 pt 2), 1977–1995. https://doi.org/10.1111/j.1475-6773.2005.00477.x

Institute for Healthcare Improvement. (2009). Improving the patient experience of in patient care evidence. http://www.ihi.org/IHI/Topics/PatientCenteredCare/Patient CenteredCareGeneral/EmergingContent/ImprovingthePatientExperienceofIn patientCare.htm

Kleinpell, R., Vasilevskis, E. E., Fogg, L., & Ely, E. W. (2019). Exploring the association of hospice care on patient experience and outcomes of care. *BMJ Supportive & Palliative Care*, 9(1), e13. https://doi.org/10.1136/bmjspcare-2015-001001

Linetzky, B., Jiang, D., Funnell, M. M., Curtis, B. H., & Polonsky, W. H. (2017). Exploring the role of the patient–physician relationship on insulin adherence and clinical outcomes in type 2 diabetes: Insights from the MOSAIc study. *Journal of Diabetes*, 9(6), 596–605. https://doi.org/10.1111/1753-0407.12443

Nelson, K., Hanson, G., Boyce, D., et al. (2022). Organizational impact on healthcare workers' moral injury during COVID-19. *JONA: The Journal of Nursing Administration*, 52(1), 57–66. https://doi.org/10.1097/NNA.0000000000001103

Quigley, D., Reynolds, K., Dellva, S., & Price, R. A. (2021). Examining the business case for patient experience: A systematic review. *Journal of Healthcare Management*, 66(3), 200–224. https://doi.org/10.1097/JHM-D-20-00207

Saad, L. (2020). U.S. Ethics ratings rise for medical workers and teachers. Gallop. https://news.gallup.com/poll/328136/ethics-ratings-rise-medical-workers-teachers.aspx

Siddique, M., Procter, S., & Gittell, J. H. (2019). The role of relational coordination in the relationship between high-performance work systems (HPWS) and organizational performance. *Journal of Organizational Effectiveness: People and Performance*, 6(4), 246–266. https://doi.org/10.1108/JOEPP-04-2018-0029

Silvera, G. A., Wolf, J. A., Stanowski, A., & Studer, Q. (2021). The influence of COVID-19 visitation restrictions on patient experience and safety outcomes: A critical role for subjective advocates. *Patient Experience Journal. 8*(1), 30–39. https://doi.org/10.35680/2372-0247.1596

Song, S., Fonarow, G. C., Olson, D. M., Liang, L., Schulte, P. J., Hernandez, A. F., Peterson, E. D., Reeves, M. J., Smith, E. E., Schwamm, L. H., & Saver, J. L. (2016). Association of get with the guidelines-stroke program participation and clinical outcomes for medicare beneficiaries with ischemic stroke. *Stroke, 47*(5), 1294–1302. https://doi.org/10.1161/STROKEAHA.115.011874

Steger, M. F. (2017). Creating meaning and purpose at work. In L. G. Oades, M. Steger, A. Delle Fave, & J. Passmore (Eds.), *The Wiley Blackwell handbook of the psychology of positivity and strengths-based approaches at work* (pp. 60–81). John Wiley & Sons.

Stevens, E. L., Hulme, A., & Salmon, P. M. (2021). The impact of power on health care team performance and patient safety: A review of the literature. *Ergonomics, 64*(8), 1072–1090. https://doi.org/10.1080/00140139.2021.1906454

The Joint Commission. (2022). Accountability measures. https://www.jointcommission.org/resources/news-and-multimedia/fact-sheets/facts-about-accountability-measures/

Uhl-Bien, M., Meyer, D., & Smith, J. (2020). Complexity leadership in the nursing context. *Nursing Administration Quarterly, 44*(2), 109–116. https://doi.org/10.1097/NAQ.0000000000000407

Veazie, S., Peterson, K., Bourne, D., Anderson, J., Damschroder, L., & Gunnar, W. (2022). Implementing high-reliability organization principles into practice: A rapid evidence review. *Journal of Patient Safety, 18*(1), e320–e328.

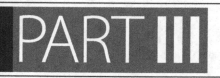

PART III

Leading and Learning in Quality-Caring Health Systems

CHAPTER 10

Leading Quality Caring

"The main thing is to keep the main thing the main thing."

—Stephen R. Covey

CHAPTER OBJECTIVES:

1. Explore the context of clinical practice.
2. Describe the role of appreciative leadership in contemporary healthcare systems.
3. Evaluate the similarities between the caring behaviors in the Quality-Caring Model and contemporary leadership terms.
4. State three challenges of contemporary nursing leaders in a remodeled health system.

THE CONTEXT OF CLINICAL PRACTICE

The delivery of healthcare in the United States is dependent on a workforce that includes multiple health professionals, each operating under unique regulatory guidelines or policies. In addition, there are many assistive personnel who provide necessary services within the system and who contribute to clinical practice. Add to this, the primary customers (patients and families with unique attributes), practice settings (and their varying characteristics), and suppliers (e.g., pharmaceutical companies, device manufacturers, and technology companies). Finally, consider associated organizations responsible for workforce training (universities), research (funding agencies), reimbursement (insurance companies and federal agencies), and system oversight (regulators and accreditors). The multidisciplinary healthcare workforce is but one component in the overall context of healthcare, albeit one that is crucial to its performance.

Although context in health systems is inconsistently defined (Rogers et al., 2020), it is a dynamic concept that includes not only the internal physical setting but also the social environment (Pfadenhauer et al., 2015). Some contextual factors that impact performance have been identified and include organizational culture and climate, leadership, various external factors (e.g., health policy), interpersonal relationships, available resources, patient and health provider characteristics, and workflow (how the work gets done; Rogers et al., 2020). In nursing, "healthy work environments" has become a buzzword for an optimistic context that leaders strive to cultivate and sustain. A healthy work environment for nurses includes "having the appropriate autonomy, adequate staff and resources, and good working relationships with physicians and management" (Schlak et al., 2021, p. 1) and is perceived as a shared responsibility between leaders and those who follow. Yet, unhealthy work environments continue to exist (Kester et al., 2021) and are especially challenging for leadership and employees alike.

Thus, context in healthcare is increasingly complex but is, to a great extent, linked to high-quality clinical outcomes (Hall et al., 2016). Within this complex network of persons, technology, and organizations, there is enormous variation in terms of how the workforce delivers services. Take, for example, the present nursing workforce. As of January 2022, national workforce data on nurses (RNs and licensed vocational nurses [LVNs]) was reported (based on data collected between February 2019 and June 30, 2020; Smiley, 2021). Findings showed the total number of active RN and licensed practical nurse (LPN)/LVN licenses in the United States were 4,198,031 and 944,813, respectively. The median age of RNs was 52 years and that of LPNs/LVNs was 53 years. The nursing workforce was more diverse than in any other study year, and findings suggested the nursing workforce was also more educated and experienced compared to previous years. A mean of 83% of licensed nurses were employed in nursing with roughly two-thirds working full-time. Hospitals and nursing/extended care facilities continued to be the primary practice setting, but nursing incomes were reported flat over time. More than one-fifth of all nurses in the sample reported they plan to retire from nursing over the next 5 years (Smiley et al., 2021). Although encouraged by the rising diversity and educational levels of the nursing workforce in this report, future workforce challenges, specifically related to projected retirements, were anticipated; and many nursing leaders were finding difficulties in recruiting and retaining new nurses as well as challenges engaging existing nurses in the workforce.

For example, numerous studies had previously described differences in hospital RN staffing and concluded that better RN staffing was associated with more favorable patient outcomes, including lower mortality in certain populations (Needleman et al., 2011; Blegen et al., 2011; Griffiths et al., 2016). During the weeks before the first wave of COVID--19, hospital nurses, in particular, were reported to be burned out and working in understaffed conditions (Lasater et al., 2021a). Furthermore, a systematic review found that lower nurse-to-patient ratios and higher nurse workloads were linked to high levels of RN burnout, needlestick and sharps injuries, absenteeism, and intention to leave the job (Assaye et al., 2021). Another systematic review and meta-analysis of 13 published reports conducted between 2000 and 2016 reported that higher nurse-to-patient ratios were linked to higher degrees of burnout, increased job dissatisfaction, and higher intent to leave (Shin et al., 2018). Thus, by 2019, the nursing workforce was reported to be in short supply, stressed, and somewhat detached. Such conditions suggested that despite the modest increase in the nursing workforce in the years prior to COVID-19, it was insufficient to meet the projected demand for professional nursing services.

Add to this an overriding culture in hospitals in which nurses who sign up to work extra, did not complain about regularly missed bathroom or lunch breaks, and who frequently took on unrealistic patient assignments were those who were the most often rewarded. The COVID-19 pandemic has made this draining work environment more unhealthy and often intolerable for many nurses.

Important in this discussion of context is that prior to COVID-19, the demand for nurses also included a more sophisticated workforce: more knowledgeable, technologically savvy, and relationally skilled. This maturing nursing workforce was gradually evolving *prior* to COVID-19 in order to meet increased patient needs for high-quality, complex services. In particular, proficiency in new technologies, including adequate use of the electronic health record (EHR), special monitoring equipment, mobile, wearable technologies, and participation in evidence-based improvements and other professional governance activities was expected of direct care RNs. In summary, the working conditions and increased expectations of RNs were negatively affecting how health services, particularly those in acute care, were provided *prior* to COVID-19.

During the first wave of the pandemic, reports proliferated about the heroic efforts of healthcare professionals, particularly frontline personnel. However, as the pandemic lingered, it exposed and intensified the already longstanding unhealthy work environment issues that have encumbered nurses for years. It was not until 2021 and early 2022 that we began to see peer-reviewed papers correctly reporting on these conditions. Over the course of the pandemic, worsening workloads; lack of appropriate supplies, equipment, and services required to deliver adequate patient care; and the ethical dilemmas common to COVID-19 contributed to existing nurses' burnout and added the dimension of moral suffering and even moral injury (Lake et al., 2021; Nelson et al., 2022). Unfortunately, many health systems leaders responded with modified staffing and/or resilience building programs that concentrated on the nurses themselves versus modifying ongoing infrastructure policies and practices (Schlak et al., 2022). For example, in one acute care hospital, non-clinical workers were encouraged to provide "supplemental staffing" as "nurse extenders" by supporting the RN's ability to serve more patients. Unfortunately, this program backfired because, although their intentions were good, the extenders needed a lot of direction and could not assist in isolated areas or with direct patient contact. The RNs found the program "more trouble than it was worth." Another health system created a resiliency committee with multiple nurse leaders and a few staff nurses. After several months of meetings, they decided to create "time-out rooms" so that nurses (and other clinical employees) could take a few quiet minutes to "regroup" during stressful moments. Although this was a great step, it again only addressed the nurses' resilience and failed to address the systems' responsibilities.

On the other end of the spectrum, however, some health systems have created much-needed employee wellness programs. For example, at Rush University Medical Center, wellness rounds, a wellness consult service, an advanced mental health intervention program, and a central wellness resource hub with wellness rooms on frontline floors were rapidly established (Adibe et al., 2021). Although several hurdles had to be overcome, over time, the program came to be well received and used with more staff interacting about their anxieties and worries. An important lesson learned in this program was the need for a senior level champion who provided system-level focus, support, recognition, and advocacy for the program.

Nonetheless, according to Schlak et al. (2022), if changes to address nurses' well-being solely target changing the individual in the absence of supportive policy and administrative improvements, they are likely to further contribute to the demoralization of the workforce. An example of this is the continued supplementation of nurse staffing with contract nurses. Such actions, over time, frustrate permanently employed staff nurses who cannot earn the same salary and may have additional duties compared to their traveling counterparts. Ultimately, this short-term fix only encourages more turnover among permanently employed nurses who only want to feel valued, safe, and recognized for their expertise related to quality patient care. To put it another way, leveraging this time in history to re-evaluate nursing work (and its conditions) and create moral communities (Wocial, 2018) where employees and leaders together

- engage in deliberations and negotiations about the right course of action,
- demonstrate supportive relationships,
- embrace honest mistakes as opportunities to learn, not reasons to punish,
- build relationships with intention and founded on respect,
- engage in discussions together to resolve conflicts, remaining focused on the issue and not the people, and
- feel free (and safe) to explore emotionally charged issues.

(Wocial, 2018)

As the healthcare delivery system continues to rebound from the changes caused by COVID-19, creating the conditions where nurses are genuinely affirmed for their contributions and included in system-level decision-making, hold realistic assignments and responsibilities, receive adequate and timely continuing education matched to their roles, are fairly compensated, and are able to confidentially participate in system-sponsored wellness programs without blame or stigma is crucial. Supporting the context of nursing work in this way encourages and reinforces the commitment to humanity that health professionals are called to honor and boosts the workforce, enabling its endurance. Authentically practicing nursing leadership is key.

LEADERSHIP AS A PRACTICE

Nursing as a practice responds to societal needs for health and wellness services, is based on ethical principles, and provides safe, quality care in accordance with disciplinary standards. Furthermore, nursing is holistic in that it considers the whole person, including the environment. In the social realm, nursing's human-interactional capacity uniquely situates nurses to advance interactions, to reinforce relationships between health professionals and patients, to find solutions, and to foster positive experiences for patients and health professionals. Such actions are proactive, inclusive, and, oftentimes, innovative. Ethical principles guide this practice that is provided by competent individuals with advanced knowledge, skills, and attitudes. Patient–nurse relationships are the primary context of nurses' practice and a core part of the nurses' role (Duffy, 2018; Hartley et al., 2020).

Just as nurses repeatedly apply their expertise directly in clinical settings, nurses in leadership positions *practice* by performing recognized leadership behaviors (processes) that support and advance clinical nursing practice. Using the lens of practice, the focus of leadership is on the *actions* of leaders, rather than on their traits or skills. In particular, relationships between leader(s) and employees, including helping to derive meanings from reality, developing a collective identity, and enabling actions are paramount. Repeated relational leadership actions provide experiences that improve leader performance, refine knowledge, build confidence, and facilitate advanced skills such as group presentations or facilitating interprofessional meetings. As well, regularly applying leadership actions in this manner helps nurse leaders gain confidence in their leadership abilities. Translating leadership theories and evidence into practice yields *best* practice. Thus, nursing leadership practice includes the application of best leadership evidence, disciplinary and system values, and relational processes to facilitate innovative responses to ongoing challenges, shaping ongoing advancement. In so doing, nurse leaders champion, defend, advocate for, and reinforce excellence in clinical nursing practice, ultimately advancing health systems' goals.

BOX 10.1: As leaders of nursing (and oftentimes nurses themselves), nursing administrators are guiding a practice whose first responsibility is to patients and families, that bears responsibility for providing competent, high-quality services, and that is uniquely qualified to advance relationships that improve the human experience. Appreciating, strengthening, and expanding these unique attributes of nursing practice is the first priority of nursing administration!

However, in the spirit of improving patient experiences, well-intentioned health systems' executives and some nursing leaders have adopted customer service models to promote better relationships between clinicians and patients. Examples include the practice of scripting nurses' patient interactions, consultation agreements, or hardwiring interactional procedures into the workflow, such as intentional hourly rounding. This structured process whereby nurses conduct hourly checks on patients using a standardised protocol and documentation, was imagined to improve compassionate care. However, one qualitative study of 33 nurses, 17 senior nurse managers, 34 patients, and 28 family carers using individual, semi-structured interviews in England found little evidence that intentional rounding enhanced the comfort, safety or dignity of patients or increased the delivery of compassionate care. The systematised approach, together with check-off documentation of its completion, was deemed more transactional or task-oriented rather than relational or individualised to patient needs (Sims et al., 2020). Such an approach does not encompass real caring relationships that include mutual problem solving, human respect, attentive reassurance, encouragement, appreciation of unique meanings, fostering of a healing environment, attending to basic and affiliation needs—that is, the caring behaviors. Rather, in this customer service–oriented approach, the connections established between patients and health professionals are functional, often superficial, and represent "one more box to check off."

In the world outside of healthcare, *customers* are generally healthy individuals who are often purchasers of products or services. They are considered equal or similar to the merchant. Patients, on the other hand, are generally unhealthy, vulnerable, and/ or seeking better health. In such a state, they are oftentimes dependent on clinicians (less than equal), are frequently fearful and in pain, and somewhat confused (see Chapter 4). Furthermore, a critical knowledge gap exists between health professionals and patients/families, creating further imbalance. Patients are seeking better health and relief from suffering and trust health professionals to keep them safe, ensure their dignity as worthy humans, effectively providing relief from discomfort, and inclusion in decision making. Using a customer-service approach changes the fundamental nature of clinical practice from a moral, relational, and therapeutic practice to a prearranged, structured series of interactions and tasks. In essence, the customer service–oriented approach, including forced scripting and structured tasks, may actually distract nurses even further from interacting in the authentic manner that characterizes caring patient relationships—the key to positive patient experiences.

Unlike retail services, healthcare involves a deeper level of human interaction with less predictable outcomes and in which multiple choices exist. "Nurses encounter patients in their most vulnerable moments, sharing an intimacy found in few other human relationships" (Chambliss, 1996, p. 1). Such intimacy is associated with self-disclosure, touch, emotions such as trust and empathy, and closeness (Kirk, 2007) and is a professional behavior (based on the professional code of conduct) nurses use in the context of therapeutic patient-nurse relationships; it balances the private work they do to meet patient needs at the bedside with the more technological or scientific work they do. Professional intimacy is a "professional" behavior in that it is founded on deep values about the worth of humans and includes respecting another's privacy. It is a learned professional skill that develops over time. As Antonytheva et al. (2021) put it, "Intimacy in nursing fosters closeness, trust, self-disclosure, and reciprocity through emotional and/ or physical forms that can influence both patient and nurse outcomes" (p. 158). Furthermore, professional intimacy requires knowledge, relational skills, and ethical comportment. It is significant to patients and families and may influence the patient experience.

BOX 10.2: Genuine intimacy is integral to professional nursing practice and requires authentic engagement and advocacy on patients' behalf. Such care demands a closeness and relational quality that, without an organizing framework, can get lost in the workflow of endless priorities. The intimacy contained in the patient–nurse relationship is an expectation that shapes patients' experiences but becomes marginalized when delegated to caregivers who are trained only in task completion or when nurses themselves do not embrace its professional nature. Safeguarding the patient-nurse relationship, including its intimacy, is an obligation of nursing leadership.

Consider this example:

A 45-year-old female was admitted to a large Magnet® designated hospital for a spontaneous pneumothorax. With a chest tube in place, she had daily chest x-rays and was ordered a routine EKG as well. A male technician from another country approached the woman to perform the EKG. He could not speak the language well, but used a script to explain what he was going to do. He proceeded to open the woman's gown, exposing her fully. He placed the leads on her chest and began the EKG machine all the while assuming he was doing his job correctly. He did not close the curtains or safeguard the woman's privacy, but continued on as though nothing was amiss. Although the procedure only lasted about 8 minutes, the woman was extremely embarrassed and felt humiliated having a male technician who did not advocate for her basic human need for privacy, but rather considered his job so matter-of-factly—as a task or procedure that needed to get done.

A professional nurse would have understood the importance of this woman's privacy to her human worthiness and the overall hospital experience and would have safeguarded it while performing the EKG. After all, it falls under the caring behavior, human respect, and is linked to human dignity! Despite the commercialistic or business-like approach to healthcare, nursing's fundamental commitment to persons in their care remains constant. This devotion to patients is the basis for nursing's codes of ethics and standards of practice (see Chapter 2) and is protected through various state practice acts.

BOX 10.3: As leaders of a professional practice, nursing leadership is morally obligated to ensure that patients' privacy and confidentiality are protected by preserving the foundational caring patient–nurse relationship that gives nursing its identity, ensures ethical and legal services, and provides individual nurses with meaning.

The American Organization of Nurse Leadership (AONL) describes numerous competencies required of nurse leaders (AONL, 2015a, 2015b). Examples include the following: to ensure compliance with the State Nurse Practice Acts, State Boards of Nursing regulations, regulatory agency standards, and policies of health systems; to champion patient care; to ensure quality and nursing professionalism; to hold self and others accountable for actions and outcomes; to uphold ethical principles; to allocate nursing resources based on acuity; to involve nurses in decisions that reflect their practice; and to create environments that facilitate teams to initiate actions that produce results. Setting expectations, upholding ethical principles, and holding each other accountable strike this author as particularly aligned with the caring patient-nurse relationships (as described above). These competencies call for leaders who have the courage to "go against the grain" and intentionally focus on the fundamental work of the organization—quality patient care—as their number one priority. Appreciating and preserving caring relationships, foundational to nursing, provides the opportunity to enhance quality and showcase the value of nursing to the overall healthcare enterprise.

Interestingly, many of the AONL leadership competencies call for the performance of relational leadership strategies. For example:

> ... build collaborative relationships, exhibit effective conflict resolution skills, create a trusting environment by following through on promises and concerns, establishing mechanisms to follow up on commitments, balancing the concerns of individuals with organizational goals and objectives, engaging staff and others in decision making, communicating in a way as to maintain credibility and relationships, establish an environment that values diversity (e.g., age, gender, race, religion, ethnicity, sexual orientation, and culture) ... (AONL, 2015a, 2015b)

Thus, the practice of nursing leadership includes actions that are performed "in relationship" that uphold the ethical principles, scopes of practice and standards of performance that undergird professional nursing practice. Especially now, in this crucial time of remodeling the healthcare system, the practice of nursing leadership must focus on creating the conditions for promising and meaningful nurse work. This includes facilitating genuine interprofessional teamwork, demonstrating with data the contributions of nursing to patient outcomes (allowing nursing to be viewed as an asset versus an expense), leveraging technology to reduce burden, noticing and reminding nurses often of the meaningful work they do, and using leadership evidence to mutually make decisions. Nursing leadership as a practice requires the cessation of ineffective, isolated, top-down decision-making; increased clinical presence; the use of best leadership evidence; serious reflection and competency-development; increased emphasis on the well-being of all persons; and increased attention to relationships, specifically those rooted in the caring behaviors!

CONTEMPORARY LEADERSHIP IN A REMODELED HEALTH SYSTEM

The world today seems so much more complex and needy compared to just a few years ago! This altered, unique, and strange state of affairs rules out clear answers or quick fix solutions. Rather, it demands rapid adaptation by leaders that embrace fresh relational approaches, particularly those that include joint learning (grasping or understanding challenges in their entirety) and rapid innovation (novel and sometimes unfamiliar ideas and behaviors).

Better understanding of complex adaptive systems (CAS) has invigorated the meaning of leadership in recent years. Complex adaptive systems rapidly adapt and change (self-organize) in response to complex conditions or challenges in order to ensure their long-term survival (see Chapter 3). Leadership, therefore, is not situated in a person; rather, it represents the ability to successfully respond to ongoing ambiguity and its resulting insecurity. Known as *complexity* leadership (Uhl-Bien & Marion, 2009), adaptation and innovation require process-oriented, contextual, and interactive (shared and relational) leadership approaches. In this more complex way of leading, both leaders and followers engage by asking tough questions or having difficult conversations about existing tensions or challenges and then co-create adaptive responses that enable creative shifts in behavior or new services (emergence), all in a protective *safe space* created by the leader (Uhl-Bien, 2021). The subsequent new behaviors and patterns emerge not from the deliberate choice of the agents, but rather as a result of the combined characteristics occurring in the systems and/or the behaviors of the agents within it. Leaders, working collaboratively with followers and others, enhance the overall adaptability and capacity of health systems to help them operate better (Uhl-Bien et al., 2020). The role of a leader is to facilitate the process of emergence by enabling the conditions (safe space, flow of information and knowledge, capturing creativity from the ground up, and fostering the multiple interactions and interdependencies among agents) that influence organizational innovation.

For example, RN retention in today's world cannot be *resolved*; rather, it can only be *addressed* by understanding the relationships and challenges that permeate places where nurses work; health systems administrators; nurse leaders; other health professionals; clinical workflow; work environments; and by understanding how individual nurses interact in these spaces. It is a complex problem requiring a comprehensive and innovative response that is developed through adaptive processes. In short, tweaking policies, adjusting salaries, marketing gimmicks and other quick fixes will not address nurse retention without a good understanding of how these resources will be enacted locally. Through ongoing interactions among leaders, followers, and stakeholders, a better understanding (learning) of how nurses work within health systems may activate new creative ideas or behaviors to unfold (rapid innovation). Positive relational approaches may advance organizations and people even further.

According to Porter-O'Grady & Malloch (2021), "*Appreciative* leadership is a positive mental model and framework for leadership practices that is an expression of the response to complexity" (p. 18). The leader's role is appreciative as it enables the contribution of persons who participate in the work of the system, adding value to it (Porter-O'Grady & Malloch, 2021). To that end, five principles guide the work of appreciative leaders:

- relational capacity to mobilize accountability
- a significant level of self-awareness and self-confidence
- exceptional skills in the expression of leadership language and leader role obligations
- authoritative competence and performance in the role that results in a definitive and intentional impact
- consistent and continuous integrity and inclusion

(Malloch & Porter-O'Grady, 2022)

Leadership, specifically nursing leadership, responds to the complexity of contemporary health systems by practicing responsively and ethically to meet society's needs for safe, quality care. Using appreciative leadership principles, practicing leadership is more about facilitating the progress of health systems toward a robust future, while simultaneously upholding disciplinary values. Noticeably, the key to leading in this manner is relationship competence.

Relationships (particularly those characterized as caring) provide an untapped resource for organizational advancement, growth, and/or renewal. Seen from this perspective, continuous interactions and relationship building form a paradigm for leadership that frames it as connected, interdependent, organic, alive, creative, and whole. It is from this standpoint that the health system continuously recreates itself. Moreover, as described in Chapter 9, the quality of relationships within health systems often counters the stresses and burdens of complexity and constant change.

Leadership centered on relationships as an essential competency acknowledges the interdependent nature of human beings and recognizes that self-advancement (individual and system) occurs naturally in complex systems, but spreads more effectively and efficiently if the leadership attends to relationships. The leader's role is to cultivate an ethos of inclusion, create safe space for genuine dialogue and the voicing of ideas, facilitate information and ongoing learning, hold up professional standards, and allow health professionals to adapt their practice in ways that are meaningful to them. As Brown (2017) states, "If leaders really want people to show up, speak out, take chances, and innovate, they have to create cultures where people feel safe—where their belonging is not threatened by speaking out and they are supported when they make the decision to brave the wilderness, stand alone, and speak truth" (p. 93). Such leadership sees the human person in the employee and vulnerability in the eyes of patients and families. It recognizes the inherent caring nature of health professionals and honors the special relationships they have with patients, families, and each other. Authentically caring for others provides leaders with the permission to give people direction, help them align with organizational purpose, and provide the affirmative and positive energy to get the job done.

Most health systems' leaders are aware of the importance of relationships—on balance, healthcare is built on relationships. However, amid the hectic demands of day-to-day work, persistent crises, and the unyielding pressure to perform and innovate, leaders often act in ways that even they know are uninspiring or less than compassionate. The rationale or excuse given at the time is, "They know I care," or "I don't have the time," or "They are professionals—they can deal with it." The effect of such reasoning contributes to a downward spiral of interactions and patterns of behavior (avoidance and working to the job description) that diminish further relationships and eventually retard forward progression—self-advancement.

BOX 10.4: Nurse leaders who appreciate the caring relationships that nurses have with patients and families understand and work hard to preserve them; after all, these relationships provide the life lessons and ongoing renewal that inspire clinical nurses to continue their important work!

As a practice, nursing leadership is a process that occurs in context—the context of clinical work and the environment where it is delivered as well as in the interactions and bureaucracies that shape the work. Relationships are central to these processes—attending to them with vigor (using caring processes) stimulates openness, innovative solutions, and adaptation to change. With this perspective, leading is always a process of relating; creating meanings (or sense-making), sharing responsibilities, collective dialoguing, moving forward interdependently, and co-evolving new patterns. Collectively, such processes enhance the capacity of systems to advance. Leadership, then, occurs at the relationship level—not at the individual authority or supervisory level. This revised version of leadership practice is more horizontal (versus vertical or top-down) and enhances, through relational responses, the forward movement of the system. Such a way of being recognizes the crucial role that all individuals play in health systems and uses this recognition to exploit their creativity. In times of conflict, appreciative leaders use evidence and a "person-centered-ness" ethic to enable viable solutions or decisions. Practicing in this manner demonstrates the value of individual health professionals and the discipline of nursing, is inclusive, and generates a positive impact on the health system.

The practice of leadership in a remodeled health system then requires systems thinkers who optimize human interactions/relationships, enabling "feeling cared for" to fuel a common purpose and interdependent actions, allowing change/innovation to emerge. They are authentic, empower others, and consider caring relationships the foundation of their work. This type of leader views decision making from a relationship-focused versus a power-based perspective. Using personal and disciplinary values, tomorrow's nursing leadership challenges many impulsive, reflexive actions and often takes the appropriate time to reflect on how potential options will impact others. Appreciative leaders are approachable, strive for harmony among their employees, and focus on interaction, conversations, and dialoguing while working to build trust. They also admit when they are wrong and seek constructive criticism. Most importantly, they act in ways that connect and re-connect nursing to disciplinary values. Consider the following leadership example as relayed to this author by Dawn Johnson, a nurse practioner and former student in the Indiana University School of Nursing nurse practitioner program:

One of the most amazing leaders I had the privilege to learn under was the vice principal at a special needs school where I worked with autistic children. She was authentic! She was intelligent, always available, and knowledgeable about the children and the system. She navigated personalities above and below her with amazing grace and resolve. She loved the children, loved her job, and was confident in her role with no excuses. She would apologize when she was wrong and be outspoken when necessary. What I was most impressed with was when I first met her, she was on the ground holding a child in a basket hold, keeping him from banging his head against a concrete wall. She was not a big lady by any means, and she was in her dress suit for a meeting. All the while, she was directing staff on removal of the other children. As soon as the child calmed down, she gave him a big hug and told him she loved him. He was big enough that he could have hurt her if she had not gotten the upper hand. It all happened very quickly. I thought to myself, now this is a lady I could follow to hell and back.

Or this example:

One night I was on fire watch in Afghanistan, which is late night watch while everyone else sleeps. I heard footsteps walking up to my post ... it had to be 0100. I look up, and it's the battalion commander. I quickly stood up straight and greeted him. He said, "Relax, I wanted to come stand watch with you for a bit." This was amazing to me as I didn't think he even knew my name—he oversaw approximately 1,000 Marines. He proceeded to ask me about my background and why I wanted to serve. I could tell that he really wanted to get an idea about who I was and how I felt about the mission. He commended me often and made me feel bigger than I was. He told me something that I will never forget; he said, "Son, the best advice I can give you is as you advance in leadership, never ask someone to do something that you wouldn't do." He won me that night as he let me know that I mattered, and I felt appreciated.

(Benjamin Hanenkratt, PMHNP-BC, former student, Indiana University
School of Nursing, and U.S. Marine)

What aspects of appreciative leadership are present in these examples?

Appreciative leaders are visible, engage often, are passionate about the work, lead by example, solicit input, make the time to dialogue and understand employees, facilitate "feeling cared for," and encourage employees' feedback. Regularly interacting with employees (not just at evaluation time) to discuss new challenges, what is working and what is not, and identifying upcoming complexities is key.

Although we have more immediate access to information than ever before, it can never replace the real human connection of in-person recognition, ongoing communication, including listening, sharing, and coming to know one another. Such actions by leaders engage, empower, respect, build up, and reassure, providing the affirmative ("I matter") fuel necessary for co-creating success. This ongoing presence with employees (how tomorrow's leaders will spend their time) also enhances the leader's relationship skills—that is, relational capacity—a critical attribute of successful leadership and organizational advancement.

In summary, relationally centered nursing leaders care about themselves as humans, about the values and purpose of the health systems in which they work, about the persons they work with (employees, clinicians, and administrators across the system), about the patients and families (customers) they serve; about safe, high quality health services (excellence), and about the community. Examples of caring relationships and contemporary leadership behaviors used by relationally centric leaders are presented in Table 10.1.

At the heart of appreciative leadership is a different employer–employee relationship that de-emphasizes status (e.g., dress, offices, position, and power) and reemphasizes colleagueship and innovation by providing interesting and meaningful work in healthy environments. Such leaders stay present to self and others and remain steadfast during crises and periods of doubt. Doing so requires leaders who lead from within, that is, halting the "thinking and doing"

TABLE 10.1 Caring Relationships and Contemporary Leadership Behaviors

Caring Relationships	Contemporary Leadership Behaviors
Self	*Appreciate self as a relational human being *Remain self-aware; maintain presence; practice self-reflection *Honor the self by regularly practicing self-caring (see Chapter 4) use the caring behaviors with self *Role-model self-caring *Share vulnerabilities *Integrate "being" and "doing"
Patients and families—excellence in safe, high quality health services	*Interact regularly with patients and families using the caring behaviors *Engage those closest to the patient in performance improvement activities *Maintain robust and transparent systems of feedback about patient outcomes *Recognize excellence, reward creativity and innovation in patient care *Create safe space (*just cultures*) for performance improvement *Set expectations for excellence in accordance with nursing standards of practice and state nurse practice acts, accreditation and regulatory agencies, and organizational policies *Ensure that organizational clinical policies and procedures are reviewed and updated in accordance with best evidence *Ensure the ethical practice of nursing, including patient confidentiality, the protection of human subject rights, and safety in clinical research *Promote systems thinking
Health systems: align with values & purpose	*Place patients and families first *Assume accountability for own performance in line with the organization's values and purpose *Create expectations and safe space for routinely connecting to organizational values and purpose—attending to, dialoguing, and centering on at every level *Hold people accountable for their performance in alignment with organizational values and purpose *Support enabling conditions for aligning with purpose
Human persons	*Assume people are capable of growth and change; demonstrate belief in them *Use the caring behaviors with all individuals *Remain visible—interacts often and effectively *Engage all (outside of staff meetings) for dialogue about clinical work, including assignments, workflow, targets, ideas, improvements and challenges *Encourage contributions *Recognize that engagement increases when persons are regularly included in decision-making *Enable learning—fosters sensemaking *Cultivate a culture of inquiry; ask and encourage questions *Translate the work of nursing into familiar terms to demonstrate how it contributes to patient and health system value.

(*continued*)

TABLE 10.1 Caring Relationships and Contemporary Leadership Behaviors (*continued*)

Caring Relationships	Contemporary Leadership Behaviors
Community	*Maintain openness, honesty, transparency, inclusion, and equity *Solicit feedback *Assess "feeling cared for" regularly and responds accordingly Support collaboration across disciplines Challenge uncivil bahavior *Build networks & relationships *Practice inclusion *Consider social determinants of health and equitable services *Engage with community to address health issues; e.g., substance use, vaccinations, wellness clinics *Serve on community groups *Facilitate employee contributions to community

mode long enough to reflect, become aware, "to be," and cultivate the self. As an executive leadership practice, the capacity to care for self, comprising one's physical health, including diet and exercise, adequate sleep, and the social, emotional, and spiritual self is necessary. However, nurse leaders at all levels need time for renewal to continuously remain in relationship mode! Department-level leaders (clinical nurse managers) in particular, are pivotal to the success of health systems through their ongoing appreciation for healthy work environments (i.e., caring cultures).

The department-level leader who is self-aware brings staff members together, keeps them informed, and helps them learn about and use challenges to innovate. Using caring relationships as the foundation, departmental nurse leaders foster inclusivity and encouragement to promote the emergence of novel ideas and behaviors. Department-level leaders have a central position in health systems that reinforces their "broker" roles in creating value. Ultimately, such middle-level leadership is a precious resource in steering health systems toward self-advancement.

BOX 10.5: Reinforcing the purpose (what we are here for) and translating that purpose to the bedside through caring relationships sets the tone of a department. Through visible and hands-on leadership, department-level leaders look for and encourage the practice improvements that health professionals construct. Acting as resources for frontline health professionals and peers, they actively pose questions, provide feedback, and help employees find meaning in their work. Maintaining a constant focus on the centrality of caring relationships, department-level leaders encourage employees to contribute and over time, individuals interact, learn, and innovate.

Executive nurse leaders, on the other hand, preserve cultures of caring across health systems by upholding a focus on caring relationships, demonstrating their high priority. Responding to challenges, activating accountability, and consistently reminding employees how they contribute influences positive interactions that fuel advancement. Especially during times of conflict, staying "in relationship" by keeping an open mind and continuing to dialogue leads to deeper connections that, over time, may bring about new patterns or responses.

The largest challenge facing all nurse leaders today is the demand for competent nurses in a world where scarce resources limit availability. Some are saying the current model is "not sustainable" and are demanding new practice models that use less RNs and more unlicensed personnel. Others have already moved in this direction. Without carefully thinking this through, however, a rush to create new practice models, especially those with fewer RNs, may, in turn, negatively impact the quality and safety of care. Sustained evidence has shown that more RNs are associated with better patient outcomes (Lasater et al., 2021b; Al-Amin et al., 2022). Difficult decisions regarding capacity, staffing ratios, job descriptions, and training are already starting to be made. Taking an appreciative (relational) stance to better understand and dialogue, rather than acting quickly and reflexively, however, may be the necessary ingredient for a more successful, long-term innovation (Table 10.2).

TABLE 10.2 Benefits and Challenges of Contemporary Leadership in a Remodeled Health System

Benefits	Challenges
Accountable employees who positively contribute to ongoing challenges	*Requires relational capacity, presence, listening skills, vulnerability, inquiring stance (asking relevant questions), authentic dialog
Engaged professionals	*Requires time and training
	*Uncomfortable/sometimes painful encounters
	*May advantage persons with assertive personalities
	*May take longer for action (but produce better outcomes)
Enhanced professionalism	*Requires activating accountability
Healthy work environments	*Unpredictable situations may disrupt
	*Increased costs
	*Requires thorough understanding of safe practice, patient care delivery systems, clinical workflow
	*Requires adequate resource management & nurse autonomy over practice
Teamwork	*Requires effective communication, conflict resolution and interprofessionalism skills
	*Some may receive a benefit without adequate contribution
Refined leadership skills	*Requires balancing separateness and ongoing interaction
	*May lead to overconfidence
Source of pride	*Requires placing clinical practice (focus on patients and families) first
	*Requires recognition of contributions
Positive patient experiences Improved patient outcomes	*Requires time and investment, use of data to inform decisions, dissemination strategies, & ongoing feedback
Self-caring employees	*Requires resourcing strategically
	*Ensuring meaningful work
	*Safeguarding persons' health

ACCELERATING LEARNING AND INOVATION IN HEALTH SYSTEMS

The present and upcoming technological advancements, together with the workforce effects related to COVID-19, has left many health systems and nursing educational programs unprepared to confront significant challenges. Developing, implementing, and evaluating new ways of doing nursing work in health systems is a significant nursing leadership challenge (Cassidy et al., 2021). One example is the difficulty implementing evidence-based practice in hospitals. After considerable years promoting evidence-based practice through education and other programs, nurses still are not regularly implementing evidence in practice (Dagne & Beshah, 2021). Another example is the integration (or lack thereof) of professional practice models into clinical workflow.

First, much confusion still exists concerning what a professional practice model is and how it is similar or different from nursing theory, shared governance, patient-care delivery systems, and the like. Within the AACN Magnet model component of exemplary nursing practice, professional practice models are considered a pivotal element with the expectation that they will be incorporated into practice and eventually tied to important achievements, for example, positive or improved patient and nurse outcomes. However, busy health systems have found it challenging and costly to embrace new processes and responsibilities, resulting in the inability to effectively move these models into practice (Duffy, 2016). This phenomenon is a leadership and systems issue that contributes to wasted resources and produces disappointed users. More importantly, the disparity between an acknowledged professional practice model and its use in everyday practice obstructs the advancement of nursing and delays the attainment of important patient health outcomes, negatively affecting organizational costs and quality of services. Nursing leaders create the environment, mobilize staff, attach the resources, and provide guidance to integrate such models into health systems. Why is their implementation and evaluation still so fragmented? Does it have anything to do with the relational aspect of nursing leadership?

Dialoguing about the roles and responsibilities of nurses and those who support them, various communication mechanisms, resources, and the environment in which nurses work are foundational to nursing leadership roles. Yet, somehow, learning together about how nursing work might be assigned, planned, implemented, and evaluated, determining accountability for care completion, appropriate staff mix, responsible numbers of staff, how members communicate, what the environment looks like, and so on remains threatening enough to prevent the engagement required to operationalize some professional practice models. The impact of professional practice models to improve nursing-sensitive processes and outcomes relies on how well they are embedded within or translated into the culture and practices of nurses (Mensik et al., 2017). Thus, evidence of the impact of professional practice models remains underdeveloped, further limiting the demonstration of nursing's impact! (Joseph et al., 2022).

The present demands for safe, high quality healthcare amidst a disconcerting nursing shortage requires rapid adaptation that hopefully takes advantage of nursing's expertise. Without nursing's expertise, it may become someone else's role to facilitate nursing practice changes! In this situation, nursing leaders no longer have the time to wait until "we are over this crisis" or "we hire a new educator" or "we have more resources." Accelerating practice changes requires implementation and evaluation approaches that are appreciative.

Using the example of professional practice model integration, careful consideration of the model and how nursing work gets done might be better understood (learned) after collaboration and dialogue among clinical nurses, nursing assistants, nurse educators, and nursing leaders. Ongoing learning in this manner allows new ideas generated from the model to inform practice changes. Following up with an implementation schedule and an evaluation plan that are carefully designed to take advantage of the newly generated ideas and the people who will implement the change locally will help assure its operationalization. Essential components to consider include how members will be included in the implementation and the change evaluated , what the indicators of success will be, ongoing education and support required, regular feedback, and the evaluation process.

Accelerating how evidence-based ideas and practices are integrated into nursing work across health systems is a leadership responsibility that has been somewhat relaxed and under-resourced. This time in history, however, is a unique turning point in nursing; one that requires courage, boldness, and rapid but thoughtful action. Nursing's expertise and deep understanding of clinical needs offer nurse leaders the advantage of accelerating learning, innovation, adaptation, and innovation. Clinical nurses know how to improve efficiency, optimize workflow, and safeguard safety and quality, but need support and assistance to bring forth their ideas. With a relational stance, nurse leaders can facilitate the reimagining of existing systems and processes through brainstorming together, creating prototypes, and evaluating their benefit. Inspiring and supporting nurses to adapt to the current complexity through appreciative leadership will ensure that the caring relationships grounding the discipline will endure.

USING THE QCM TO LEAD

Exemplary nursing leadership is "relationship-oriented and understands the wisdom of actively involving others and investing in partnerships, trustworthy cooperative relationships and team-building" (Forrester, 2016, p. 14). Although this quote is several years old, its author wisely offered readers an understanding of the relational approach that has been the focus of this chapter. It includes appreciating the significance of caring relationships, holding them close, and actively working to strengthen them through inclusion and connection—the secret to local changes that eventually allow larger self-advancing innovations to emerge.

Although the caring behaviors are most often thought of in relation to direct patient care (see Chapter 5), examining them in a leadership context is helpful for they can also serve as guides for administrative professional practice. In fact, the caring behaviors are analogous to many contemporary leadership terms (see Table 10.3).

For example, mutual problem solving is a caring behavior that facilitates decision making. As leaders provide information, help staff members see the bigger picture, explore alternatives, brainstorm together, and validate perceptions, they provide a safe and inclusive atmosphere for planning a future course of action.

TABLE 10.3 Comparison of Caring Behaviors, Contemporary Leadership Terms, and Relevant Leadership Competencies

Caring Behaviors	Contemporary Leadership Terms	Relevant Nursing Leadership Competencies
Mutual problem solving	Shared visioning Translating evidence into practice Shared leadership Reframing Conflict management Budget development Variance analysis Performance improvement Decision-making	Relational capacity Brainstorming skills Soliciting feedback Maximizing information flow Educating Engaging Clarify and validating Adaptation
Attentive reassurance	Appreciative inquiry Circular leadership Recognition MBWA	Availability Optimistic/convey possibilities Authentic presence Noticing Maintain belief in employees Use of humor and celebrations Temporarily postpone action
Human respect	Ethical behavior according to established standards	Acceptance, value Recognition of rights, responsibilities, ethics, standards, legalities Patients first Solicit feedback, listen Awareness of non-verbal behavior Call people by name Eye contact
Encouraging manner	Evaluation/performance appraisals Empowerment Human resource management Remuneration and rewards	Encouraging demeanor Enthusiastic Provide support and training Congruent verbal and nonverbal communication See patterns Build relational capacity

(continued)

TABLE 10.3 Comparison of Caring Behaviors, Contemporary Leadership Terms, and Relevant Leadership Competencies (*continued*)

Caring Behaviors	Contemporary Leadership Terms	Relevant Nursing Leadership Competencies
Appreciation of unique meanings	Systems thinking Meaning/sensemaking in work Inclusion	Appreciate frames of reference Point out meaning in the work Acknowledge the subjective Point out unique contributions to purpose Preserve the uniqueness of the patient-nurse relationship
Facilitating a healing environment	Behavioral interviewing Hiring and selection process Human resource management Remuneration and rewards Evaluation/performance appraisal Safe staffing Organizational culture Culture of safety/"just" cultures	Respect privacy and confidentiality Create a unit culture of caring Foster teamwork Design manageable workflow Safe environment
Basic human needs	Resource management	Attend to personal and employee's physical, emotional, and spiritual health Recognize higher level needs for achievement, self-esteem
Affiliation needs	Work-life balance Networking; membership in professional organizations	Responsive to belonging needs

BOX 10.6: Leaders who accept feedback and use it to make decisions convey mutual problem-solving. Implicit in performing in this manner is comfort "in relationship;" an open, engaging stance and reciprocal, shared dialogue. An example of this caring behavior would be engaging staff in planning, organizing, directing, and evaluating a new patient care delivery system.

Consider this recent scenario:

The patient in room 326 said he did not like Asian nurses and did not want any [expletive deleted] taking care of him. The patient, D.L., a 60-year-old white male in the primary care unit (PCU), had been hospitalized for acute stroke for two days. During this time, D.L. had been insulting the bedside nurses, racial epithets peppering his outbursts. To accommodate him, the charge nurses had changed several shift assignments. The nurses were frustrated and conflicted: tired of putting up with the abuse in the interest of putting the patient's needs first, offended by the personal attacks, and wanting to preserve their own dignity. Still, the nurses were acutely aware of their ethical obligation as professional nurses and the policy of our academic medical center to put the patient's care and comfort first. The charge nurse on the day shift was on the phone now, frustrated that she had followed our organization's new policy for addressing racist language and behaviors and had gotten nowhere. She was now appealing to me, the nurse manager, for resolution.

Demeaning behavior from patients in the PCU is not out of the ordinary. The nurses understand the psychological and physiological duress of illness and injury and that pain, medication, frustration, fear, and attention seeking may all underlie outbursts like D.L.'s. But to expect our nurses to rise above bad behavior or to change shift assignments to accommodate prejudice is a disservice, making their hard job even harder. In the past, we had responded to situations like D.L.'s by explaining to the patient that all nurses were competent and then changed shift assignments. Neither intervention addressed the human relationships at the crux of the problem. Our new policy for addressing racist language and behaviors spells out specific steps in a decision tree. The charge nurse was now at the second step; the nurse had alerted risk management and a supervisor. Following our protocol, I would engage with the patient directly, then debrief with the charge nurse.

I went to see D.L., accompanied by a peer, and a mix of conflicting feelings. As a nurse leader, I was close to my staff, knew how hard they worked, and wanted to protect them. As a woman and person of color, I resented a white male directing his verbal abuse to female nurses of color. However, patient-centered care is the nursing credo at our medical center; and as such, my obligation was to put patient's comfort and needs first. I entered D.L.'s room still processing all this and thinking about the fragility of human relationships.

I introduced myself and sitting a comfortable and unimposing distance away, asked "How is your stay so far?" D.L had little to say at first. I reassured him that our talk would stay between us. "Something's bothering you," I offered. "Want to get it off your chest?" "They talk about me at the nurses' station," he said. "I hear those [expletive deleted]." I asked him to tell me more, but without cursing. He apologized, admitting his "choice of words" was not ideal. He expressed a few more concerns, but not about the nurses. He didn't like being in the hospital, the stay was too long, too noisy at night, then shrugged and leaned back into his pillow. I told him I'd investigate his concerns and would be back to check on him throughout the day. A "thumbs up" from him would mean everything was fine.

I debriefed with the bedside nurses involved with his care and the charge nurses. They felt defeated from having to deal with "these types" of patients more frequently and feeling ill equipped to handle the verbal abuse. They resented being treated badly when they were "just trying to do their jobs." They talked and I listened, then we discussed mutual problem solving with patients in a patient-centered environment. The discussion centered on the difference between "the old way of caring as more clinical; every nurse was competent to care for every patient" and the uncomfortableness of contemporary relationships. It was easy to see how racist behavior could be construed both as a personal insult and an attack on competency, both toxic to the relationship between a nurse and a patient. To just say "don't take it personally," or "put the patient's needs first," diminishes the seriousness of racist behavior and patronizes our nurses.

What tools can we give nurses to deal with unwarranted requests and/or racist language? In our medical center's case, we developed a policy to describe biased behavior and provide a clear decision-making pathway for staff to respond to a patient's discriminatory behavior. The policy describes an appropriate response for staff when patients or their families display discriminatory behavior and sets the organizational expectation that all patients will be considerate of the rights of others. As such, the first step was to reassure the staff that reporting an incident in order to resolve it would not come back to hurt them. From there, we could proceed step-by-step.

The policy begins with human relationships. A patient's medical needs guide the medical team's decisions when staff encounter discriminatory behavior. In some cases, a patient's request for reassignment based on a staff member's social characteristics can be honored. However, reassignment requests motivated by bigotry are problematic and will do harm. In the case of D.L., several staff changes had already been made in attempts to accommodate him, yet his behavior persisted. The policy guides the supervisor of the affected staff member to "create a therapeutic alliance" with the patient in an attempt to de-escalate the conflict. De-escalation is a negotiated interaction; the offender is to be made aware of the biased conduct and instructed that it must stop. The supervisor may choose to refer to the medical center's "Patient's Rights and Responsibilities," and "Principles of Community" to reinforce the expectation of mutual respect.

D.L. was unhappy about being in the hospital and chose an inappropriate way to express his frustrations. He wanted attention and accommodation, both understandable, but demeaning the staff was the wrong way to go about getting either one. His outbursts backfired as he thought the staff were now speaking badly of him at the nurses' station. The staff nurses did not want to feel powerless in the face of personal humiliation. They wanted to know the medical center "had their backs" and recognized the difficulty and value of their work. In the simplest sense, both patient and staff wanted to feel cared for.

The policy helped us to reorient to caring relationships by providing structure for the occasions when they will inevitably break down. With the policy to guide them, the nurses were able to engage with each other and with me, to agree on the appropriate approach with D.L. The problem was solved mutually with D.L. as well. He was satisfied that someone was checking on him frequently. One day, I stood at the door while the bedside nurse was passing meds to D.L. He saw me, gave me a quick "thumbs up" and a wink, and I moved on to continue rounding on the floor.

—Dawn Carroll, DNP, NE-BC, WHNP

Wow—this exemplar highlights leadership's use of *mutual problem-solving* in a very difficult situation! However, notice that the leader began with *attentive reassurance*. She was available and present, noticed the clinical staff and charge nurse's struggles, and before applying the policy, she reassured the staff that reporting an incident in order to resolve it would not come back to hurt them!

She also used *human respect and appreciation of unique meanings* as she communicated with the patient trying to understand his unique needs. She valued him as a worthy human being by recognizing him, giving of her time, actively listening, recognized his rights but also his responsibilities, solicited his feedback, and I am guessing here, that she was aware of her non-verbal behaviors and used eye contact in her interaction with him. She acknowledged his concerns and relayed that she would follow up.

Later, she followed up by listening to the nurses, heard their concerns and frustrations again, while also acknowledging the patients' needs for attention and accommodation. Using the well thought-out policy, decisions were eventually made *mutually* between staff members and the leader; and when applied, D.L. indicated his satisfaction.

When using traditional leadership language, this case could have been described as one of conflict management; however, it can also be considered mutual problem-solving, a *caring* behavior, that demands relational capacity, brainstorming skills, the ability to solicit feedback, providing information, educating, engaging, clarifying and validating, and adapting practice. Likewise, the use of attentive reassurance demands leadership availability, an optimistic stance, authentic presence, noticing, belief in the employees, and temporarily pausing action long enough to reassure and work this situation out. This leader appreciated the significance of caring relationships (a universal human need) to both the patient and the staff members, held them close, and actively used them through inclusion and connection, allowing a shared and professional decision to evolve that resulted in an acceptable practice adaptation.

Attentive reassurance—being physically present often with an optimistic outlook—is nurturing to employees and conveys the leader's recognition. Noticing and listening to nurses, acknowledging changes or improvements and their caring behaviors, or a gentle affirmative touch shows nurses that they matter and builds confidence in the system. Using appropriate humor to lighten stressful situations and taking the time to appreciate someone's effort can be transforming. Of course, practicing this caring behavior requires frequent interaction, so regular rounding, assistance with certain patient care activities, or joint projects can provide the means to enact this behavior. Called "management by walking around" (MBWA) by Peters & Waterman (1982), put in plain words this factor implies "being there" and with a hope-filled attitude.

Human respect conveys the worth of the unique person who is an employee, a health professional, a stakeholder, another leader, or a patient. Not only does it signify value for the person, but in this case it creates an appreciation for the contribution of the individual. Remembering and calling employees by name and conversing about appropriate personal issues (such as children's sports, birthday celebrations, or marriages), using eye contact, and allowing safe space for dialogue can remind employees that they are inherently worthy and valuable to the organization. Upholding rights and responsibilities in an ethical manner, expecting high standards, and appropriately following legal statutes conveys unconditional acceptance and high regard for patients and families as well as employees.

Using an encouraging manner when interacting both verbally and non-verbally provides support for nurses that can lead to empowerment and risk-taking. Pointing out the good along with the challenging behaviors, especially during formal disciplining, helps others learn and advance in their roles. For nurses who take risks on behalf of patients or the organization, formal recognition is appropriate. For those who offer to chair a council or lead a meeting, being there with them especially for the first meeting promotes the confidence required to volunteer the next time. An example of this behavior occurs when a nurse who has never written an abstract or proposal for a professional conference, volunteers to do it, but hesitates because it is the employee's first attempt. Supporting them through the writing process, artfully critiquing the work, and offering praise where appropriate are supportive behaviors that encourage the employee to finish the task. Showing up for the resulting poster or presentation further demonstrates how the employee is valued!

Appreciating the unique context of employees recognizes the importance of culture, past and current experiences, and other unique meanings that impact the work life of the employee. Attuning to these meanings and allowing them to influence decisions at times are affirming for the individual. For example, a nurse with a specific cultural worldview might be allowed to explain the origin of a certain nursing action that is pertinent to his or her culture. Followed by discussion and a search of the literature, this action might be adopted for use, upholding this individual's personal worldview.

Facilitating a healing environment is one of the most important leadership roles that may be tied to RN job satisfaction and patient outcomes. Such an environment includes the surroundings in which nurses work, including their privacy and safety. It also includes the organizational culture or the norms and behaviors that characterize a patient care department. Relationship-centered cultures enhance one's sense of worth and encourage one to take risks. They focus on frequent interaction, open communication, and flexibility. Making sure that the body, mind, and spirit are in optimal condition for patient care is a role of the leader that often is tied to resources. A healthy work environment includes regular periods of relaxation, availability of healthy food choices, special quiet places for reflection and renewal, and uplifting continuing education. The leader who is focused on a caring–healing–protective environment will arrange the resources to support these activities. Making sure the night shift gets access to decent food is an example. This gesture relieves many who work nights from the hassle of "ordering out" or unhealthy eating from machines.

Consider this example:

Nurses from UC San Diego Health created a mission, vision, and motto specific to nursing that speaks to what it means to be a UC San Diego Health nurse. These were inspired by the organization's adopted professional practice model. They are:

Nursing Mission: To deliver safe, high-quality care to all patients throughout their UC San Diego Health experience. Caring relationships are at the core of our nursing practice. We nurture patients, families, the healthcare team, and ourselves. We are accountable for evidence-based practice in alignment with national standards. Through shared governance we are encouraged as nurses to advocate, educate, and be lifelong learners. We create an innovative and healing environment that leads to stellar outcomes.

Nursing Vision: To create a healing environment where feeling cared for is an everyday experience.

Nursing Motto: We care.

To enculturate these new statements at the bedside, I created an implementation bundle that included acts of appreciation, midshift reset and recharge moments, and creation of a relaxing space on the unit. At the core of the bundle was my objective to create a healing environment for my colleagues to care for each other and feel cared for in return.. I knew that if my colleagues practiced in a healing environment, they would be able to better care for and create a healing environment for our patients.

I started by asking my coworkers to write a sentence about why they appreciated specific team members. I then gave this anonymous positive feedback to everyone on the team. It was amazing to see even the most guarded staff members smiling when they received their expressions of admiration. I also created a space in our break room where posting of shout outs for our colleagues to celebrate one another after a tough shift or for lending a helping hand was displayed. It has been amazing reading how we support each other every day.

In addition to anonymous praise and authored shout-outs, I also introduced leadership and team members to reset and recharge moments using essential oils in the middle of the shift. These moments have really helped the nurses take a step back and relax.

One of the last things in the bundle was the creation of the "Zen Den," a relaxing space for staff to visit during breaks. The space has two massage chairs, different sleeping areas, yoga mats, diffusers, and calming music.

To help introduce this healing environment, I invited a healing touch practitioner and a massage therapist to care for my coworkers. As nurses, we pride ourselves in making sure we create a healing environment for our patients and their families. I have always thought that it was equally important to create that same healing environment for each other. I encourage all nurses to take time to reach out to their colleagues and support each other.

—Kristina James MSN, RN, CNL, PCCN

Other examples of healing environments include peaceful artwork, artifacts that respect persons' privacy and confidentiality, teamwork in the form of deliberate rounding and interprofessional group meetings, ensuring safety, as well as professional continuing education programs focused on relaxation and mindfulness practices.

Attending to basic human needs, such as not only those described above but also those higher level needs for group activities and self-esteem, keeps us connected to one another and generates the confidence so necessary for a safe and effective practice. Finally, affiliation needs recognize humans' need for belonging and honors the extended family of employees, other leaders, and stakeholders and includes them in celebrations and other work initiatives. Their special needs can also be noticed in staffing and scheduling practices.

In summary, leadership practice that is based on caring relationships requires leaders who *live* the caring behaviors and use the unique network of relationships that define health systems to energize staff, stakeholders, and other leaders. Interestingly, using the caring behaviors in leadership practice provides a living model of relevant behaviors for health professionals to emulate! By integrating professional practice with the mission of the organization and holding each other accountable, nursing leaders elevate the unique patient–health professional relationship as the most fundamental aspect of professional work. Helping to develop caring knowledge, behaviors, and attitudes and making decisions based on a caring ethic/philosophy are facilitated through a PPM that clearly delineates roles and responsibilities. Using the caring behaviors as a guide for leaders is congruent with expectations of employees, sustaining passion for the work, and expert care to the vulnerable persons who deserve safe and quality healthcare.

With the underlying philosophical beliefs (assumptions) clearly articulated and the concepts defined, the QCM has provided the foundation for nursing practice that honors the holistic nature of humans and the caring relationships essential for high-quality outcomes in many organizations. Because the QCM views independent and collaborative caring relationships as a responsibility of professional nurses and "feeling cared for" as a crucial intermediate outcome sensitive to nursing, nurse leaders who embrace it may find more meaning in their own work as it is aligned with disciplinary values.

SUMMARY

The context of clinical practice varies and currently is challenged by disengaged employees, high stress, and limited resources in a complex and changing external environment. Furthermore, the physical and emotional stress resulting from the COVID-19 pandemic has demoralized many in healthcare, leading to a discouraged and limited nursing workforce. Nursing leaders, in their support of health professionals, have a moral obligation to uphold the professions' ethical standards, including the intimate caring relationships so necessary for high-quality care. With performance pressures rising and other external forces mounting, healthcare leadership is being remodeled to a practice that is more horizontal, inclusive, and relational, enabling adaptation and innovation. Caring relationships serve to ground nurse leaders in their practice and can be tapped as resources for advancement. Leadership based on caring relationships acknowledges the connections among humans and upholds the special relationship nurses have with patients and families. In fact, caring leaders set the tone for health professionals, generate confidence in their staff, and shape the infrastructure that supports them. Use of the caring behaviors personally and with others energizes organizations and their employees toward self-advancement. Finally, the caring behaviors provide leaders with specific approaches and behaviors to effectively ensure caring relationships remain at the center of health professionals' work.

CALL TO ACTION

Health systems, comprised of people who live and work in relationship, are living systems that are complex, dynamic, and vary in context. Sustaining caring relationships energizes employees, stakeholders, other leaders, and health systems and influences their ability to be self-caring. **Get up, walk around**, and **engage** to appreciate the contributions being made. Protecting the caring relationships that professional nurses cultivate with patients and families is a responsibility of nurse leaders. At the end of the day, it is the patient–nurse caring relationship that provides the inspiration that drives staff nurses to continue their important work! **Safeguard** patient–nurse relationships. **Review** your leadership, including your relational competencies and the shared leadership structures created at your organization. Living the caring factors enables nurse leaders to make better use of the unique network of relationships that define health systems. **Cultivate** caring relationships.

REFLECTIVE QUESTIONS/APPLICATIONS

For Professional Nurses in Clinical Practice:

- Reflect on a leader who greatly influenced your work life. Who was it, what did they do, how did they do it, when did they do it, where did they do it?
- Does your health system have forums for informal dialoguing about current challenges? What occurs in them? Who leads them? Where are they held? Are they used? Have they ever been evaluated?
- Do nurses in your health system regularly interact with frontline leaders? How about executive-level leaders?
- What caring behaviors does your nurse leader display? How often? Does it make a difference to you?

For Professional Nurses in Educational Practice:

- Design a case study around the concept of relationship-centered leadership.
- Critique the discussion of complexity and appreciative leadership presented in this chapter. Are these forms of leadership evident at your university?

- What teaching/learning strategies do you think will best guide graduate students to apply the caring behaviors to leadership practice?
- Is the integration of evidence-based nursing approaches across health systems (e.g., use of EBP and professional practice models) part of your curriculum? Why or why not? What would it take to include it?

For Professional Nurses in Leadership Practice:

- As a leader of a caring profession, relate how you care for yourself. How do you relieve/cope with job stress? Who can you point to that listens to your concerns about work-related matters?
- When was the last time you enjoyed an evening out with friends? What practices do you routinely perform to help you feel a sense of harmony with yourself and your work life? How do you care for your body, your mind, and your spirit?
- Examine your calendar for the past month. Where did you spend most of your work time? What does this say about what you value? What do your actions reveal about your fundamental beliefs about caring relationships? How might your actions affect the results you are getting?
- Create a calendar for self-care that includes time for physical, reflective, and expressive practices. Be specific, including dates, times, and frequency. Now *do it*!
- Think about the patient care delivery system at your institution. Is it relationship centered? Is caring for self and others a predominant theme? Using the QCM, design a patient care delivery system that fits with the system's mission and addresses RN roles and responsibilities (what will they be held responsible and accountable for), resources (what staffing, scheduling is necessary), communication (how will RNs communicate with each other and the healthcare team), and the environment (what is necessary to create a healthy work setting for patients and staff)?
- Draw a diagram depicting the congruence between the QCM and the patient care delivery system developed in number five.
- Discuss approximately how much time nurses spend "in relationship" at your organization. What activities do nurses perform that interfere with time spent "in relationship"? Offer some innovative ways to eliminate or decrease these activities so more time can be spent "in relationship" with patients and families.
- Explain the approach of nursing leadership to professional nursing care at your institution. What is their involvement? How do they ensure nursing care is performed in accordance with professional standards? Or better yet, how does nursing leadership demonstrate the impact of nursing to the organization?

PRACTICE ANALYSIS

A departmental-level nurse manager who is smart, ambitious, and committed moved quickly from staff nurse to charge nurse to nurse manager. She had a stellar clinical track record but was recently reported by the staff nurses as not being "visible or engaged." In fact, staff nurses characterized her as not only distracted but also domineering and fast-paced, while other managers were worried about how she was representing nursing in the organization. So, her immediate supervisor, the Director of Medical Nursing, took her aside (in the middle of the evaluation year) and sat with her to relay needed feedback. Together, the director and the departmental manager reflected on the gap between how others viewed her and how she viewed herself as leader. The middle manager acknowledged her fast-paced approach and nonverbal reactions. She also reported feeling stressed and "drained out," but remained energetic in meeting system outcomes.

Accepting this feedback was difficult, for the nurse manager, who prided herself on excellence, and she seemed to be ambivalent and a little defensive about it. But the director pursued and together they developed a plan for behavior change. It included:

- reminders for "big picture" framing
- recognizing anxieties
- slowing down long enough in tense situations to pay attention to physical sensations
- practicing mindfulness
- being clinically present
- reorganizing routines for high energy
- relaxation techniques

The departmental nurse manager practiced these techniques over the next two months and has integrated many of them into her routine. She is more aware now, taking her time to engage colleagues and ask questions rather than doing, doing, doing. She takes the time to "sense" the tone of the unit prior to taking action and, in so doing, has built more genuine connections with her employees. In essence, she has learned that appreciative leadership requires a relational approach that requires ongoing self-awareness.

- Did the nursing director's behavior prompt the departmental nurse leader's behavior change? If yes, how?
- How would the nursing director guarantee lasting or sustained behavior change in the departmental nurse leader?
- Why do you think the departmental nurse leader accepted the guidance of the nursing director?

REFERENCES

Adibe, B., Hebert, D., Perticone, K., & Dowd, S. M. (2021). Creating wellness in a pandemic: A practical framework for health systems responding to covid-19. *NEJM Catalyst: Innovations in Care Delivery, 2*(2), 1–8. https//doi.org/10.1056/cat.20.0218

Al-amin, M., Islam, M. N., Li, K., et al. (2022). Inpatient covid-19 mortality rates: What are the predictors? *medRxiv.* https://doi.org/10.1101/2022.01.07.22268906

American Organization of Nurse Leadership. (2015a). Nurse executive competencies. https://www.aonl.org/system/files/media/file/2019/06/nec.pdf

American Organization of Nurse Leadership. (2015b). Nurse manager competencies. https://www.aonl.org/system/files/media/file/2019/06/nurse-manager-competencies.pdf

Antonytheva, S., Oudshoorn, A., & Garnett, A. (2021). Professional intimacy in nursing practice: A concept analysis. *Nursing Forum, 56,* 151–159. https://doi.org/10.1111/nuf.12506

Assaye, A. M., Wiechula, R., Schultz, T. J., & Feo, R. (2021). Impact of nurse staffing on patient and nurse workforce outcomes in acute care settings in low- and middle-income countries: A systematic review. *JBI Evididence Synthesis, 19*(4), 751–793.

Blegen, M. A., Goode, C. J., Spetz, J., Vaughn, T., & Park, S. H. (2011). Nurse staffing effects on patient outcomes: Safety-net and non-safety-net hospitals. *Medical Care, 49*(4), 406–414. https//doi.org/10.1097/MLR.0b013e318202e129

Brown, B. (2017). *Braving the wilderness: The quest for true belonging and the courage to stand alone.* Random House.

Cassidy, C. E., Flynn, R., & Shuman, C. J. (2021). Preparing nursing contexts for evidence-based practice implementation: Where should we go from here? *Worldviews on Evidence-Based Nursing, 18*(2), 102–110.

Chambliss, D. (1996). *Beyond caring: Hospitals, nurses, and the social organization of ethics.* University of Chicago Press.

Dagne, A. H., & Beshah, M. H. (2021). Implementation of evidence-based practice: The experience of nurses and midwives. *PloS ONE, 16*(8), e0256600. https://doi.org/10.1371/journal.pone.0256600

Duffy, J. R. (2016). *Professional practice models in nursing: Successful health system implementation.* Springer Publishing Company.

Duffy, J. (2018). *Quality caring in nursing and health systems: Implications for clinicians, educators, and leaders.* Springer Publishing Company.

Forrester, D. A. (2016). *Exemplary nursing leadership—Nursing's greatest leaders: A history of activism.* Springer.

Griffiths, P., Ball, J., Drennan, J., et al. (2016). Nurse staffing and patient outcomes: Strengths and limitations of the evidence to inform policy and practice. A review and discussion paper based on evidence reviewed for the National Institute for health and care excellence safe staffing Guideline development. *International Journal of Nursing Studies, 63,* 213–225.

Hall, L. H., Johnson, J., Watt, I., Tsipa, A., & O'Connor, D. B. (2016). Healthcare staff wellbeing, burnout, and patient safety: A systematic review. *PloS One, 11*(7), e0159015. https://doi.org/10.1371/journal.pone.0159015

Hartley, S., Raphael, J., Lovell, K., & Berry, K. (2020). Effective nurse–patient relationships in mental health care: A systematic review of interventions to improve the therapeutic alliance. *International Journal of Nursing Studies, 102,* 103490.

Joseph, M. L., Nelson-Brantley, H. V., Caramanica, L., Lyman, B., Frank, B., Hand, M. W., Parchment, J., Ward, D. M., Weatherford, B., & Chipps, E. (2022). Building the science to guide nursing administration and leadership decision making. *JONA: The Journal of Nursing Administration, 52*(1), 19–26.

Kester, K., Pena, H., Shuford, C., Hansen, C., Stokes, J., Brooks, K., Bolton, T., Ornell, A., Parker, P., Febre, J., Andrews, K., Flynn, G., Ruiz, R., Evans, T., Kettle, M., Minter, J., & Granger, B. (2021). Implementing AACN's healthy work environment framework in an intensive care unit. *American Journal of Critical Care, 30*(6), 426–433.

Kirk, T. W. (2007). Beyond empathy: Clinical intimacy in nursing practice. *Nursing Philosophy, 8*(4), 233–243. https://doi.org/10.1111/j.1466-769X.2007.00318.x

Lake, E. T., Narva, A. M., Holland, S., Smith, J. G., Cramer, E., Rosenbaum, K., French, R., Clark, R., & Rogowski, J. A. (2021). Hospital nurses' moral distress and mental health during COVID-19. *Journal of Advanced Nursing, 78*(3), 799–809. https://doi.org/10.1111/jan.15013

Lasater, K. B., McHugh, M., Rosenbaum, P. R., Aiken, L. H., Smith, H., Reiter, J. G., Niknam, B. A., Hill, A. S., Hochman, L. L., Jain, S., & Silber, J. H. (2021a). Valuing hospital investments in nursing: Multistate matched-cohort study of surgical patients. *BMJ Quality & Safety, 30*(1), 46–55.

Lasater, K. B., Aiken, L. H., Sloane, D. M., French, R., Martin, B., Reneau, K., Alexander, M., & McHugh, M. D. (2021b). Chronic hospital nurse understaffing meets COVID-19: An observational study. *BMJ Quality & Safety, 30*(8), 639–647.

Malloch, K., & Porter-O'Grady, T. (2022). *Appreciative leadership: Building sustainable partnerships for health.* Jones & Bartlett Learning.

Mensik, J. S., Martin, D. M., Johnson, K. L., Clark, C. M., & Trifanoff, C. M. (2017). Embedding a professional practice model across a system. *JONA The Journal of Nursing Administration, 47*(9), 421–425. https://doi.org/10.1097/NNA.0000000000000508

Needleman, J., Buerhaus, P., Pankratz, V. S., et al. (2011). Nurse staffing and inpatient hospital mortality. *New England Journal of Medicine, 64*, 1037–1045.

Nelson, K. E., Hanson, G. C., Boyce, D., et al. (2022). Organizational impact on healthcare workers' moral injury during COVID-19: A mixed-methods analysis. *JONA Journal of Nursing Administration, 52*(1), 57–66. https//doi.org/10.1097/NNA.0000000000001103

Peters, T. J., & Waterman, R. H. (1982). *In search of excellence: Lessons from America's best run companies.* Harper and Row.

Pfadenhauer, L. M., Mozygemba, K., Gerhardus, A., et al. (2015). Context and implementation: A concept analysis towards conceptual maturity. *The Journal of Evidence and Quality in Healthcare, 09*(2), 103–114. https//doi.org/10.1016/j.zefq.2015.01.004

Porter-O'Grady, T., & Malloch, K. (2021). The emerging principles and practices of appreciative leadership. *Nursing Management, 52*(9), 16–22.

Rogers, L., De Brún, A., & McAuliffe, E. (2020). Defining and assessing context in healthcare implementation studies: A systematic review. *BMC Health Services Research, 20*, 591. https://doi.org/10.1186/s12913-020-05212-7

Schlak, A. E., Aiken, L. H., Chittams, J., Poghosyan, L., & McHugh, M. (2021). Leveraging the work environment to minimize the negative impact of nurse burnout on patient outcomes. *International Journal of Environmental Research and Public Health, 18*(2), 610.

Schlak, A. E., Rosa, W. E., Rushton, C. H., Poghosyan, L., Root, M. C., McHugh, & M. D. (2022). An expanded institutional- and national-level blueprint to address nurse burnout and moral suffering amid the evolving pandemic. *Nursing Management, 53*(1), 16–27. https//doi.org/10.1097/01.NUMA.0000805032.15402.b3

Shin, S., Park, J. H., & Bae, S. H. (2018). Nurse staffing and nurse outcomes: A systematic review and meta-analysis. *Nursing Outlook, 66*(3), 273–282.

Sims, S., Leamy, M., Levenson, R., Brearley, S., Ross, F., & Harris, R. (2020). The delivery of compassionate nursing care in a tick-box culture: Qualitative perspectives from a realist evaluation of intentional rounding. *International Journal of Nursing Studies, 107,* 103580.

Smiley, R. A., Ruttinger, C., Oliveira, C. M., Hudson, L. R., Allgeyer, R., Reneau, K. A., Silvestre, J. H., & Alexander, M. (2021). The 2020 national nursing workforce survey. *Journal of Nursing Regulation, 12*(supp 1), S1–S96.

Uhl-Bien, M., & Marion, R. (2009). Complexity leadership in bureaucratic forms of organizing: A meso model. *The Leadership Quarterly, 20,* 631–650.

Uhl-Bien, M., Meyer, D., & Smith, J. (2020). Complexity leadership in the nursing context. *Nursing Administration Quarterly, 44*(2), 109–116. https//doi.org/10.1097/NAQ.0000000000000407

Uhl-Bien, M. (2021). Complexity leadership and followership: Changed leadership in a changed world. *Journal of Change Management, 21*(2), 144–162.

Wocial, L. D. (2018). In search of a moral community. *OJIN: The Online Journal of Issues in Nursing, 23*(1), Man02. https://doi.org/10.3912/OJIN.Vol23No01Man02

CHAPTER 11

Learning Quality Caring

"The goal of all learning is action, not knowledge."

—John C. Maxwell

CHAPTER OBJECTIVES:

1. Describe the preparation required for contemporary professional nursing practice.
2. Evaluate "effective" nursing education.
3. Describe caring pedagogies.
4. State two approaches for learning "how to care."

PREPARATION FOR CONTEMPORARY PROFESSIONAL NURSING PRACTICE

A practice involves the performance of specific activities or behaviors and is usually based on some standards (or rules) that occur in particular contexts. Practices can be performed well or poorly (e.g., one who regularly practices yoga can do it properly, satisfactorily, skillfully, badly, or inadequately). In nursing, bio-psycho-socio-cultural-spiritual concepts are pondered and learned and then expressed behaviorally in the practice environment to assess, plan, implement, and evaluate health services. We also use those same concepts to communicate about the practice so that over time, familiar language about the practice evolves, making it meaningful and even regulating its conduct.

Nursing as a practice refers to nurses' understandings, perceptions, interpretations, and actionable decisions used in healthcare situations for the benefit of those in need (individuals, populations, and communities). It is a complex practice that encompasses knowledge-based actions within a complex, scientific, and continuous changing context. In fact, what specifically constitutes nursing practice and how it is learned continues to be debated, especially in light of the pandemic-induced workforce variations.

In 2021, the shared and unified *New Essentials for Professional Nursing Education*, representing a revised approach to nursing education in the United States (US), was born (American Association of Colleges of Nursing [AACN],

2021a). This collective understanding between academia and clinical practice about the preparation for professional nursing practice viewed the discipline wholistically as one that practiced from a caring-healing base; was interconnected to the larger community; practiced within a social, political, and economic context; and was focused on well-being for all, including those who nurse. The document also proposed that although nursing is a unique discipline, it functions in an interdisciplinary world that requires attention to contemporary trends and influences (e.g., team-based care, advanced technology, inclusion, diversity, health equity, and lifelong learning).

The resulting competency-based framework advocates person-centered care, where the individual with health needs is a full partner and the source of control, requires the intentional presence of the nurse seeking to know the totality of the individual's lived experiences and connections to others (family, important others, community), and where nurses employ a relational lens that fosters mutuality, active participation, and individual empowerment. In fact, AACN (2021a) acknowledged that the core purpose of nursing as a discipline is person-centered care (p. 29).

Furthermore, as a *professional* practice, nursing is founded on a set of ethical standards and has specific social/public responsibilities (see Chapter 2). Finally, as a caring practice, it is undergirded by an awareness of human persons who are worthy, are capable of growth and change, who exist in relationship to themselves, others, communities, or groups, and who are influenced by the larger environment (including the workplace), and the larger universe— see Assumptions of the QCM in Chapter 3. Nursing's specialized knowledge, skills (behaviors), and attitudes ultimately converge in the clinical setting with professional actions or behaviors that advance the health and well-being of individuals, populations, and communities while upholding human dignity.

This union of knowledge, skills, and attitudes results in professional behaviors or actions similar to that of a performing art, such as playing the piano. In this case, music theory must be understood, psychomotor exercises (scales and chords) are repetitively carried out to perfect the practitioner's technique, and musical pieces are rehearsed over and over again in order to culminate in a beautiful performance. The value of music as a social good by the musician underlies their performance. The feedback obtained from the audience informs future musical performances. Nursing practice is similar. It has discipline-specific knowledge that must be comprehended, psychomotor techniques that must be perfected, and professional behaviors that must be internalized, experienced, and repeatedly performed in order to perform in an excellent fashion. Nursing practice is also dynamic and contextual, demanding an awareness of how the self, others, and the larger systems in which it is performed responds, ultimately informing future practice.

BOX 11.1: Most importantly, excellence in nursing practice focuses first on those requiring health services—their experiences of health and illness, their safety or protection from harm, their participation in the process of receiving care, their "feelings of being cared for," and their progress toward health and/or advancement. Excellence in nursing practice integrates being and doing; executes high-level clinical judgement; is interprofessional; evidence-based; aware of its contextual surroundings; and is always professional. Furthermore, excellent nursing practice requires a curious nature that slowly and continuously reflects upon questions such as "What am I observing about this patient and family?" "What am I learning about me?" "What am I learning about nursing?" Listening for answers to these questions over time helps one discern what is relevant or salient about clinical situations and guides responses accordingly.

Embodying excellent nursing practice, however, requires exceptional academic preparation combined with strong nursing service leadership to better align the reality of practice with disciplinary expectations. Investments of time, repeated experiences, and ongoing support provide needed reinforcement.

In the learning environment, the pressure to learn everything—from theories; disease and pathophysiology; treatments, including medications and specific interventions; technical and interpersonal skills; safety precautions; interprofessional teamwork; leadership and delegation; evidence appraisal to increasingly difficult cognitive applications in short periods of time is distressing for many nursing students. The separation of clinical courses from their associated didactic counterparts has not made it easy to connect theory with practice. The recent pandemic-related changes to prelicensure preparation (less clinical hours and more online learning formats) revealed nursing student concerns, such as being unprepared for practice, worries about passing the NCLEX, concerns that the quality of their care would be affected because of the alternative teaching strategies, and their desire for direct patient care versus simulation (Feeg et al., 2021; Emory et al., 2021; Michel et al., 2021). Comparably, in a mixed methods study of new graduates who were hired during the pandemic ($N = 295$), many reported very limited direct clinical time and feared being overwhelmed or unsafe in their practice (Smith et al., 2021). Further research on the impact of COVID-19 related to new graduates' competency, confidence, resiliency, and retention was recommended. Thus, in the last couple of years, undergraduate nursing students, although excited about career possibilities, have had little time for reflection and focused application (necessary for a developing practice).

At the graduate level, most students were already working (many full time) while simultaneously supporting families. Many courses were being held online before COVID-19 and although this format continued to accommodate the students' busy schedules during COVID-19, many students worked overtime to support their peers in practice, leaving little time for online dialoguing. Furthermore, the hectic lives of faculty members and their equally busy students can compromise nursing student–teacher relationships, representing lost opportunities to form and cultivate the necessary caring relationships that allow for ongoing role formation (i.e., learning about the real practice of nursing).

Nursing education is also constrained by academic progression issues, lack of adequate clinical experiences, changes in learning strategies to accommodate innovative new approaches, and the integration of new competencies. Beyond that, there continues to be concerns about the differences and similarities between doctor of nursing practice (DNP) and doctor of philosophy in nursing (PhD) programs in terms of the scholarly project, progress in translating evidence for practice, outcomes, course content, and rigor (Bergren, 2022).

Moreover, the ongoing faculty workforce issues continue to plague nursing education, ultimately limiting the number of qualified students who can be admitted to nursing programs (McFadden et al., 2021). Educational programs tend to fill this faculty gap by relying on "adjunct" or clinical faculty members. Oftentimes, this practice is met with less-than-ideal orientations, mentoring, support, salary, and connection (McPherson, 2019). Thus, the current nursing education milieux is complex and evolving. How these academic-related issues impact student learning and/or transition to practice is unknown.

On the positive side, however, there appears to be increased interest in nursing as a career and in 2020, there was a 5.6% rise in enrolment in baccalaureate programs (AACN, 2021b). However, the gaps from education to practice continue to challenge the professional practice of nursing, prompting concerns about practice readiness.

EFFECTIVE NURSING EDUCATION

Similar to effective clinical nurses and nurse leaders, effective nursing educators have well-developed knowledge, skills, and attitudes that allow for adaptation to the demands of the profession, students, and practice settings for learning and competency development. In fact, nursing educators are considered experts in their field and are expected to incorporate certain behaviors that facilitate student learning and increased clinical proficiency. In addition, nursing faculty members are also expected to be creative, successful researchers, provide service to the university and the profession and act as national/international leaders in their field. Nursing education, therefore, is a practice (process) that unfolds each day as nurse educators repetitively extend their knowledge, skills, and attitudes through specific activities (in classrooms, online, in chat rooms, and in clinical settings). It is a creative practice that influences others with the actions that are displayed, the shared ideas that are communicated, the skills that are employed and the values and beliefs about nursing that are transmitted both overtly and covertly. The nurses who work in professional development or continuing education in practice settings play similar crucial roles in continuing to develop professional nurses for future practice, including helping them *use* evidence, improve practice, plan for career advancement, and cope with the ever-changing healthcare environment.

Importantly, nursing education is an exceptional form of practice that profoundly impacts the discipline and future of nursing as well as health systems. As such, the performance of nursing educators with respect to professionalism, caring relationships, accountability, and ongoing self-advancement are significant and set the tone for students' professional careers!

While there is no consensus on what specific behaviors effective nursing faculty members should display, one study of both faculty and students reported that faculty performance should be knowledgeable, enthusiastic, approachable/personable, creative/interesting, and promote critical thinking in students (Groccia et al., 2018). Despite a small sample size, another study used the Teacher Behavior Checklist (Geier, 2022) to investigate faculty perceptions of effective teaching. Results showed some similarity among respondents; however, the number one effective faculty behavior identified was knowledgeable, and the second most chosen behavior was approachable/personable (Noll, 2021). In addition, faculty members expected educational content to be delivered in an enthusiastic and thought-provoking way. The authors postulated that faculty members who do not adequately understand the content they are teaching or who are unapproachable may not effectively facilitate student learning and may fail to build rapport, further delaying learning.

Unfortunately, many currently employed nursing faculty members have not been prepared in effective teaching (Bullin, 2018) and must learn how to be an educator *on the job*. Clinical faculty development, in particular, has been hampered by limited resources, poor participation, and some resistance to change, possibly contributing to the informal (hidden) curriculum (Pownall et al., 2022) that may influence students' socialization processes (Raso et al., 2019). Yet, effective clinical education is foundational for student learning at all levels in most health professions. An integrative review of students' perceptions of nurse faculty teaching characteristics revealed that nursing students value nursing faculty's competence and interpersonal skills over their personality traits (Labrague et al., 2020). Furthermore, the review highlighted the general lack of evidence on this and recommended future studies aimed at the correlation of faculty teaching characteristics and student learning outcomes.

Scientific evidence for teaching efficacy is slim, but generally, advanced understanding of the science of nursing, including current clinical practice, and knowledge of teaching and learning principles, including curriculum development, implementation, and evaluation are recognized as crucial. It is this last portion that is concerning as these content areas are not usually incorporated into most of today's graduate nursing programs.

The National League for Nursing (NLN) has developed core competencies and a certification program for nurse educators (National League for Nursing [NLN], 2022). They describe academic nursing as a process of facilitating learning through curriculum design, teaching, evaluation, advisement, and other activities undertaken by faculty in schools of nursing (p. 2) and acknowledge that nurse educators have a number of roles and functions, reflecting the core competencies of nursing faculty. The broad major competency areas are to:

- facilitate learning
- facilitate learner development and socialization
- use assessment and evaluation strategies
- participate in curriculum design and evaluation of program outcomes
- pursue continuous quality improvement in the academic nurse educator role
- engage in scholarship, service, and leadership

■ function as a change agent and leader

■ engage in scholarship of teaching

■ function effectively within the institutional environment and the academic community

(NLN, 2022, p. 6).

Additionally, within each broad area, there are several sub-content areas that are levelled according to the faculty role and are assumed to be present when one is practicing in the full scope of the educator role. How many current nursing faculty members (and those working in health systems) can claim competency in these areas? Who is responsible for assessing and assuring them?

Once in the role of faculty member, student evaluations, peer review of teaching, and evidence of scholarship have become commonplace at many universities around the world to evaluate faculty ongoing competency. However, some of these forms of evaluation, although meaningful, are not standardized, are subjective, require faculty acceptance of the feedback, and follow through. In the clinical environment, evidence of a return on investment (ROI) related to professional development in terms of successful practice transitions, improvements in nursing practice, increased nurse engagement, and other nursing outcomes are increasingly tied to the performance of nurse educators. However, there are few robust studies on these forms of evaluation to improve educational performance.

The other area related to educator effectiveness is relational. In fact, positive learning outcomes have been linked to the quality of the student–teacher relationship. For example, in a systematic review, findings indicated that students' perceptions of faculty caring impacted their intent to graduate and were instrumental in motivating them to continue learning (Henderson et al., 2020). Another study using Q methodology with prelicensure students assessed students' perceptions of faculty caring. The largest factor that emerged from the findings was confident faculty who were experts in the course content and could explain complicated concepts while sharing their clinical experiences. They also found that faculty members who were "cheerleaders" and who genuinely helped students achieve their goals (academic success, graduation, and passage of the NCLEX exam) were perceived as caring. These findings were consistent with the caring behaviors in the Quality-Caring Model© (Barbour & Deline, 2021). Similarly, another qualitative study (N=31) of college students enrolled in a state university showed that students articulated the importance of "caring" to their engagement in the class, assessment of the course, their likelihood to succeed, and their willingness to work (Miller & Mills, 2019). As one student in the focus group put it, "If they don't care, I don't care." The participants in this study represented a variety of majors, including the arts, humanities, STEM fields, education, and healthcare were divided almost equally between white and black racial groups and had a mean cumulative grade point average of 2.75. Finally, students in the study described ways in which they worked harder and were more motivated in situations where they believed faculty members cared.

Thus, the capacity of faculty "to care" may play a significant role in nursing students' success!

Caring relationships between faculty members and students are occasions to be nurses *together*, understand patients' perspectives, mutually consider the context of patient situations, decide on a course of action and associated priority setting, think about the rationale or evidence base for actions, and together evaluate performance.

BOX 11.2: Being attuned to students' needs, reassuring them of their abilities, supporting them through hard times, being receptive to suggestions and feedback, understanding the pressure from their family and peer groups (being there), and sometimes doing for—such as specific helping behaviors that enable and empower students to be more self-reliant or successful—are examples of caring student–teacher relationships.

Consider the following:
A busy 39-year-old DNP student, who worked as an NP in an outpatient facility, was in her final course, working on completing her DNP project. In addition to her full-time job as an NP, this student had multiple personal issues (she was a recent divorcee and a mother of two) and was barely getting by, rushing with most of her assignments at the last minute. Although the project was already under way with data collection completed, the remaining data analysis, interpretation, and formal written and poster presentations were going to demand lots of thought time. As her faculty member for the course and project director, a professor sat down with her and in a very firm but caring manner relayed her concern that the student may not finish on time. She listened as the student told her about her problems and then suggested that the student extend her time in the program in order to complete the DNP project well. The student, however, resisted the idea as she could not afford to pay another semester's fees. She begged the professor to work with her to get the project completed. The professor, knowing the student, didn't think there was much hope to complete the project during the final semester, but after listening to the student, she agreed to work with her for a few weeks to give the student the benefit of the doubt that she could do the work.

She sat with the student, and together they made a detailed plan for completion with weekly assignments. The student was told that she would need to work hard, spend time thinking and brainstorming, be receptive to feedback, and turn in her assignments on time. The professor agreed to quick turnaround times for providing feedback and "being there" for ongoing support. Although the professor was quite busy teaching two other courses, directing dissertations, and conducting her own research, she kept her commitment to this student despite the time it took to read and reread multiple drafts. There were times during the semester when the professor had to impose stricter timeframes, give uncomfortable feedback about the work, and ask the student to redo sections of her paper multiple times. The poster required five revisions before it was in a good enough shape to present! Each time, the professor provided some guidelines about how to do the revisions but required the student to do the work. The professor provided the student with websites, assistance with interpreting data, and implications for practice, each time asking the student "What do you think about... ?" A few times throughout the semester, the professor had her doubts about the student's ability to complete the project on time. However, the student was committed to completion, worked very hard, and in the end, did successfully complete the project on time, surprising and delighting the professor.

In the course evaluation, the student wrote, "Dr. XXX was the best thing that happened to me. She knew exactly what I needed and pushed me to succeed. I couldn't have done it without her. Her caring wisdom guided me to project completion."

The professor was pleasantly surprised at the evaluation because she had pushed the student hard, provided some very detailed and hard-to-take feedback, and never received much in the form of reaction from the student during the process. The professor did, however, integrate "being with and doing for" by being attuned to the student's need for structure and setting priorities, by demanding times for dialogue in person, by providing frequent, detailed feedback, by showing the student how to interpret data so that it has meaning for advanced practice nursing, and helping the student present data in a way that others could understand. In the end, the student was proud of her project, learned how to be more self-confident and resourceful, and discovered much about how to contribute to the *real* practice of nursing.

BOX 11.3: As educators of nurses, nursing faculty members are shaping a clinical practice whose first responsibility is to patients and families that bears responsibility for competent and quality services and that is uniquely qualified to advance relationships that improve the human experience. Facilitating the lifelong development of these responsibilities inherent in the clinical practice of nursing is a priority of nursing educators!

Nursing educators are tasked with facilitating knowledge, skills, and attitudes in students using a distinct disciplinary perspective. Although nursing's theoretical base continues to evolve, its practice is clearly relational with the intended goal of advancing health and/or well-being, that is, promoting self-advancing systems. Relating to students in a caring manner (using the caring behaviors wisely), aligns nurse educators' practice with the values, focus, and ideals of nursing as a discipline. Practicing this way requires self-caring and continued learning activities as well as frequent reflection on the discipline.

LEARNING HOW TO CARE

Most health professional students learn a lot about assessing patients, diagnosing health problems, pathophysiology, chemistry, and microbiology, and have specialized skills ranging from taking blood pressures to appraising scientific publications. Fewer have been vulnerable hospitalized patients. Lacking this experience, young health professional students may not fully appreciate what it feels like to be in chronic pain, wait endlessly in doctors' offices or emergency rooms while taking precious time off from work, hear conflicting advice from several different health professionals, take multiple medications (with countless side effects) or assess one's glucose levels daily, have emergency medication and/or alerts on hand at all times, or deal with impossible billing personnel.

BOX 11.4: Yet comprehending the human person's experience of health and illness, including the adjustment to a new or changing illness, disruptions in social roles and family responsibilities, and the many personal losses inherent in illness is necessary to adequately respond to peoples' health needs. A deep understanding of these experiences grounds health professionals in providing expert care.

Nevertheless, the continued focus on biological systems, diseases, or diagnostic-related patient populations is what typically organizes the thoughts of health professionals, and it starts early in educational programs, continues during clinical courses, and, most often, is the basis for preparing for state licensing examinations.

In schools of nursing, for example, students complete the familiar medical–surgical, family (obstetric and pediatrics), mental health, and community health clinical rotations, where they are assigned to patients and preceptors in the clinical site. They participate in supervised patient care for several hours; and when the assignment has ended or patients are transferred/discharged, their relationships with those patients and staff are over. Patients and their families, however, continue their illness and require ongoing education, motivation, and comfort measures. How often do pre-licensure nursing students coordinate home care services, make referrals, give report to extended care facilities, make discharge phone calls, or participate in transitional care teams? I wonder how their clinical experiences would be enriched if they followed patients' illness trajectories? Or, if during the experience, they participated in clinical rounds or staff meetings? Or better yet, led a brief learning activity with the staff? Sometimes, these occasions do occur, and students have remarked to this author that they made all the difference! How could we build more participative activities that mimic the reality of clinical nursing practice into student experiences?

Likewise, nursing students typically spend a little time in specialty areas (e.g., the operating room, critical care, cardiac catheterization labs, or interventional radiology) and have no relationship with patients, but rather just observe. Would it not be better to go to these areas with a real patient to learn how the situation was experienced by the patient and how the care teams worked together? Or simply to learn more about the physiology involved? How does this form of learning prepare students for systems thinking (seeing the bigger picture), improving the health of populations, including the complexities of illness, how it impacts individuals' way of life, including various treatment regimens? How does it foster professionalism? How does it help students learn how to initiate, cultivate, and sustain caring relationships while at the same time perform highly technical procedures and make important judgments, which is the reality of nursing practice?

Interestingly, when people with health needs are asked about their healthcare experiences, they often speak about the interactions they have had with healthcare professionals, whether their needs for comfort or pain relief were met, and whether they were treated with respect. Of course, they also discuss what illnesses or problems they have and how much healthcare costs. Most often, however, their focus is on the interactions they have with healthcare professionals.

BOX 11.5: Focusing on the health experience of patients through mutually relating and helping students adopt interventions that are meaningful to patients and families may be more beneficial than completing checklists of procedures or skills that do not impart person-centered care. Such a focus, however, requires new learning strategies focused on patients as drivers of care, a renewed emphasis on the clinical aspect of learning (including revamping and elevating clinical courses), and a revised evaluation structure.

Although caring relationships are implicit in nursing education and occur over time, making them explicit in terms of course objectives or program outcomes, tying them to cognitive and behavioral domains of learning, and following their development and eventual competency achievement over the course of a program may help bridge the practice–education gap. AACN's new essentials domain of person-centered care includes the subconcept of engaging with individuals in establishing a caring relationship (AACN, 2021a). This domain of nursing competencies also includes the integration of accountability, communication, coordination, promotion of self-care, and the actions associated with the nursing process. This learning approach contains defined performance expectations based on observable behaviors that require frequent assessment through the course of an educational program. It is expected that such performance-based learning translates easier into practice and advances professional identity.

To better meet the needs of tomorrow's patients and families, designing a curriculum using the enduring disciplinary concepts articulated in the revised AACN *Esssentials* such that they are learned in depth and evaluated for competency provides the formula for easier transitions to the clinical setting (of course, robust implementation and evaluation are yet to be seen)! Caring relationships embedded in person-centered care is one of those enduring concepts.

The profession of nursing has long considered caring relationships fundamental to quality practice. Caring relationships are critical to person-centered care, have been linked to improved patient outcomes (Epstein & Street, 2011), and are considered critical to meaningful nurse work (Duffy, 2018). It is often cited as one of the central concepts in nursing curricula and is frequently observed through faculty role modeling or "taught" by embedding it in classes on therapeutic communication and is often evaluated through faculty observations during clinical courses. One would deduce that a concept considered so crucial to a practice would be extensively taught, modeled, and learned in a rigorous manner with multiple ways of evaluating its competence!

Still, prelicensure students are often more focused on biological processes, and graduate students have even more limited exposure, as it is presumed that graduate nurses already have the requisite knowledge, attitudes, and skills to care. Thus, the teaching and learning of caring relationships is fraught with discrepancies at a time when the ongoing needs of health systems and patients for nurses with the relational knowledge, skills, and values that comprise inclusion, interaction, equity, connection, collaboration, teamwork, communication, big-picture (systems) thinking, and reflective awareness have never been greater!

In reality, nurses perform what they know and value "in relationship"; likewise, learning about nursing occurs "in relationship" (between students and faculty members, among groups of students, between students and self, or between students and preceptors [clinical role models]). Why not use this medium to teach students "how to care (and therefore, to nurse)?"

BOX 11.6: Understanding nursing as a caring practice is fundamental to advancing the health/well-being of individuals, groups, and communities. Appreciating that ongoing caring relationships between patients (and families) and nurses is needed to achieve therapeutic relationships where patients can trust, be comforted, feel understood, engage, become empowered, and prepared to make health decisions is significant to the practice and health systems. Understanding the development of caring competence as a process that builds over time and often involves struggle, discovery, repetition, encouragement and optimism, humility, and spirituality (Purnell, 2009, p. 115) is paramount. Discovering the meaning of nursing in innovative learning environments and translating this knowledge to clinical courses emphasizes its significance.

Transforming the learning environment (both didactic and clinical) to one that is authentic, connected to the real world, supportive, and mutually beneficial (in terms of learning) helps students share meanings, elicit relevant data, listen, notice cues, establish rapport, and develop mutually caring interactions that may increase caring capacity from admission to graduation. Monitoring such progression or evolving caring capacity is a faculty responsibility. Furthermore, sustaining caring relationships with students may be considered a moral responsibility of nurse educators so that caring interactions as the basis for professional practice can be affirmed and operationalized, facilitating students' internalization of the concept (Adamski et al., 2009). It is worth remembering here that students in the health professions often learn from the informal or hidden curriculum (what they see us do); thus, how professional caring is learned (whether we intend it or not) is influenced by what students perceive the faculty does with respect to clinical practice or by how they behave in learning situations. It bears asking: Are we preparing professional nurse doers or professional nurse beings or both?

CARING PEDAGOGIES

Pedagogy refers to specific learning methods, strategies, and instructional technologies used in the learning process. A caring pedagogy uses the caring behaviors (see Chapter 3) to create environments of engagement and inclusion that are genuine and person-centered. *Caring*, as one of the core values of professional nursing, is honored, given high regard, and lived out through the behaviors of faculty members and staff in a school or work environment. In other words, teaching and learning caring begins with faculty members themselves who create a "caring milieu" first, by using the caring behaviors with students, and second, by facilitating developing caring competence by repetitively noticing, recognizing, and providing feedback on the caring behaviors used by students.

BOX 11.7: Faculty members who continuously reflect on the nature of nursing and its enduring concepts, the experience of learning, and integrate the caring core of nursing with their words and actions set the tone for a school and become powerful role models for students.

Caring pedagogy emphasizes relationships as primary and implies that both subjective and objective components of learning are valued and used to adequately develop and evaluate the knowledge base. Simply put, caring knowledge is partially learned didactically through innovative teaching strategies, followed up in the simulation laboratory, and evidenced as performance in clinical courses. For example, a classroom or online activity directed at understanding caring collaborative relationships (among health professionals) may involve readings, reflective questions, discussion forums, and a culminating case study that includes elements of the affective domain. In the simulation lab, a difficult scenario involving deep conflict among a physician, a nurse, and a respiratory therapist concerning the course of treatment for a ventilator-dependent patient could be presented to an interdisciplinary group. The students would be directed to work with the team and the patient in making a safe and quality health decision about ongoing treatment. Behaviors such as focusing, active listening, clarification, assertiveness, gathering of facts, readiness to engage, acceptance of feedback, optimism, confidence, deep breathing, congruence between verbal and nonverbal messaging, and use of humor might be observed by peers and faculty members to assess the student's skill in relating to others, including the patient's view, use of the caring factors, and ultimately collaborating in decision making. Finally, in associated clinical courses, faculty members could expect students to engage in and even lead such collaborative discussions with those in other disciplines. Using this method of learning, the emphasis is on the collaborative nature of relating and ultimate decision making (including the patient/family) versus on the respiratory disease or ventilator. The concepts so central to the profession in this case (caring, person-centeredness, collaborative relationships) are more likely to remain foremost in the minds of students. Cognitive, psychomotor, and affective domains of learning were all apparent, and students were exposed to the concept multiple times with gradually increasing expectations of performance.

Evaluation of learning should examine deep understanding versus superficial knowledge of core concepts in an effort to develop competency. Using the traditional domains of learning (Bloom, 1956), cognitive, psychomotor, and affective caring practice is best translated by learner-centered activities/experiences that facilitate depth, connection, and contextual awareness. The faculty member's role is to design, facilitate, and evaluate the learning experiences of students for effective translation to practice.

The caring behaviors provide the groundwork for student–teacher relationships and create the context for learning. *Mutual problem-solving* assists students in understanding how to approach and think about clinical situations. Providing some information, reframing students' perceptions, brainstorming together, and using back-and-forth active discourse with appropriate feedback, faculty members help shape students' comprehension of specific content. The faculty member caringly uses the relationship as the basis for learning by engaging and encouraging student-led participation. In addition, faculty members who can share stories about clinical practice that relate to the content being learned facilitate student understanding. Using the "flipped classroom" approach (Murphy et al., 2022) to enable students' best use of "class" time for meaningful activities, such as case studies, peer role playing, or standardized patients is a form of mutual problem-solving. Both teachers and students together are actively engaging in new knowledge and applying it to clinical practice examples. Faculty members who conduct short formative assessments during the "classroom" portion of the flipped learning can better evaluate students' engagement and developing confidence.

Attentive reassurance requires availability along with a positive outlook on student performance on the part of the educator. Availability of faculty members is always an issue for students and faculty alike because demanding work lives and lifestyles often interfere. It is important for faculty members to take a look at how often and in what ways they allow students access to them. In some cases, office hours may not be enough, especially for those students who often do not come to campus. Multiple ways to ensure regular student access to faculty are paramount; faculty members who make a point to "check in" or initiate conversations with students (using various means) demonstrated caring. Paying attention to students' progress requires faculty members to slow down enough to listen and notice students' behaviors. Noticing particularly positive behaviors in students and following up with recognition is an important aspect of this caring factor. Likewise, noticing behaviors that threaten patients' safety and remediating early is crucial. Struggling students, in particular, need special time and an open and confident stand. Occasionally, students will fail; faculty members who offer students other hopeful futures (suggest alternative courses or career pathways) can help students find meaning and strength in the process.

Human respect, or honoring the inherent worth of individuals and accepting them unconditionally, is a fundamental caring factor that conveys that persons matter. All individuals want to feel significant; therefore, when faculty members acknowledge students by name, use eye contact, maintain appropriate nonverbal behaviors, and remember that students are members of families and larger communities that they value, students learn the importance of maintaining human dignity. Approaching patients and families in this manner also conveys the importance of this factor.

Using an *encouraging manner* refers to the demeanor of the faculty member. It consists of the congruence between verbal and nonverbal messages, showing enthusiasm for student activities, cheering for students, attending and supporting student functions, and providing appropriate positive feedback. This last behavior is frequently missed as faculty members often assess examinations (particularly multiple-choice tests) and scholarly papers looking for mistakes or weaknesses in the student's work. Taking an alternative approach, choosing essay-type or other more reflective evaluation methods, and assessing them for strengths, pointing out the good aspects of students' work, takes more time but promotes confidence and builds independence.

Appreciating the unique meanings or what is important to students is a caring factor that requires intention on the part of nursing faculty. This factor honors the individuality of each student and his or her background, culture, and life experiences. At the graduate level, using the varied nursing experiences of students in seminar discussions recognizes the expertise of students and enhances learning. Directing attention to students or staying student-centered is a purposeful behavior that is especially difficult when faculty members have large class sizes or online courses. Yet recognizing the unique frame of reference of students, acknowledging their subjective perceptions, and using these to devise meaningful learning experiences avoids speculation and enhances further interactions.

Creating and maintaining a caring, healing environment in schools of nursing or care delivery environments is a vital role for faculty administrators and individual faculty members who, together, are co-creators of that environment as they go about interacting with students, staff, and other faculty members. Surroundings that are conducive to learning are comforting to students and may reduce their anxiety. Such actions as maintaining a safe and confidential student lounge, providing adequate lighting, reducing noise, keeping safety a priority, resolving conflicts or disputes early, and bringing together experts or resources that augment classroom activities provide students with a caring milieu that enhances learning. The organizational culture or tone of the school, including the teamwork among faculty and staff, the vibrancy of employees, certain behavioral norms, and traditions add to the circumstances surrounding learning and have an impact on student performance. For example, faculty members in one school of nursing host a journal club once a month. By hosting this scholarly activity, faculty members demonstrate the importance of research by taking the time to coach a student leader who chooses and distributes an article and leads the discussion. The faculty member advises the student in the process and provides a safe space for dialogue. Another example is the emphasis that clinical faculty members place on the safety culture of the school and/or a patient care unit. A caring faculty member will consistently scan the environment for risks, attend to them, and provide safe space to discuss, inquire about, and share concerns. Maintaining student confidentiality is another aspect of this caring behavior that is important to future interactions and creates one of the conditions necessary for high-quality learning.

Meeting students' *basic human needs* is a caring behavior that, on the face of it, does not seem pertinent to healthy persons. Yet, as individuals, physical, safety, social/relational, and self-esteem needs are important. It is critical that faculty members remember that basic human needs provide the motivation for behavior (Maslow, 1943). Adequate fluid and nutrition, rest and sleep, and exercise are physical needs that remain important during the educational process. Maintaining social relationships such as including students in group activities preserves belonging needs, whereas a sense of security provides order. In clinical situations, making sure students get to lunch or dinner, are recognized for their achievements, and are not manipulated by employees meets basic human needs. Helping students learn to meet their own human needs through self-caring activities such as specific health promotion activities contributes to the students' future self-caring capacity.

Keeping in mind that students have *affiliation needs* and belong to larger family and community groups is also caring in nature. When faculty members allow students to remain engaged in these groups through specific behaviors (e.g., allowing a student in a community health course to complete a project for her own community), students may find more significance in their assignments and acquire more in-depth knowledge. Using the full range of caring factors provides quality learning experiences that may have profound consequences in student learning outcomes.

CLINICAL LEARNING: INTEGRATING COGNITIVE, PSYCHOMOTOR, AND AFFECTIVE DOMAINS

Learning in a clinical context is foundational to the education of health professionals, and health professional students want these experiences (personal observations). However, significant challenges in clinical learning environments exist, especially in this overtaxed pandemic-related health system. Understaffing, workload pressures, the work environment of the health system, including how nursing is focused, and unsupported, uncivil behaviors displayed toward students threaten clinical learning. In addition, some students have voiced that they often feel unprepared for clinical courses (Günay & Kılınç, 2018), although clinical experiences with real patients and families in need are key to successful practice transitions from student to clinician (Arkan et al., 2018).

Within the framework of the QCM, the cognitive and psychomotor learning domains are rather easy to articulate. However, the need to translate this learning into clinical practice is the ultimate goal of learning a practice; thus the affective domain or the feelings, emotions, values, beliefs, responses, and attitudes of students must be integrated with the cognitive and psychomotor activities in the performance of nursing. For example, assuming responsibility for a patient's discharge occurs through the interplay of cognitive and psychomotor activities that manifest in a distinct series of caring interventions, together with affective characteristics such as motivation, attitudes, perceptions, and values surrounding the performance of patient discharge. With the goal of successfully transitioning a patient from one level of care to the next in a safe manner, nurses usually prepare cognitively for this process by reviewing the patient's medical record for orders, including potential drug interactions, determining whether the patient has an adequate support system, can follow discharge instructions, and adequately perform activities of daily living. In the psychomotor aspect of care, nurses coordinate with the interprofessional team to assure the patient's readiness for discharge and complete medication reconciliation. On the day of discharge, nurses educate the patient and family using specific instructional strategies to review medications, warning signs, follow-up appointments, and so forth. Affectively, however, the inclusion of the patient and family as full partners in the process, listening to and honoring their goals and preferences, providing support through appropriate referrals, using educational styles congruent with patients' characteristics, dialoguing about the safety/healing nature of the home environment, helping to alleviate worries by highlighting the positive aspects of the discharge, acknowledging any emotions that arise, and demonstrating ongoing interest and concern by allowing enough time for understanding to occur (e.g., teach-back methods) may facilitate the confidence and motivation required by patients to properly follow instructions. Upon reflection, these behaviors may also contribute to nurses' ongoing sense of professional identity and raise important new perspectives of clinical practice that may spark practice changes. Translating all domains of learning into clinical practice is a role of a nursing educator; clinical teaching and learning is the medium for this learning.

BOX 11.8: The affective dimension of learning is best supported in a person-centered environment with full use of the caring behaviors, observed and evaluated in the clinical setting by expert practitioners, and reinforced through reflection, either group or individual. Reflection, an essential activity of self-caring, helps one see more clearly how experiences shape future thoughts and behaviors.

Expecting students to be self-aware, lifelong learners is an outcome of most nursing programs that can be integrated throughout nursing curricula, including clinical courses. Integrating the patient's perspective in group reflection during post conferences helps students "see" how a clinical experience can provide meaningful insight into future practice. For example, students who can relate emotionally to other nurses and their work are influenced to act in certain patterns. Emotions experienced in clinical courses such as a feeling that one belongs, can facilitate confidence, motivate one to return, and increase one's sense of professional identity. Students who feel psychologically safe are more apt to recognize such emotions and integrate them into their learning.

Acknowledging the importance of this setting for learning professional nursing practice is essential. In the clinical setting, where theory and practice converge, caring professionalism is internalized, teamwork is learned, safety and quality is ensured, accountability is developed, and an appreciation for the larger health system is formed" (Duffy, 2018).

BOX 11.9: Thus, the richness of clinical experiences for students (and faculty members) cannot be overemphasized for it is in this environment that students learn what is important to pay attention to, how to react safely, and to adopt caring values. Caring experiences with patients and families during clinical courses help students appreciate their influence on health outcomes and their own growth as caring persons. Designing such experiences, shepherding students through, and reflecting on them afterward is a significant role of faculty members.

At the graduate level, clinical experiences for learning advanced practice nursing are equally important. Clinical faculty who work with preceptors and graduate students set the tone for learning through their thoughtful supervision of the learning experience. Ongoing meetings among students, preceptors, and faculty members; mutual evaluation of student performance; regular visits to clinical sites; use of site and preceptor evaluations in course revisions; and faculty participation in clinical site activities advances student learning.

In summary, clinical education is an innovative form of education that is not routinely given its rightful status in nursing academia today. In fact, it is pretty routine to see lower-ranked or part-time faculty members as clinical course instructors/coordinators and higher-ranked faculty members as separated from clinical practice, tackling research, or administrative responsibilities. This is precisely where students are most impressionable, where the practice is evidenced, and where health systems need highly qualified professional nurses!

BOX 11.10: Health professional faculty members who are separated from clinical practice are missing out on the opportunity to align education with real-world clinical practice, emphasize enduring concepts that are central to their discipline, influence employees to advance their education, participate in ongoing clinical research, and renew their own passion for their chosen profession.

Despite course and program revisions, the structure of nursing clinical education remains constrained by older models, role strain among faculty, limited sites and opportunities, and the limited involvement of senior faculty. Healthcare information, patients, interventions, and payment models are rapidly changing, requiring new graduates to promptly transition from students to practicing nurses. To meet these challenges, pilot studies, nurse residency programs, and dedicated education units have begun; and evidence related to these is emerging. One area of promise is the cultivation of strong academic–practice partnerships that share resources, provide research opportunities, increase the availability of clinical preceptors, facilitate the transfer of knowledge from the classroom to the clinical setting, increase student and staff satisfaction, and improve patient outcomes (Jones et al., 2021; Stamps & Smith, 2022; Zlotnick & McDonnell-Naughton, 2022). Although this is a good first step, nursing faculty members are currently busy revising their curricula, dealing with faculty shortages and expected retirements, contending with fewer clinical placements, and changing student characteristics. At present, the organization, sequencing, and time spent in clinical courses for the most part remains stagnant with student experiences still based on geographic locations versus patient populations and little time actively practicing within healthcare teams.

Radical change is needed in traditional nursing education to meet the demand for nurses who can relate in a caring manner, engage in real-time practice improvement, use evidence, collaborate with others to ensure safe, quality outcomes, and honor patient experiences. In addition, the next generation NCLEX exam focuses more on interactions between nurses and patients and the resulting nursing decisions that are required for safe practice in today's world. It uses unfolding case studies and a detailed measurement model that can be incorporated into nursing education settings, particularly clinical courses with real patients (e.g., debriefings, post-conference sessions, group reflections). Additional recommendations for improvement of clinical courses include:

- Designing clinical learning experiences that highlight caring relationships (with self, patients and families, other health professionals, and the community served)
- Facilitating learning about disease and illness through patient experiences of health and illness—case studies, rounding with the interprofessional team, patient and family "guests" in the classroom, nursing grand rounds
- Embedding caring relationships over the course of a chronic illness or health event (pregnancy and child-rearing or palliation and death) versus a specific clinical setting or a specific timeframe to facilitate learning from the patient's perspective
- Providing ongoing feedback about performance (practice) through observation and group reflection; expect practice revisions in real time
- Reconceptualizing faculty roles, elevating the status of clinical teaching
- Dialoguing about the wisdom of innovative models where students from all levels and associated faculty work together in teams with health system employees to provide care for small groups of patients and families—assume assigned roles, allowing students to learn how different nursing roles contribute to patient outcomes in health systems
- Including students in the design and evaluation of feasibility studies in clinical innovation centers with interprofessional faculty members
- Using existing partnerships between academia and service to better integrate clinical learning with provision of services

Clinical education is a crucial faculty assignment that offers the opportunity to role model, invite thinking, create safe space for exploration, evaluate effectiveness of various teaching methods, and stay close to the patient. Facilitating student learning while honoring patients and families by asking questions such as, "What is happening in this relationship?" or "What seems to be important to this patient?" or "How can I engage this patient and family?" places caring relationships at the center of clinical learning, better preparing today's students for the realities of *real* clinical practice. There is no greater privilege. Preparing a sustainable, agile, resilient, competent, diverse nursing workforce requires bold, transformative innovations, and reimagined nursing education models.

RENEWING NURSING EDUCATION

Since the publication of "Educating Nurses: A Call for Radical Reform," a Carnegie Foundation study that examined the state of nursing education, presented results, and offered recommendations in light of changing nursing practice and health systems (Benner et al., 2010), nurse educators have continued to dialogue about curricular revision. The report highlighted the need for clinical practice assignments that are contextual and relevant, use of postclinical conferences and small patient-care assignments to allow for in-depth learning, clinical reasoning, follow up, "thinking like a nurse," and reflection on practice. The report also advocated for student development in the areas of ethical comportment, change management, and clinical inquiry using multiples means of assessing student performance. Multiple forms of faculty development, including advancing contemporary clinical expertise, and the addition of teacher preparation in graduate schools was also recommended. Since the report, concepts such as genomic knowledge, professional identity, disaster-preparedness, palliative care, precision-nursing, along with new teaching strategies such as the flipped classroom and others have dominated the nursing education literature. Ten years later, how many nursing programs have had clinical courses that follow patients and families across time? How many nursing educators had current expertise in a clinical practice area? How many of these educators' assignments were aligned with this practice expertise? How many forms of student evaluation were being used, especially at the prelicensure level? How many graduate nursing programs incorporated teacher preparation into their curricula? And how many clinical practice assignments were relevant, allowing for in-depth learning, including reflection on practice?

Reports from 2021, however, suggested a continuing decline in the initial preparedness of new nurses (AACN, 2019; Kavanagh & Shaprnack, 2021) and spearheaded the development of the essential preparation for 21st century nursing. And, in 2022, the influence of the COVID-19 pandemic transitioned greater amounts of student learning to virtual environments. At this point in time, we have to ask ourselves, "How have nursing educators made substantive changes in the rigorous preparation of nursing students?"

Today's practice environment has been forever changed by the convergence of the pandemic and technological advances. This unforeseen consequence requires a new kind of nurse (a systems thinker, i.e., a professional not bound by procedures and tasks and who perceives the big picture), one who draws on knowledge (research and performance improvement), incorporates knowledge of self, adapts quickly to changing situations, and, most importantly, possesses exceptional relational skills and attitudes. Such characteristics call for mature professional nurses who understand nursing science, the natural sciences, social sciences, technology, and the humanities, *and* who:

- prioritizes caring relationships
- effectively responds to changing conditions
- recognizes the patient/family as the decision maker
- protects patients and families from harm
- identifies self as a significant health professional who practices in accordance with ethical standards
- leads/inspires
- accesses information and uses evidence as the basis for practice
- activates patients, families, and health professionals
- contributes to policy development and implementation
- gathers and uses data to make decisions
- regularly evaluates self (including self-reflection and the development of clinical wisdom) and revises practice accordingly
- cares for self
- takes pride in their contribution to the nation's health
- contributes to communities, including prevention of illness

These professional characteristics are not an exhaustive list; however, they do require a renewed educational system that works in tandem with service to support learning for a high-level scope of practice that continues across a professional career. Strong leadership, mutual collaboration, robust and connected didactic and clinical curricula, and regular assessment of competencies, all in the context of professionalism and accountability, provides the basis for such change. This opportunity necessitates a shift in education that moves nursing education to more adaptive forms of learning that are personalized and provide just-in-time feedback focused on competency-development.

BOX 11.11: The response of nursing educators to the New Essentials (AACN, 2021a) that are focused on nursing's enduring concepts will determine whether strong learning experiences centered on persons and attuned to the learner will advance the profession. Incorporating learning competencies that are assessed with rigor, elevating the importance of clinical courses, using and evaluating contemporary learning strategies, and including relational approaches that strengthen student engagement and readiness for practice are indispensable.

Structuring the delivery of content to the profile of the learner, using active learning approaches, such as case methods with innovative questioning techniques, ongoing faculty coaching and role modeling to keep students engaged and helping them understand the importance of various clinical situations as well as the bigger picture will also be necessary. These approaches might best be accomplished through interactive faculty members who use a combination of e-learning techniques combined with robust and connected clinical courses. Embracing pedagogies relevant to new generations of nursing students that are relevant, sensitive, help students see the impact they can make, and keep students connected to the emotions associated with learning and practicing nursing is crucial. Implementing simulations based on nursing's enduring concepts, increasingly providing depth throughout the curriculum, providing *real* leadership opportunities, not observations of leadership, and requiring multiple interprofessional clinical experiences will strengthen students' experiences of the actual practice world. Applying professionalism through one's own demeanor and throughout the curriculum, designing and using a system of ongoing inquiry at the university so that students internalize the value of lifelong learning and use of evidence (e.g., regular journal clubs, grand rounds, improvement, and research), renewing and elevating pre- and post-clinical conferences, and redesigning how students are evaluated adds depth to the learning experience that hopefully will translate to the practice environment.

Such widespread recommendations give both nursing faculty and educational leaders heartburn! With the faculty shortage apparent, educational revision of this magnitude carries many risks. Yet the health system requires fully educated professional nurses who can practice at the top of their license in a highly charged world. In fact, some are already advocating for re-designed care delivery systems with fewer nurses who work in teams supervising others (Weston, 2022). Sounds like "back to the future," doesn't it? Those nurses who work in professional development are tasked with similar pressures to redesign nursing continuing education using robust methods that complement those in academe. Nurses in all types of educational practice and their leaders must rise to this challenge!

Accepting that students cannot learn everything and selecting those concepts that best drive contemporary professional practice is the first step. Designing curricula geared toward teaching these concepts *in depth*, using meaningful readings, and multiple group sharing and reflective opportunities that include affective dimensions of nursing are key. It will be important not to teach to a particular textbook or test but rather use multiple readings from the current literature, real case studies, and group dialogue to help students master knowledge, versus memorizing. Evaluation techniques must move away from primarily using multiple-choice tests; although these serve their purpose, they do not easily allow for application of knowledge, responding to changes, clinical reasoning, or adequate assessment of the affective domain—all essential for professional practice. Finally, progressively begin treating students as they would be treated in clinical practice—as professionals with disciplinary values, including accountability, who must engage with others, practice teamwork, use evidence, communicate effectively, and lead.

Lastly, nursing faculty who are aligned with current clinical practice and are able to move easily between practice and academia build relationships with service partners and other health professionals. This ensures quality experiences for students. An example of this is the use of true joint appointments where faculty members serve their health system partners in specific roles. Doing so leads to better understanding of the current requirements of staff nurses (e.g., Magnet® criteria, various reportable nursing-sensitive quality indicators, delegation and follow through, joint rounding, committee work, shared governance). Likewise, it enables clinical and advanced practice nurses opportunities to engage in clinical teaching and learning.

Mobilizing now to prepare future nurses for successful, lifelong careers is not an option; the future of nursing is at stake! The initiatives proposed by AACN provide an opportunity for nursing educators to respond to the pace of change and the evidence of obvious gaps in nursing readiness for practice. This unprecedented opportunity to advance nursing education calls for relationship-building that conveys an ongoing passion for the practice of nursing.

EVALUATING CARING RELATIONSHIPS

Assuring Individual Caring Capacity

Caring capacity is a complex phenomenon referring to an individual's expertise and ability to engage in caring relationships. As such, its measurement is daunting and requires multiple approaches. It is best accomplished through formative and summative approaches that help prepare health professionals "to be" as well as "to do" work in their respective disciplines. Attending to all three domains of learning is essential (e.g., an increase in knowledge, for example, does not ensure adequate performance of caring behaviors or internalization of caring values in the practice setting). Despite the fact that graduates of nursing programs are expected to initiate, cultivate, and sustain caring relationships with themselves, their patients, members of the healthcare team, and the community served (Duffy, 2018), caring competency in nursing is rarely measured in the academic setting and even less so in the practice environment.

Starting with crafting specific course competencies related to caring relationships encompassing all domains of learning and increasing in complexity over the progression of a program will build proficiency. For example, while a sophomore student might "establish caring relationships with patients and families," a senior student may "independently monitor and modify their caring relationships with patients and families." Multiple evaluation techniques, such as written essays, critical analyses, concept mapping, role playing, peer review, simulations followed by reflective analysis, video observations of behaviors, and patient feedback administered over time versus the traditional multiple-choice testing approach, allows for more comprehensive evaluation of developing caring capacity. At graduation, summatively assessing caring competence will demonstrate readiness for practice. Using multiple approaches (e.g., valid and reliable measurement tools from the students' perspective, peers' perspectives, patients' perspectives, faculty evaluations; final reflections; portfolio) are available for this; however, the key is that they are completed and used to assess student competence as well as revise curricula. Such a rigorous summative evaluation approach provides a comprehensive perspective of overall caring ability and assures faculty that students are prepared for this aspect of practice. After all, clinical settings are expecting nursing graduates "to care" in all their interactions.

After graduation and in the clinical setting, assessing the caring capacity of staff nurses can be done using a novice-to-expert approach (Benner, 1984) in which multiple perspectives (self, patient, supervisor, and peers) provide evidence of progression. Evaluation of caring capacity from the patient's perspective offers unique insights into how patients view professional nursing practice and can assist nurses to better understand how to improve their practice. For example, Duffy & Brewer (2011) used a collaborative quality improvement approach with 12 hospitals to assess patients' perceptions of nurse caring and provided feedback for use in practice revision. On a more individual level, Duffy et al. (2012) pilot tested the feasibility of assessing hospitalized older adults' perceptions of nurse caring using an electronic format during hospitalization. Using a mobile device, 86 older adults provided feedback on RNs' caring relationships. The study demonstrated feasibility and is intended to be applied to provide data for real-time practice improvement. Using the wisdom of multiple sources and perspectives to provide this important feedback is a generative approach that is less threatening to individual nurses and allows for patient participation.

Feedback from patients in both academia and the clinical setting keeps the focus on human persons needing healthcare and can be used creatively to:

- encourage more open dialogue about caring professional practice
- reinforce the importance of caring processes (or behaviors)
- reflect back to students and/or clinical nurses how significant their caring relationships are to patient outcomes
- identify strengths and areas for development
- raise awareness of how the curriculum or the practice environment might be influencing caring practice

Assuring Educational Program Success

Formative and summative evaluation of concepts considered central to a program's curriculum and based on that program's philosophy and objectives provides important evidence of the program's success. Such evaluation helps meet the mandate of producing competent clinicians who can fulfill practice expectations (in this case, caring competency). In the second domain of person-centered care (AACN, 2021a), examples of caring competencies (see below) are included:

- demonstrates qualities of empathy
- promotes caring relationships to effect positive outcomes
- demonstrates compassionate care
- fosters caring relationships
- establishes mutual respect with the individual and family
- demonstrates relationship-centered care

- applies nursing knowledge to gain a holistic perspective of the person, family, community, and population
- engages the individual and the team in plan development
- assists the individual to engage in self-care management
- employs counseling techniques, including motivational interviewing to advance wellness and self-care management.
- respects individuals and families' self-determination in their healthcare decisions.
- promotes collaboration by clarifying responsibilities among individual, family, and team members

(AACN, 2021a, pp. 29–32)

In the educational environment, caring relationships is one of several enduring nursing concepts; thus, it would follow that a quality program evaluation would encompass caring-based performance indicators. Using the major concepts in the QCM as a guide, identification of student and faculty variables that contribute to learning processes and resulting competencies could be assessed. Evaluating curricular processes, such as instructional methods, relationships between students and faculty, including values, attitudes, and behaviors that faculty members carry out in partnership with students during the learning process provide important formative evaluation of the program. Including collaborative relationships with other departments or practice partners also provides valuable information. In fact, such relationships undergird and facilitate student learning, leading to specific educational outcomes.

The third major component of the QCM, "feeling cared for," can be considered an intermediate program outcome that is the immediate result of the educational process. "When one feels 'cared for,' a sense of security develops making it easier to learn, change behaviors, and take risks" (Duffy & Hoskins, 2003, p. 83). Undergraduate students who feel cared for while in the learning environment have reported better academic outcomes (Ingraham et al., 2018). Several tools and other methods are available for this purpose. "Feeling cared for" in students and faculty leads to similar outcomes as those in patients—feeling safe, empowered, respected, listened to, encouraged, connected—that ultimately result in self-advancement.

Creating caring environments during the educational process and role modeling caring relationships raise awareness of its importance and facilitate learning. Assessing students' perceptions of faculty caring can yield important data about the structure and processes of an educational program. The Caring Assessment Tool-Educational Version (CAT-edu) is an example of an instrument used to evaluate this variable (Duffy, 2007). Students can complete this assessment formatively or summatively, and the results can be used by faculty members to revise their interactions with future students. Although this discussion has centered on quantitative program evaluation, using qualitative approaches such as reflective journaling, narratives, portfolios, focus groups, and other methods adds valuable information to the quantitative assessment.

Finally, transparent and ongoing feedback and curricular revisions are consistent with educational practice improvement.

BOX 11.12: A self-advancing educational system reflects forward progress that enhances the systems' well-being. It evolves naturally without external control, provided attention is paid to the relational components of the model.

Self-advancing educational systems can be evaluated through empirical indicators (summative learning outcomes, evaluated by demonstration of those skills. faculty productivity, system utilization, and resources used), and are used to provide ongoing evidence for process changes.

With a foundational model as a guide, a program's evaluation plan should reflect the faculty's decisions about responsibility, frequency of assessment, specific measurements, and acceptable criteria. Multiple perspectives applied formatively over the course of the curriculum culminating in end-of-program summative evaluation are recommended. In this case, assessing those relationships inherent in educational processes and relational learning outcomes is crucial.

Assuring caring competence from the perspective of the student, the faculty, and, most important, the recipients of caring (patients) is worthy.

Patients' perceptions of student nurse caring capacity better assesses whether students are actually conveying caring to patients and families. To prevent faculty and patient burden, a limited number of these evaluations is recommended at key points in a program. Using valid and reliable instruments, faculty can design how students will best select patients and administer the instrument. Scores from such evaluations should be shared with students and used by faculty (along with the other evaluations) to provide feedback about performance and make judgments about the effectiveness of the curriculum in preparing caring graduates.

Although subjective, student self-reports of nurse caring can provide a baseline assessment at program entry and then be followed annually (or more frequently) to determine improvement. This allows for trending by program level and over time. Clinical evaluation tools that include both subjective and objective measures of nurse caring that are consistent across the program can be used from a faculty perspective to assess students' progress in caring competence. Such measures can be as simple as one item with higher scores expected as students progress in the program or composed of multiple items that are summed for a total score. Faculty evaluation of students' caring competencies can then be easily assessed across program levels and compared for progression across the program.

Taking advantage of lessons learned during the past few years requires nursing faculty members and continuing education professionals to shift their thinking (and resulting actions) towards more collaborative learning, practice readiness, integration of more meaningful clinical experiences, and different ways of learning and evaluation. At the same time, ensuring excellence by measuring key competencies related to nursing performance while co-creating more robust interactions with service partners may help to bridge the theory–practice gap.

SUMMARY

This chapter focused on teaching and learning the practice of nursing. In particular, nursing practice was likened to a performance integrating "being" and "doing" simultaneously. Learning how to care was described as a repetitive process that occurs over time and in a context requiring relational learning strategies, renewing emphasis on clinical courses, and revising how one evaluates learning. Person-centered caring pedagogies using the caring processes (or behaviors) and encouraging openness, risk-taking, and engagement facilitate the design of meaningful learning experiences that contribute to self-advancement (positive learning outcomes). Incorporating aspects of these factors into learning objectives across the curriculum best integrates the concept of caring as a significant ingredient in professional practice.

Emphasizing the affective domain of learning in the performance of nursing is key to quality clinical education. Best evidenced in clinical courses, nursing faculty have multiple opportunities to role model, facilitating student learning while honoring patients and families. The importance of a revised curriculum to meet complex health systems' needs for professional nurses is stressed with recommendations for curricula and faculty members. Finally, assessing developing caring capacity throughout educational programs at graduation and within the practice environment is discussed. Nursing educational programs can incorporate caring-based instruments to formatively and summatively evaluate individual students' developing caring capacity and to ensure that this important and enduring concept is embedded throughout the curriculum and the learning environment, allowing for fully prepared and caring graduates.

CALL TO ACTION

Student–faculty caring relationships combined with rich experiential learning in the clinical setting is the best possible way to help students learn professional caring. *Evaluate* your relationships with students. Using the context of caring relationships to design and implement learning experiences assists nursing students to understand complex phenomena. Faculty members who connect caring nursing situations to the larger whole enable graduates to adjust to the complex healthcare system and transfer their knowledge to a variety of nursing situations. *Increase* the amount of time you spend with students this week.

The performance of nursing is best demonstrated during clinical education. In the clinical situation, faculty members have the opportunity to encourage opinions, shape ideas, establish a secure system for inquiry, and assess the usefulness of their teaching. *Sign up* for a clinical course. Noticing students' attitudes and actions, actively listening to verbal and behavioral cues, and showing interest in their work is necessary to gauge student progress. It requires faculty members to remain unhurried, focused, and deliberate enough to pay attention. *Acknowledge* the strengths of students' work.

Professional nurses are better able to advance their practice (and resulting caring capacity) when they receive feedback from multiple sources, including from the patient's perspective. Such detail offers unique insight directly from the source and suggests specific ways to improve. **Rewrite** your last lecture to include the patient's perspective.

In the context of caring relationships, nursing faculty members have the responsibility to design, facilitate, and evaluate learning experiences that positively impact student learning and enhance patient outcomes. **Revise** your student evaluation method(s) to enhance student learning. **Employ** valid and reliable tools to evaluate students' perceptions of faculty caring and use the data to improve.

REFLECTIVE QUESTIONS/APPLICATIONS

For Professional Nurses in Clinical Practice:

■ Do you engage in student learning activities—as a preceptor or clinical instructor? How does affective learning bring together knowledge and psychomotor skills? What will you do to foster this domain?

■ Analyze the education–practice gap. How would you recommend it be narrowed?

■ What is your stand on "caring can be learned"? Why?

■ Are you surprised to hear that patients report that caring relationships with nurses and person-centeredness was a need? Why or why not?

For Professional Nurses in Educational Practice:

■ Does your educational program still use the traditional methods for clinical courses? Are they separated from didactic content? How much clinical time do students get? Are they experiencing *real* nursing practice?

■ Appraise the phrase *caring pedagogies*. How is it operationalized in your curriculum?

■ Appraise the sentence *"Clinical education is an advanced form of education that is not routinely given a rightful status in nursing academia."* What challenges or conflicts are implied by this?

■ List baccalaureate and graduate student demands that limit authentic relationships in the educational environment. How could these be eased or the environment revised to enhance relationship building?

■ What caring and non-caring faculty behaviors do you observe at your institution?

■ Analyze the core concepts that undergird your curriculum. Are they enduring? How are they learned in depth and advanced over the program? What evaluation methods do you use to ensure profound understanding of these concepts?

- What innovative strategies can you identify to ensure that the three domains of learning related to caring relationships are threaded throughout your curriculum?

- How would you implement a 360-degree student evaluation program in your curriculum?

- Reflect on your role as a faculty member. How do *you* role model caring? What self-caring practices do you regularly carry out? Are you certain that meaningful (i.e., breadth and depth of the content) learning occurs in your classroom? What ways can you identify to integrate caring pedagogies into your teaching style? How can you better integrate didactic and clinical learning?

- Make a list of the caring factors and describe how you enact them in relationships with baccalaureate and graduate students. Do they differ based on level? Should they?

- Consider an online course with graduate students. Develop at least three learning objectives each for the cognitive, psychomotor, and affective domains that include caring relationships with patients. How would you ensure by your interactions with students that caring was conveyed?

- Consider a course that you currently teach. Design a caring learning experience that includes five small (three to five students) groups, each with its own activity that blends into one larger caring concept.

- What ideas do you have to help baccalaureate students develop deep meaning in the caring relationships they have with patients and families? How would you implement them? What practice experiences could best provide opportunities for students to know and connect with patients and families?

- What strategies might you use with graduate students to help them develop deep meaning regarding the caring relationships they should cultivate with the healthcare team? How would you implement them?

- What type of faculty members can best use caring pedagogies? Are there some who cannot? What are the characteristics of those who are successful?

- Describe how you are able to transfer humanness from the simulation lab to the clinical area.

- Is your educational program currently in the process of revising its curriculum? How many of the competencies from the New Essentials (AACN, 2021a) have you used to revise the curriculum? Be honest.

- How do you assure caring capacity in your students?

- Does your program use a conceptual framework to guide evaluation? How could you influence that?

- How do you partner with a clinical service?

For Professional Nurses in Leadership Practice:

- What do you see as the major factors of concern between academia and service? What is your part in this process?

- How does the new graduate experience at your institution affect caring professional practice?

- What continuing education activities at your institution promote caring professional practice? How do you know?

- How are professional development nursing educators in your system evaluated? Should it be changed?

- Are nurse caring behaviors integrated into the required annual competencies at your institution? Could they be integrated? How would you go about integrating them?

- How would you suggest professional development nursing educators in your system continue the trend toward competency-based learning?

- How do you partner with schools of nursing? What competencies in new graduates do you expect? Have they been discussed and agreed to?

PRACTICE ANALYSIS

After multiple attempts at teaching nurses the value of high-quality patient experiences at a large community hospital, the nurse educators were frustrated. Over the last 2 years, they had developed online learning modules, in-class lectures, and annual competency assessments to help RNs improve their practice. These learning activities were required, and over 85% of the hospital RNs had attended at least one of the above classes; however, patient experience scores had not improved. They concluded that simply having the knowledge and skills did not ensure that behaviors would change.

During a series of discussions with a faculty member at a local nursing school, they decided to turn their attention to the actual practice environment where RNs' work in collaboration with other health professionals who interface with patients and families. They developed and implemented a team-based training approach, ensuring that it was integrated into the actual work environment, and followed with an assessment of both individual and team competencies related to patient experience.

As a first step, the educators exposed healthcare teams to the value of positive patient experiences using video clips of real patients, stories, and brainstorming techniques to raise awareness. They then used a case-based exercise based on a real patient currently receiving care on the unit to engage the team in active review of a real situation. Evaluation of this activity included active participation in the co-creation of an ideal patient experience diagram. In the next learning activity, during AM huddles, the educators observed team members for voluntary expressions of the value of positive patient experiences and called them out to reinforce their importance. During interprofessional rounds attended by an educator, team members were challenged to ask participating patients to comment on how the interactions with the team influenced whether they felt "cared for." The educators reviewed the comments with the team, providing pointed feedback that showed the link between any new practice behaviors and positive patient experiences.

Continued observation of clinical teams on the units by the educators was completed looking for evidence of "advocating" for positive patient experiences. Reinforcement and advanced facilitation techniques (e.g., coaching, conflict management) for consistent performance were provided by the educators. Finally, tracking the teams' behaviors over time to continue their development through self-assessments and observations were conducted. In this review, a self-assessment was tied to the value of positive patient experiences, and links to other important patient outcomes were pointed out. Encouragement and positive rewards as well as opportunities for sharing their newfound expertise were offered.

- What did the educators do differently after they met with the university professor? What did the clinical aspect of this learning experience accomplish? How do you think the RNs accepted this form of learning and why?

- How do you think the educators should evaluate this learning experience?

REFERENCES

Adamski, M., Parsons, V., & Hooper, C. (2009). Internalizing the concept of CARING: An examination of student perceptions when nurses share their stories. *Nursing Education Perspectives*, 30(6), 358–361. https://doi.org/10.1097/HNP.0b013e3181dd47bc

American Association of Colleges of Nursing. (2019). AACN's vision for academic nursing. https://www.aacnnursing.org/News-Information/Position-Statements-White -Papers/Vision-for-Nursing-Education

American Association of Colleges of Nursing. (2021a). The essentials: Core competencies for professional nursing education. https://www.aacnnursing.org/Portals/42/AcademicNursing/pdf/Essentials-2021.pdf

American Association of Colleges of Nursing. (2021b). Student enrollment surged in U.S. schools of nursing in 2020 despite challenges presented by the pandemic. https://www.aacnnursing.org/News-Information/Press-Releases/View/ArticleId/24802/2020-survey-data-student-enrollment

Arkan, B., Ordin, Y., & Yılmaz, D. (2018). Undergraduate nursing students' experience related to their clinical learning environment and factors affecting to their clinical learning process. *Nurse Education in Practice*, 29, 127–132.

Barbour, C., & Delene, V. (2021). Nursing students' perspective of faculty caring using Duffy's quality caring model: A Q-methodology study. *International Journal of Caring Sciences*, 14(1), 18–28.

Benner, P. (1984) From novice to expert: Excellence and power in clinical nursing practice. *American Journal of Nursing*, 84, 1480. http://dx.doi.org/10.1097/00000446 -198412000-00027

Benner, P., Sutphen, M., Leonard, V., & Day, L. (2010). *Educating nurses: A call for radical transformation*. Jossey-Bass, Higher and Adult Education Series.

Bergren, M. D. (2022). Call for doctor of nursing practice project manuscripts: Closing the knowing-doing gap. *The Journal of School Nursing*, 38(2), 124–125. https://doi.org/10.1177/10598405211073867

Bloom, B. S. (Ed.) (1956). *Taxonomy of educational objectives, the classification of educational goals—Handbook I: Cognitive domain*. McKay.

Bullin, C. (2018). To what extent has doctoral (PhD) education supported academic nurse educators in their teaching roles: An integrative review. *BMC Nursing, 17*(1), 1–18.

Duffy, J. (2007). Caring assessment tools. In J. Watson (Ed.). *Instruments for assessing and measuring caring in nursing and health sciences* (2nd ed.). Springer Publishing Company.

Duffy, J. (2018). *Quality caring in nursing and health systems: Implications for clinicians, educators, and leaders*. Springer Publishing Company.

Duffy, J., & Brewer, B. (2011). Feasibility of a multi-institution collaborative to improve patient–nurse relationship quality. *Journal of Nursing Administration, 41*(2), 78–83. https://doi.org/10.1097/NNA.0b013e3182059463

Duffy, J., & Hoskins, L. (2003). The quality-caring model©: Blending dual paradigms. *Advances in Nursing Science, 26*(1), 77–88. https://doi.org/10.1097/00012272-200301000-00010

Duffy, J., Kooken, W., Wolverton, C., & Weaver, M. (2012). Evaluating patient-centered care: Feasibility of electronic data collection in hospitalized older adults. *Journal of Nursing Care Quality, 27*(4), 307–315. https://doi.org/10.1097/NCQ.0b013e31825ba9d4

Emory, J., Kippenbrock, T., & Buron, B. (2021). A national survey of the impact of COVID-19 on personal, academic, and work environments of nursing students. *Nursing Outlook, 69*(6), 1116–1125. https://doi.org/10.1016/j.outlook.2021.06.014

Epstein, R. M., & Street, R. L. (2011). The value and values of patient-centered care. *Annals of Family Medicine, 9*(2), 100–103. https://doi.org/10.1370/afm.1239

Feeg, V., Mancino, D. J., Mooney, C., Catanese, S., & Buonaguro, R. (2021). The COVID-19 nursing student self-reported education and personal experiences during the early months of the pandemic. *Deans Notes, 42*, 1–7. https://www2.ajj.com/sites/default/files/services/publishing/deansnotes/spring2021.pdf

Geier, M. T. (2022). The teacher behavior checklist: The mediation role of teacher behaviors in the relationship between the students' importance of teacher behaviors and students' effort. *Teaching of Psychology, 49*(1), 14–20.

Groccia, J. E., Ismail, E. A., McConner, M., Ford, C. R., & Noll, K. (2018). Perceptions of excellent teachers: International, HBCU, and health professions perspectives. *New Directions for Teaching and Learning, Winter 2018*(156), 85–94.

Günay, U., & Kılınç, G. (2018). The transfer of theoretical knowledge to clinical practice by nursing students and the difficulties they experience: A qualitative study. *Nurse Education Today, 65*, 81–86.

Henderson, D., Sewell, K. A., & Wei, H. (2020). The impact of faculty caring on nursing students' intent to graduate: A systematic literature review. *International Journal of Nursing Sciences, 7*(1), 105–111.

Ingraham, K. C., Davidson, S. J., & Yonge, O. (2018). Student-faculty relationships and its impact on academic outcomes. *Nurse Education Today, 71*, 17–21.

Jones, K., Burnett, G., Sztuba, L., & Hannon, R. (2021). Academic practice partnerships: A review of a statewide population health nursing leadership initiative. *Public Health Nursing, 38*(1), 64–76.

Kavanagh, J. M., & Sharpnack, P. A. (2021). Crisis in competency: A defining moment in nursing education. *OJIN: The Online Journal of Issues in Nursing, 26*(1), Man 02. https://doi.org/10.3912/OJIN.Vol26No01Man02

Labrague, L. J., McEnroe, P. D. M., D'Souza, M. S., Hammad, K. S., & Hayudini, J. N. A. (2020). Nursing faculty teaching characteristics as perceived by nursing students: An integrative review. *Scandinavian Journal of Caring Sciences, 34*(1), 23–33. https://doi.org/10.1111/scs.12711

Maslow, A. H. (1943). A theory of motivation. *Psychological Review, 50*, 370–396. https://doi.org/10.1037/h0054346

McFadden, T., Keyt, J., & Fang, D. (2021). Special survey on vacant faculty positions for academic year 2021–2022. https://www.aacnnursi ng.org/Portals/42/News/Surveys-Data/2021-Faculty-Vacancy-Report.pdf

McPherson, S. (2019). Part-time clinical nursing faculty needs: An integrated review. *Journal of Nursing Education, 58*(4), 201–206.

Michel, A., Ryan, N., Mattheus, D., Knopf, A., Abuelezam, N. N., Stamp, K., Branson, S., Hekel, B., & Fontenot, H. B. (2021). Undergraduate nursing students' perceptions on nursing education during the 2020 COVID-19 pandemic: A national sample. *Nursing Outlook, 69*(5), 903–912.

Miller, A. C., & Mills, B. (2019). 'If They Don't Care, I Don't Care': Millennial and generation Z students and the impact of faculty caring. *Journal of the Scholarship of Teaching and Learning, 19*(4), 78–89.

Murphy, N., Strong, C., & Jones, G. (2022). Flipped learning: A shift in graduate nursing education. *Journal of the American Association of Nurse Practitioners, 34*(1), 135–141.

National League for Nursing. (2022). Core competencies for academic nurse educators. http://www.nln.org/professional-development-programs/competencies-for-nursing-education/nurse-educator-core-competency

Noll, K. (2021). Effective teaching qualities as identified by nursing faculty. *Nursing Education Perspectives, 42*(4), 243–245. https://doi.org/10.1097/01.NEP.0000000000000744

Pownall, M., Harris, R., & Blundell-Birtill, P. (2022). Supporting students during the transition to university in COVID-19: Five key considerations and recommendations for educators. *Psychology Learning & Teaching, 21*(1), 3–18.

Purnell, M. J. (2009). Gleaning wisdom in the research on caring. *Nursing Science Quarterly, 22*(2), 109–115. https://doi.org/10.1177/0894318409332777

Raso, A., Marchetti, A., D'Angelo, D., Albanesi, B., Garrino, L., Dimonte, V., Piredda, M., & De Marinis, M. G. (2019). The hidden curriculum in nursing education: A scoping study. *Medical Education, 53*(10), 989–1002. https://doi.org/10.1111/medu.13911

Smith, S. M., Buckner, M., Jesse, M. A., Robbins, V., Horst, T., & Ivory, C. H. (2021). Impact of COVID-19 on new graduate nurses' transition to practice: Loss or gain? *Nurse Educator, 46*, 209–214. https://doi.org/10.1097/NNE.0000000000001042

Stamps, D. C., & Smith, C. M. (2022). RN-to-BS transition: An academic–practice partnership focused on quality and safety. *Journal for Nurses in Professional Development, 38*(1), 33–39.

Weston, M. J. (2022). Strategic planning for a very different nursing workforce. *Nurse Leader, 20*(2), 152–160. https://doi.org/10.1016/j.mnl.2021.12.021

Zlotnick, C., & McDonnell-Naughton, M. (2022). "Thinking outside the box": Social innovations emerging from academic nursing-community partnerships. In C. Păunescu, K. L. Lepik, & N. Spencer. (Eds.). *Social innovation in higher education: Innovation, technology, and knowledge management*. Springer Publishing Company.

CHAPTER 12

The Value of Quality Caring

"Knowledge is of no value unless you put it into practice."

—Anton Chekhov

CHAPTER OBJECTIVES:

1. Evaluate examples of sustained theory-based clinical practice.
2. State four products/services that will impact the future of healthcare.
3. Describe characteristics of healthy clinical, leadership, and educational work environments.
4. State two approaches for advancing the science of caring relationships.

ENVISIONING THE FUTURE: 10 YEARS, 50 YEARS, AND BEYOND

Futurists speculate on how people will live, work, die, be educated, pay for, and experience healthcare 50 to 60 years from now—and in some cases, in the next few months! The COVID-19 pandemic has exposed the fact that rapid deployment of novel products and services is possible and has expedited several of them that were already in the pipeline for implementation (e.g., telehealth). Based on this experience, digital health is now seen as *necessary* for efficient communication, sharing of health data, monitoring and surveillance, actual provision of health services (telehealth, consultations, prescriptions), health education, and decision support (Cowie & O'Connor, 2022; Fotis, 2022; Williams et al., 2022). Artificial intelligence, robotics, epigenetics, blockchain, data mining, and other deep or machine-type learning technologies are already transforming how healthcare is learned, delivered, and evaluated (Agbo & Mahmoud, 2020; Bartosiak et al., 2022; Pinella et al., 2022; Triberti et al., 2022). New products/services such as virtual traffic control systems (to expedite hospital bed assignments), Short Messaging Service (SMS) texts used in rural areas, home-based care such as "hospital at home," a renewed focus on prevention and prediction versus disease-based care, natural language processing for nurses, and interprofessional team-based care (American Hospital Association [AHA], 2022; Clipper, 2022) are already operational.

From an economic and regulation perspective, demands for health systems and health professionals to deliver care differently, specifically in relation to increasing value and prevention continue. From a nursing perspective, practicing at the top of the license, instituting novel care delivery systems, data-informed decision making, patient/families and health care teams co-creating health, incorporation of technology, all amidst a challenged and exhausted workforce will require higher and more sophisticated levels of knowledge and optimum flexibility.

From a patient perspective, expectations for individualized services delivered at the point of care by health teams that actually collaborate with each other, active roles in decision making regarding health parameters, alternative treatment options, financing alternatives, and electronic communications, all provided within a framework of person-centeredness will significantly affect healthcare delivery and the work of all health professionals.

These varied points of view are only a small perspective of the overall context of healthcare at present. No one can predict the future with certainty; however, in general, individuals and systems tend to underestimate the pace of transformation and the resultant need for swift action. For example, from the time the first edition of this book was published until now (13 years), several of the original projections have already come true. Real-time virtual meetings including continuing education conferencing have become the norm, distance learning dominates healthcare professional education programs, virtual doctor's visits, point-of-care diagnostics and monitoring; and more transparent, integrated, electronic information systems connect hospitals, physician offices, and outpatient clinics. As has been the case for many years, healthcare costs continue to dominate the discussions around healthcare and will continue to do so.

National health spending was projected to grow at an average annual rate of 5.4% for 2019 to 2028 and to reach $6.2 trillion by 2028. Among the major payers, Medicare was expected to experience the fastest spending growth (7.6% per year), largely as a result of having the highest projected enrolment and growth (Centers for Medicare and Medicaid Services [CMS], 2020). *These CMS projections did not include the effects from the pandemic, which remain highly uncertain.* However, a more recent publication reported that US healthcare spending increased 9.7% to reach $4.1 trillion in 2020, a much faster growth rate than the 4.3% increase seen in 2019, and this acceleration was due to a 36.0% increase in federal expenditures for healthcare that occurred largely in response to the COVID-19 pandemic. At the same time, gross domestic product declined 2.2%, and the share of the economy devoted to healthcare spending spiked, reaching 19.7% (Hartman et al., 2022). In 2022, inflation is at an all-time high, and the international humanitarian crises generated by the Ukraine war climate change, and worldwide immigration is expected to create increased needs for worldwide health programs, adding to elevated costs!

How these increased projections for healthcare costs will be spread across hospitals, insurers, programs, and individuals over the next several years remains uncertain; and how they will impact health professionals in terms of income and workload is also worrisome. In fact, most agree that delivering healthcare may never "go back to normal;" rather, current world circumstances have altered forever the "work of nursing" and other health professionals (Rosenfeld et al., 2022) and demands a national "reset" (Kerfoot, 2022). There remains much uncertainty and sometimes angst when discussing this issue, leading some to express ongoing weariness and doubt. Yet, the melding of multiple events that impact health has instigated exciting possibilities to improve, grow, and support health and well-being, albeit with fundamental infrastructure modifications.

The rate of innovation expected today is novel and sweeping. It demands changes in behavior, including forward movement from from both leaders and employees that is often counter cultural to traditional health systems, The increased demand and range of services required, including increased attention to public health and social determinants of health, necessitates nonconventional thinking and different ways of working. The persistent challenges inherent in professional nursing (e.g., the workforce, the workflow, and the workload) remain at an all-time high, continuing to plague hard-working professional nurses and their leaders and educators. However, yesterday's solutions will not repair today's or tomorrow's healthcare challenges.

BOX 12.1: The future of healthcare—and the quality of patient care—depends on health professionals actively participating with the right leadership and supportive educators in a spirit of mutual problem-solving, to remodel healthcare delivery in accord with persons' needs (versus the system's needs).

Fortunately, recent nursing graduates and other health professionals are more educated and tech savvy than previous generations. Most grew up with handheld technology and understood its inner functions before they entered the educational system, giving them skills that are crucial to healthcare today. They also have ambition, embrace change, are innovative, and have a desire to keep learning, but are uncomfortable with rigid organizational structures and are turned off by information silos. They expect rapid progression, recognition, a varied and meaningful career, and encouraging, continuous feedback, and will move on quickly if their expectations are not met (Shorey et al., 2021). Such expectations require very different workplaces, those focused on individuals—employees, healthcare providers, and most importantly, patients, families, and communities.

BOX 12.2: In fact, today's nurses are multigenerational, and they hold many of the qualities needed by health systems today. Working with this talented group of nursing professionals is a privilege, *provided they are valued and empowered to practice in health systems where caring relationships dominate.*

However, most professional nurses' work structures remain the same as they were over 40 years ago! In fact, nursing work environments continue to be associated with preventable reasons to leave (Taylor-Clark et al., 2022). *The fundamental challenge facing the nursing profession today is ensuring the delivery of high-value healthcare by expertly attending to the enduring core values and responsibilities of the discipline—those that are central to professional practice. This challenge extends not only to the delivery of clinical care, but also nursing education, nursing leadership, and nursing research!* A health profession that recognizes, identifies with, and *uses* caring relationships as the basis for its work, structures its practice accordingly—focusing it on persons with health needs as they exist in relationship to others and their communities. Preserving this implicit reality as new practice models are being developed honors the centrality of the patient-nurse relationship in facilitating optimal health outcomes, including costs, while upholding longstanding disciplinary values, the key to professional and personal advancement.

RENEWED AND REVITALIZED QUALITY CARING PRACTICE

Health professionals understand the benefits of caring relationships well, but often seem timid about fully actualizing them. In many health systems and other places where nurses work, caring relationships are assumed, are not routinely recognized or honored, and are considered "soft" skills. The work environment in many health systems, particularly hospitals, is not organized with this in mind. What if nurses' work was organized such that it truly aligned with disciplinary values, professional practice models, and patients/families' needs and preferences? What if the relational aspect of nursing was overt and valued? What if clinical advancement programs were predicated on steady progress in relationship skills?

BOX 12.3: Caring relationships are fundamental to patients, health professionals, and health systems' advancement in that they provide the context for health behaviors, offer health professionals meaningful work, and are vital for safe and quality patient outcomes.

Given that all health professionals learn about, provide care within, and are expected to participate in caring relationships, the fact that they are not fully actualized is a great irony. The ability to deliver safe, high-quality services, collaborate, engage, continuously learn and be innovative, and ultimately advance *depends* on caring relationships. In fact, caring relationships are the basis for person-centered care and health professionals' own work-life satisfaction. The theorized results of caring relationships—feeling cared for and ultimately self-advancement—become obvious when we examine those health systems and health professionals who are choosing to embrace caring relationships as the basis for their work. Such systems and health professionals are committed to serving patients and families, build trust, and create value by "going against the grain" enough to make a difference. These are courageously engaged health professionals and systems who understand that meaningful human connections elevate healthcare from a commodity that can be nicely packaged and paid for to a human partnership based on professional ethics, joint knowledge of the other, and ongoing accountability. One might ask, "How can high-caring organizations—those with observable relational capacity, energy, and joy—operate in such an uncertain, metric-focused, and resource-driven world?" The answer lies in their grasp of caring relationships as the fuel that propels self-advancing systems forward. As such, nurses in these organizations continuously work on faithfully integrating quality caring principles throughout their systems.

Recently, the world has witnessed nurses on the frontline of a pandemic, responding as they always do—equitably, with caring, and expertise. They have selflessly delivered care to COVID-19 positive patients while continuing to provide services across the health and care system. Many, if not most, have done this while simultaneously raising children, completing educational programs, or conducting other family responsibilities. Their vital contribution to the health of all citizens has been demonstrated as has the care and comfort provided to families who were grieving. Unfortunately, nurses in organizations who commit to caring relationships as the basis for practice are not often highlighted in the media or exposed in newspaper articles. Yet, they quietly demonstrate differences for patient and health systems every day! Examples are presented in the following paragraphs that represent both academic and community health systems and some universities, larger and smaller (in terms of numbers of beds or students), urban and rural, diverse and homogeneous, and with differing patient populations. For many, these health systems have been quietly integrating quality caring principles throughout their organizations for some time, and in some cases, serve as national exemplars of quality caring practice. Their choice to continue the focus on caring relationships is fueling momentum—improving practice, reducing low-value care, providing evidence, and creating healthy work environments.

At Lakeland Regional Health, for example, an 864-bed, not-for-profit hospital in Florida with over 165,278 emergency department visits in 2020, leaders and health professionals continue to advance human persons by placing people at the heart of all they do, choosing to place the value of caring at the center of daily activity for the entire organization (Lakeland Regional Health, 2022). They have adopted a culture of relationships and caring that pledges certain promises to its people:

- to treasure all people as uniquely created
- to nurture, educate, and guide with integrity
- to inspire each and every one to do their very best

The promises are prominently displayed on the system's walls and website, within the elevators, and are exhibited in its people. Accordingly, they are at the heart of caregiving, decision making, and used in everyday interactions.

Impressively, this organization has stayed the course with this culture of caring, and evidence can be observed within the entire team, including the board, the departments of human resources, public relations, information technology, nursing, clinical services, support services, and financial services. Their compelling application of relationships and caring places people at the heart of their work and has shaped a unique culture that is proudly displayed in their mission statement and evidenced by multiple state and national awards.

At Lowell General Hospital (LGH) in Lowell, Massachusetts, a Magnet®-designated hospital that has been using the Quality-Caring Model© (QCM) for many years, multiple examples exist of caring relationships as the center of practice. One example includes the work of a particular clinical manager, a longstanding employee of the system. As part of an awards ceremony, the staff on the unit related how this manager leads by example, ensuring that all patients receive excellent care, and staff feel supported as well. This clinical manager was observed to be always ready to help as evidenced by the many times she assisted during rapid responses with hygiene care and by working during nights, evenings, and weekend shifts when staffing was low. Staff members relayed that she actively listens to their concerns while working to find team solutions and posts words of encouragement on the whiteboard on her office door. When COVID-19 changed the typical work flow and staff were floated, this clinical manager helped ease the transition by meeting these staff members in the lobby, bringing them to the location where they would be working, and introducing them to that team. Such actions demonstrated several of the caring behaviors, namely mutual problem-solving, human respect, attentive reassurance, and encouraging manner; and they made a big difference during an uncertain time. Results of her leadership helped staff feel inspired, attrition has decreased, staff satisfaction has improved as they were challenged to be their best, and a sense of family evolved in the department. Staff members stated, "She has united us, pushed us to be better, and lifted us up" (Lowell General Hospital, 2022). What an example of "feeling cared for"!

At Jefferson Health, a large academic health system in the Greater Philadelphia and South New Jersey area (18 hospitals, two main University campuses, and 42,000 employees), nurses began integrating the QCM *during* the COVID-19 pandemic. After a comprehensive 2-day virtual conference in early 2020, the nursing leadership team and several clinical nurses and nurse educators began integrating the model into various aspects of operations. For example, in the nurse residency curriculum, new graduates address the relationship of the QCM in their residency project, and the QCM (specifically the caring behaviors) is incorporated into the top nursing award presented during the Nurses Week Awards ceremony. An ongoing pre-post implementation assessment of patients' perceptions of "feeling cared for" is being conducted to evaluate the success of the integration effort. Interestingly, Jefferson Health nurses have continued their integration efforts *despite* the fact that they have cared for more COVID-19 patients than any other health system in the Philadelphia area!

At the South Florida State College School of Nursing, faculty members have used the QCM to guide their BSN curriculum for several years. To better demonstrate its significance, two nursing faculty members are developing a course entitled, *Caring in Nursing Practice*. The intent is to include it in the BSN curriculum and then modularize it to offer CEUs to nurses in the community. Likewise, at the University of West Georgia, the goal as stated on their website is: Academic excellence in a caring environment (University of West Georgia, 2022). The QCM is used to guide curriculum and was used to evaluate students' perceptions of faculty caring (Barbour & Volkert, 2021). Interestingly, students in this study reported that delivery of content effectively and efficiently was the most important demonstration of caring, while helping them reach their goals followed. Hopefully, faculty members will use this feedback during curricular revision.

At the Massachusetts Department of Health and Human Services Sexual Assault Nurse Examiner (SANE) program, a national nursing telemedicine center (NTC) was established several years ago to serve victims of sexual assault. Through the use of innovative video conferencing technology, the NTC continues to provide knowledge and support related to quality, trauma-informed sexual assault care. The QCM provides the foundation for the NTC clinical practice model, where it is operationalized to provide real-time guidance and support to victims as well as health professionals to assist crime victims and leadership, promoting justice and health for all (Massachusetts Department of Health and Human Services, 2017).

At the Montefiore Health System in the Bronx, New York, nurses held the 10th Annual Nursing Research Symposium virtually in October 2021, *in the midst of caring for many* COVID-19-*positive patients*. Nurses throughout the system showcased their improvement projects that continued during the pandemic. For example, nurses in the surgical ICU identified the problem that daily morning rounding was dominated by physicians/physician assistants (PAs) resulting in limited roles for nursing. The literature established that this collaborative time among the *entire* healthcare team was necessary to deliver optimal patient care. So, the team collaborated to design a performance improvement project using an evidence-based standardized rounding model that included a written report used by nurses, a "read-back of plan" by the PA, and active nursing participation. Several process variables, job satisfaction, and teamwork were assessed pre and post the "intervention" with valid and reliable instruments. Findings showed that the standardized rounding process improved both nurse and provider perceptions of teamwork and decreased the time in rounds overall. Nursing engagement in rounds increased somewhat as the intervention continued. However, job satisfaction decreased during this time and was noted to be impacted by several variables, including the difficulties associated with the pandemic.

Although this example is only one of several, it is noteworthy that interprofessional collaboration underpinned by the caring behaviors was crucial in carrying out this project. In addition, this highly impressive nursing organization continued their scholarly approach towards practice improvement *during* the pandemic and conducted a winning symposium that integrated collaboration and evidence-based patient care validated by the systematic approach to performance improvement evaluation.

At the University of California San Diego Health, the focus on cultivating caring relationships with all individuals generates a work environment where feeling cared for is an everyday experience. For example, Jacqueline Imus (Jackie), who works on the surgical oncology unit, identified a problem related to patients with ostomies.

She writes, "I have come across so many patients struggling to look at their ostomy, let alone care for it." This life-changing experience often engenders feelings of awkwardness, embarrassment, and even shame. She sensed that there must be a better way to help patients cope and transition to a more secure view of themselves while living with their ostomy. One day, while on social media, the nurse saw an ostomate wearing an ostomy cover. After thinking about it, she decided that this may be a way to reduce the stigma associated with ostomies. She decided that although she had no experience sewing, she would figure out how to make the covers. She searched the web and sure enough there was a video detailing how to make the covers step by step along with a pattern. One day, Jackie asked her grandmother, a seamstress, to watch her attempt to make a cover. Jackie states, "After watching the video countless times, and some trial and error, I DID IT!! She could not have been more excited to share her idea with her managers at the time. Her manager responded, '"This has to be a performance improvement (PI) project!" Not knowing what a PI project entailed, Jackie agreed because she "wanted to do whatever it took to increase ostomates' comfort looking at their ostomies, adjusting to them, and increase their readiness to learn about caring for themselves."

The PI project used the Plan-Do-Study-Act (PDSA) model for performance improvement with the following objectives: 1) Increase patient satisfaction and body image, 2) decrease unit supply expenditures of home ostomy supply distribution, and 3) ensure nurse satisfaction with the process. A nurse-led sewing group was formed to make ostomy covers from a variety of fabrics and patterns for patients to select from. A comprehensive support packet was created and provided to patients. An additional layer to this project was creating a new discharge ostomy supply process. Teaming up with the wound ostomy nurses (WOCN), at UC San Diego Health, a standardized discharge ostomy supply process was added.

Jackie collaborated with the nurse scientist who helped with project instrumentation, including designing some qualitative questions on patients' personal experience and selecting valid and reliable instruments. Surveys were completed by patients and nurses pre- and post-intervention. Data were collected over a 4-month period.

After receiving the ostomy cover and support packet, patients reported an improvement in comfort with looking at the ostomy, adjusting to the ostomy, and their readiness to learn about their ostomy. Seventy four percent of patients found the packet to be helpful, and 93% reported the pouch cover helped them recover. There was a statistically significant increase in adjusting to the idea of having an ostomy after the use of the pouch ($p = .00044$); a statistically significant improvement in comfort looking at the pouch after using the pouch cover ($p = .0002$); and a statistically significant improvement in readiness to learn about ostomy care after the use of the pouch ($p = .00512$). Nurses also reported that providing the ostomy covers and support packet increased their job satisfaction. Additionally, there was a significant decrease in unit supply expenditures through standardization of home ostomy supply distribution.

Jackie states, "I was fortunate to have such amazing managers at the time who were always looking to advance and support my ideas. I knew in my heart that our patients needed this, but I did not realize how much they did until after gathering and compiling all the data. I am so grateful for the support from all the people that have embraced and helped with this project to show our ostomates that We Care."

The ostomy covers and support packets are still currently available, and Jackie has disseminated the project to other units at UC San Diego Health. She remains committed to making the covers and spreading awareness of ostomates' needs, including the importance of the caring behavior, appreciation of unique meanings, for years to come.

—Jacqueline Imus, BSN, RN, Clinical Nurse II

The evidence for application of caring relationships in this health system is remarkable. The nurse herself used appreciation of unique meanings to grasp patients' perspectives, including the difficulty adjusting to a life-changing situation. More importantly, she acted on it by finding a way to help them acclimate! But, just as important, her leaders and the nurse scientist used the caring behaviors (encouraging manner, mutual problem-solving, and healing environment) to support and facilitate the nurse's growth by instigating a PI project. As a result, the nurse learned, clinical practice was enriched, and patient outcomes were improved.

As demonstrated by these courageous nurses and health systems who hold caring relationships at the center of their practice, many find reassurance, strength, and encouragement. These caring leaders, educators, and clinical nurses are creating a critical mass of health professionals that are dramatically affecting the work of nursing practice and the course of patient care. As a whole, these health systems have been visited and observed by others to learn what they are doing differently; and in the interconnected world we currently live in, their influence may be larger than they even think. Health systems that have chosen to embrace caring relationships as a central unifying strength are benefiting in multiple ways: Reduced adverse outcomes, positive patient experiences, better and faster communication and collaboration, and patient and staff engagement.

BOX 12.4: Caring relationships are an asset to healthcare systems—they are critical for person-centered care, high-functioning teams, engaged patients and employees, learning, and ultimately, the best-quality outcomes.

QUALITY CARING IN ACTION

Clinical Practice

The disruption inflicted on the health system as a result of COVID-19 continues to affect the ability of nurses and the nursing profession to recover. Some, recognizing the depletion of the health professional workforce, are warning that "We will never have the numbers of nurses we had in the past" (personal conversations with hospital chief executive officers [CEOs] and chief nursing executives [CNEs]). Based on this, many are now calling for care delivery system changes with larger team-based patient-nurse ratios, incorporating less skilled health workers, while others are more cautious, citing that hospital leadership should more effectively manage the workforce (Seegert, 2022; Weston, 2022). This is interesting given that the current evidence has repeatedly shown that increased

BSN-prepared RNs lead to decreased errors in some patient populations (Harrison et al., 2019; O'Brien et al., 2018). Either way, the underlying challenges that the pandemic revealed, but were long known beforehand, require substantive change in work environments if nursing practice is to advance. Increased reliance on public health, virtual care, and technology during COVID-19 demonstrated that when challenged, fundamental adaptation and innovation can occur. However, the continuing fallout from COVID-19 in terms of nurse employment trends and unhealthy work environments requires immediate attention. Nurses and others are demanding it.

The nursing workforce emerging today is more diverse and multigenerational than ever before—baby boomers, generation X, generation Y (millennials), and generation Z nurses are working together in rising numbers at a turning point in the healthcare history. Their unique characteristics impact the nursing profession and healthcare environments. Most are open-minded and want to work in environments with supportive leadership, reasonable pay and benefits, adequate staffing to meet patient needs, opportunities for growth, flexibility, frequent feedback and connection, recognition, and an opportunity to make a difference (personal conversations and observations). They are technologically savvy, and many have had significant experiences beyond nursing school. As such, they are knowledge workers—that is, they are prepared to make impactful decisions, want to practice to their fullest extent, and aspire to respond in caring ways to the patient, family, and their own needs. To do this, however, they need work environments that make use of their talents. The dominant disease-based, task-oriented, and shift-focused approach of today is not the structure that nourishes the soul of this workforce!

Rather, today's nurses want to work in safe, empowering, and meaningful work environments that are linked to their true nature, *caring*. In other words, nurses want to work in health systems that are congruent with their professional values and the knowledge they have accumulated.

BOX 12.5: Professional nurses are educated to focus primarily on the whole person, rather than just the disease, to mutually collaborate with other health professionals, to use the caring behaviors and best evidence, to make clinical judgments, to engage in practice improvement, to perform holistic health assessments, to advocate for patients and families, to practice safely and to be accountable, and to have an appreciation for the larger system and community in which they work. They are educated to be responsible yet flexible, see possibilities, and strive for self-improvement by accepting feedback and continuously learning.

How many nurses are routinely using these talents in everyday practice?

The essence of nursing—caring—competes with the dominant context of contemporary healthcare workplaces, creating inconsistencies with disciplinary values. The COVID-19 pandemic magnified this discrepancy. Work environments where nurses feel a sense of pride in their work, that are meaningful, inclusive, attend to their human needs, and that positively impact patient outcomes are long overdue.

Consider the following:

One of the best places I ever worked in my long career was in a coronary care unit in the Northeast. I worked on the evening shift, and we usually had a 2:1 patient-nurse ratio. On this unit, a senior charge nurse was always there, and although she was a little intimidating, I knew if I needed advice, she would instantaneously be there. One night this happened. A new MI patient, a 64-year-old male, was admitted and assigned to me. I had only been employed on this unit for one month and was still learning and orienting. My patient abruptly dropped his pulse to 46. I went in, assessed his BP (which was low), and although I knew it was an emergent situation, I couldn't remember which standing order to implement. I went to get Emily, the charge nurse, and as I was coming out of the room, she was coming in—she had seen his bradycardia on the monitor. She immediately went to the patient's bedside and got the prefilled atropine syringe and administered the correct dose IV. His pulse increased to 68. Emily stayed with the patient and me, continuously assessing us. After she was assurred the patient was stable, we walked out of the room together. All the while, I was observing her behavior with the patient—she was calm, caring, and clever. She took me into the conference room and reviewed my performance with me. She did not yell, but was firm, reminding me of the standing orders for severe bradycardia, atropine's mechanism of action, and my duty to the patient. I have not forgotten her approach, especially her focus on the patient! After that experience, I vowed to learn as much as I could from her and about cardiovascular nursing and bought several books on the topic. I read them in my spare time, and they offered many helpful approaches.

My peers on this unit were of different ages and experiences, but after about 3 months of working there, we quickly bonded and became a team. We did things together outside of work and while at work, we often brought in dinners to share with the house staff. Since this was a teaching hospital, we participated in clinical rounds every evening with the cardiac fellow and other residents. We discussed how patients were progressing (or not) and then went into the patient's room to assess— all the while, the cardiac fellow was teaching. This was a great learning experience; everyone participated, including the patients who were able–and this was over 40 years ago! Sometimes after rounds, we would gather in the lounge with a coffee and discuss topics on the spot. One night, I clearly remember we just started talking about the classes of antiarrythmic drugs on the fly. A resident did a good job classifying their mechanisms of action, all the while joking with us. Although they have been updated over the years, I still remember those drug classifications!

Later, as a group of CCU nurses, we decided we needed a patient education program for recovering MI patients. I was encouraged to participate by developing the curriculum and teaching some classes and so I volunteered. Later, as we began a joint program with the county Emergency Management System, I was taking calls from paramedics in the field who were transporting MI patients to the hospitals. (At that time, calls came directly to the CCU). This was fun, and it kept me challenged.

But what I remember most about my work there was the comradery I felt with my co-workers, the equal status I shared with the medical staff, the safe space that was the unit norm (Emily always had my back), the autonomy and support I had once I was off orientation, the fun we had together, the learning we shared, and the patient experiences I was afforded. What a great place to work—I will never forget that experience!

The professional caring delivered to me in the work environment at this health system generated a sense of security, increased knowledge (I perfected my knowledge of heart sounds on this unit and was inspired to continue my education), confidence, a recognition of the significance of my work, and hope for an amazing career. At that time, I needed this reassurance, and I still remain appreciative of the caring received from those nurses and physicians many years later! The charge nurse expertly practiced the caring behaviors by placing patients first; expecting me to learn and participate, integrated being and doing, and maintained a purposeful and inclusive manner. In so doing, she met my needs as well as those of the patients. I have no doubt that this work environment fuelled my desire for advancement in my chosen profession.

BOX 12.6: Nurses, as one of several health professionals, forge collaborative relationships with other health team members for the benefit of patients and families and actively incorporate evidence from quality improvement and research activities into their practice. In many places, the clinical nurse of today is an admired and essential member of the healthcare workforce and is included in important clinical and system decisions.

Nurses who work in such environments gain so much in terms of their own personal and professional development. The acknowledgment that their work matters generates a sense of pride in their career choice, enabling and inspiring them to engage, learn, and appreciate the personal meanings that are generated from the work.

By genuinely caring, nurses in clinical practice experience many life lessons. Recently, a nurse relayed this story:

Mr. Carey was a 52-year-old male with chronic lymphocytic leukemia (CLL). He was post two bone marrow transplants (one autologous and one allogeneic) and one round of chemo and was in the process of a second round of chemo. He was admitted to a large suburban Magnet-designated hospital on an evening in May with herpes zoster (shingles) of his left arm starting at the axilla and continuing to his fingers. He had been suffering with this for over 3 weeks. Tonight, the pain was unbearable, and he was also experiencing brief episodes of shortness of breath. His wife of 8 years had been supportive of his treatment, traveling with him cross-country twice for the bone marrow transplants. Lately, however, she was irritated by his increasing use of narcotics to ease the pain and wanted to pursue more aggressive treatment. It was in this spirit that the two appeared on the oncology unit. After the admission process, Mr. Carey had his blood drawn, was offered pain medication, and Mrs. Carey stayed with him for an hour before going home. The next morning, Mrs. Carey became irritated after the oncologist elected to stop Mr. Carey's chemo—he recognized its immunosuppressive effects as an underlying source of the increasing herpes and was not convinced it would actually prolong Mr. Carey's life. (Mr. Carey and the oncologist had discussed this together and made a joint decision.) Mrs. Carey demanded to talk to the doctor who she felt wasn't doing everything possible for her husband. The nurses assigned to Mr. Carey interacted with the couple and provided pain control, but did not address the conflict in treatment. The oncologist finally showed up at 8 p.m. at which time he took Mrs. Carey aside and discussed with her the poor prognosis of Mr. Carey, reinforcing to her that "there was no hope." Mrs. Carey went into a tailspin trying to process the fact that her 52-year-old husband would die despite all the agony he had been through during two transplantations, and she did not agree to the planned course of action.

Meanwhile, Mr. Carey was fully conscious and agreed to the physician's assessment and recommendations. The situation became tense on the unit first between the couple and then between the wife and the nursing staff. (By this time the oncologist had left.) Mrs. Carey continued to demand treatment. The night shift nurses came on, and Mr. Carey's assigned nurse was one with about 4 years of experience. She assessed the situation and understood that the wife was not ready to accept the prognosis of her husband and possibly had misconceptions of the therapeutic value of further treatment, whereas Mr. Carey had accepted his condition. Once Mr. Carey was settled, and she had assessed her three other patients, the nurse asked the charge nurse to look after her other patients, and she invited Mrs. Carey to sit with her in a private room to talk. She listened as Mrs. Carey recounted the long and unpleasant months post transplantation only to have the cancer come back twice. She stayed as Mrs. Carey spoke of her frustration, isolation, and money lost during Mr. Carey's failed treatment. The nurse's nonverbal behaviors were encouraging and unhurried. She then took Mr. Carey's chart and gently went through it with Mrs. Carey and used the laptop computer in the room to provide the current guidelines for CLL treatment to her. Mrs. Carey gradually began to comprehend that the oncologist was following current guidelines—even more so—and her attitude softened. The nurse, who was conscious of the time that had passed while her other patients were waiting, provided Mrs. Carey with a cup of tea and said she would return in an hour. Upon her return, she found Mrs. Carey sitting with her husband and talking softly with him. The following evening, she checked in with Mrs. Carey and reflected to herself, "Now I understand how to interact with my brother-in-law who is dealing with his father's colon cancer diagnosis."

Although this is an ideal situation, the nurse could have acted otherwise. Instead, she *chose* the power of a caring relationship to help this family member process a poor prognosis. She took responsibility and demonstrated an ethic of caring that is consistent with the profession. In so doing, she alleviated some of Mrs. Carey's suffering (and Mr. Carey's too), generated a sense of security in the process, and instilled hope for their ongoing relationship. But she also learned some life lessons in the process. As Swanson (2008) once stated, she was "being a nurse" versus "doing nursing." However, the nurse in this vignette would not have been able to act in this manner if the work environment was not supportive. On this evening, the unit was appropriately staffed, another nurse was willing to cover her patients, allowing her the time needed to spend with this family member, and she *chose* to "*be* a nurse." It seems to me that leadership and the norms of behavior on this unit must have also encouraged this form of interaction.

On a typical work day, most of us have opportunities for caring—instances in which we are able to cultivate, build, or extend caring relationships. Our response in those times often has a disproportionate impact:

A young nurse (this author) was scheduled to work on Christmas day (her favorite of all holy days). She purposefully chose the evening shift because she had young children and wanted to spend Christmas morning with them as they opened their presents. She was angry she had to work—after all, her entire family was gathering for a big meal, and her children wanted to play with her. But she trudged on into the coronary care unit (CCU) where she was employed. She was assigned one patient with a myocardial infarction (MI) and the first admission. It was quiet for a while, and she kept ruminating with her colleagues about why nurses always had to work holidays and weekends while other professionals were at home, having fun. Her anger increased, and she was in the midst of deciding whether she wanted to continue working as a nurse when a new admission was called up from the emergency department (ED). He was a 56-year-old man, from out of town, visiting his daughter and newborn baby granddaughter. He had chest pain and shortness of breath, was brought by ambulance to the hospital, and it was determined by ECG that he was suffering an anterior wall MI. He was stabilized in the ED and brought to the CCU on a monitor with multiple intravenous drips and an oxygen mask. He arrived pale, blood pressure was 92/50, heart rate 110, with minimal chest pain (he had morphine in the ED). The young nurse assessed him, made him comfortable, and got orders from the resident on call, all the while deliberating about her employment situation. She was not aware that his wife and daughter were in the waiting room. Within 20 minutes, the patient's heart rhythm started to decrease and he felt "queasy." When the resident arrived, it was obvious that the patient needed a pacemaker, and the nurse became even more distressed that on Christmas evening she had to spend her time in a fluoroscopy room (with no window)—it meant she couldn't call and say goodnight to her children!

Wheeling the patient to the fluoroscopy room, the nurse saw the patient's wife and daughter in the waiting room. They were distraught—no one had interacted with them since the ED, and now they saw their husband/father on a gurney going somewhere. The nurse stopped and let them know what was going on and allowed them a couple of seconds to talk to the patient. Because of his condition, they had to move fast, so she rolled him into the room. As she settled the patient on the table, he told her that he and his wife had made the trip to visit his daughter to see their new granddaughter on Christmas. He was so excited about the baby, describing her in detail. Tears appeared in his eyes as he realized that he was in a very precarious situation.

The nurse touched his arm gently and began explaining the procedure. She donned a mask and made sure the resident had his on, adjusted the monitor and all his invasive lines, and assisted the physician with the insertion, all the while monitoring the patient's vital signs—it was 5 p.m.

An hour passed and the pacemaker was in, but just would not capture (it did not generate a rhythm), and the patient's heart rhythm (Mobitz II, AV block) continued with dropped beats and a rate ranging between 48 and 55, with a BP of 90/50. The nurse went to see the family and explained what was happening and that the physician was working hard to get the pacemaker working. They thanked her. She then went to the nurses' station and asked a colleague to call the chaplain to sit with them while she went back to the fluoro room. They worked on the patient for another hour and still no pacing. Meanwhile, the patient was alert and oriented and softly speaking about his trip and the baby. He asked to see his wife and daughter, and the nurse allowed the wife and daughter in the room for about 15 minutes. They appeared to have a wonderful, loving relationship.

Gradually, the patient's blood pressure started dropping, so additional meds were added to his IV (intravenous medication). The nurse smiled at him over her mask, and he held her hand tightly. Occasionally, the nurse remembered her children at home on Christmas, but she knew her husband was taking care of them, and they were snuggled in their beds—now all her attention was focused on this patient and his Christmas night. It was now 8:15 p.m, the cardiac fellow had been called in, the pacemaker was still failing to capture, the patient's blood pressure continued to drop, and it was apparent that his prognosis was very poor. The nurse then reflected on how she had had a beautiful Christmas morning, while this man was dying on Christmas night, after only spending a few hours with his beloved new granddaughter. How lucky she was! She held onto his hand under the sheets, looked at him over her mask, and he returned the look—somehow they both knew his fate. The two physicians were conversing about the pacemaker and the drugs, while the patient and nurse were communicating silently about the meaning of this Christmas night! After multiple attempts at the pacemaker, the patient lost consciousness, arrested, and despite a full code, he died—it was 8:40 p.m. The two physicians, who were also angry that they were called away from their Christmas dinners, left, leaving the nurse to interact with the family.

She went to the waiting room to find them sitting, softly crying with a priest in attendance—the young resident had given them the news and then gone home. When the nurse entered, they immediately stood up and hugged her. Then they spoke about the patient—his quirks, his love, and his humor. The daughter mentioned how happy she was that he got to see his granddaughter, and his wife remarked about their long marriage. The young nurse was sad—after all, they had not saved him—and it was Christmas. She thought, "Every Christmas from now on, they will remember this sad, sad day." The nurse could not contain her emotions, and she cried too, thinking again of her own family. After she cleaned up the patient, the family visited him and were getting ready to go home around 9:30 p.m., when the wife said, "Thank you so much for caring for him, this was the greatest of Christmas gifts, his last hours were not alone, he spent them with an angel."

Although it has been over 44 years since this incident, this nurse can remember it like yesterday—the details, the emotions, the smells, the faces. And every Christmas since that night, the new grandpa, his wife, and daughter remind her of the real meaning of Christmas. The nurse's experience caring for this patient and family have had a lifelong impact on *her* as similar situations do for so many nurses and other health professionals. *Clinical practice is the place where health professionals find meaning and renewal.*

Too often nurses let the work just happen to them. Seizing the opportunities to *notice* what is important about nursing work and then deliberately spending time prioritizing the individual will make all the difference. It is often the subtle behaviors rooted in daily relationships that help connect values with actions. Such connections are necessary for more meaningful work and better understanding of the contributions nurses make to the healthcare system. These realizations are motivating and prompt active participation; and if reflected on, such connections will add meaning to one's life. Healthy work environments are key to meaningful nurse work!

BOX 12.7: Accordingly, in clinical practice, it's not so much about getting more things done; rather, it's about getting the *right* things done. Investing wisely in one's nursing time is a characteristic of self-caring!

Quality-Caring Leadership

Nurse executives are challenged daily to *deliver superior services in healthy work environments at the lowest possible cost.* Balancing organizational costs with the human caring processes required for superior patient outcomes and healthy work environments, however, depends on relational expertise. Moreover, that expertise must generate "feeling cared for" in others to drive self-advancement. In other words, the quality of relationships nurse executives use must be of a caring nature.

Over the years, many leadership theories have been used by nurse leaders to operationalize their work, the most recent being transformational leadership. In these theories, the role of leader was typically situated in a person with a title, who assumed authority over certain locations (or departments) in a health system, including the human, material, and intellectual resources in those locations. The leader was tasked with planning, organizing, directing, and controlling these resources in order to meet company goals. However, contemporary healthcare systems are complex with many interconnected parts and persons, all attached in some way to patients, families, and communities. Each of these parts are interdependent, and under the right conditions, generate new patterns or behaviors that are sometimes unpredictable, but eventually emerge in a self-organized fashion (i.e. complex adaptive systems—see Chapter 3).

During the COVID-19 pandemic when health systems were overwhelmed with patients, individual health professionals and groups of health professionals adapted by immediately changing their workflow to meet the needs of incoming patients. In this situation, many "leaders" came up with novel ideas and resulting actions that were quickly adopted. Some of these "leaders" were Emergency Department physicians, others were charge nurses on inpatient units, and others were clinicians who practiced differently during this time. Still others worked in communities as teachers, public health nurses, and first-responders. According to Malloch and Porter-O'Grady (2022), *appreciative* leadership is responsive and emerges where it is needed. Co-creating emerging new patterns or behaviors that spread forward throughout health systems, adapting to changing and future needs, is one such response. Appreciative leaders nurture the best in others and use relational capacity to move systems forward. They boost others up through inclusive participation and fill them with hope for a strong and inviting future. Let's see—appreciative leaders nurture, use relationships, recognize potential, are positive and inclusive—do any of these expressions sound like caring behaviors?

Health systems using the QCM employ nurse leaders who extend caring to others first and use their relational expertise to disseminate the benefits. Such leaders inspire by example, mutually relating in caring ways that generate energy and even joy, extending authentic caring works with patients and families—we have empirical data to support this. So, why can't these same results apply to employees and other stakeholders? It is the job of leadership to extend caring as it engages and motivates others. Such leaders' actions have almost a ripple effect that snowballs throughout organizations, ultimately affecting the work environment.

BOX 12.8: Caring leaders make it easy for employees to relax, do their best work, enjoy themselves on the job, engage in innovation, and maybe even share economic benefits.

Wouldn't it be interesting to evaluate absenteeism, presenteeism, and employee engagement in health systems that are led by relationally-oriented leaders?

BOX 12.9: Leaders who are observed in caring relationships with stakeholders (patients, families, employees, and providers) both in and outside the health system uphold the ethical principles and standards on which healthcare is based, demonstrating that healthcare is *not* just a service but rather a professional, accountable, intimate, and highly regarded series of professional actions that benefit society. Likewise, when leaders display caring relationships with employees, they are actively reminding them of their value to the system and creating the conditions for reciprocation.

Several nurse leaders who are experts in caring relationships in a health system collectively create *Quality-Caring Cultures* characterized by expert professional practice bounded by an open and inclusive environment that demonstrates its value (through evidence) to the health and well-being of the community served. In this way, nursing's powerful impact on people's lives is visible, documented, and celebrated.

Conversely, in an interesting ethnography, Grundy & Malone (2017) provide an explanation for nurses' continuing invisibility in health systems. As the largest proportion of health professionals who are "situated at the hub of multidisciplinary teams and focused on the prevention and management of increasingly common and costly chronic diseases" (p. E29), many nurses prefer to use their influence covertly in order to avoid conflict while maintaining their long-held insider knowledge. While this may work in individual situations, unfortunately in the wider world, nursing still is considered a cost that is seen as having limited tangible value in health systems. Yet, *quality caring leaders* are able to transcend this challenge by demonstrating how patient–nurse relationships (or the community–nurse relationship), the processes of nursing, impact organizational performance, including effectiveness, efficiency, and outcomes of care.

What keeps nursing administrators up at night are the continuing problems of *adverse events; productivity, staffing, and retention; clinical workflow; professionalism; and the leadership abilities of first-line managers*, to name a few. The cost implications of *nursing-related adverse outcomes* portray nursing not only as a health system expense, but at times, a liability. Individual nurse factors (such as experience and credentials), patient treatment related factors, missed or incomplete care (McCauley et al., 2021), and environmental factors such as interprofessional collaboration (or not), workflow, and staffing (Kakemam et al., 2021; Rochefort et al., 2022) are implicated in adverse outcomes. Increasingly, nurse presenteeism or being present at work but not fully productive (because of a variety of factors) is becoming noteworthy as a variable associated with poorer nursing-sensitive quality indicators (Rainbow et al., 2021). Although the real cost and adverse outcome burden of presenteeism in health professionals are not known, one can conjecture about some of its sources. For example, as today's health systems and their employees have encountered serious disruption and change these last few years, many employees themselves have altered their work styles. The increase in households with sick children or older adults, fear of "calling in sick," working more than one job (especially as 12-hour shifts have decreased the number of available days off), and care demands at work are examples of situations that might affect an individual's productivity and engagement while at work. Nursing administrators thus must be concerned not only with attendance (staffing numbers) but with the contributions and productivity (particularly, the ability to engage in caring relationships) of their workforce.

Clinical workflow, often used synonymously with patient care delivery models, refers to how nursing care processes are organized, sequenced, and performed for person-centered care and is a national priority. Consider how hospital nurses continue to use their time during a shift. First, they spend about 1 hour receiving report from the previous shift—often this is not comprehensive, person-centered, or relationship-enhancing. Next, they organize themselves according to the various tasks—assessments, medication administration, and treatments that need completion. Then, as they proceed down the list of tasks, they check them off one by one making sure that the electronic health record (EHR) is updated. Oftentimes, updating the EHR takes tremendous amounts of time. Finally, nurses report to the oncoming nurse. One or two disruptions or emergencies can throw the entire checklist off, necessitating overtime in order to complete the list. This process has not changed for over 40 years, with the exception of the EHR. But, during this 8- to 12-hour period, one of the patients received a cancer diagnosis, another remained in pain, another patient required a complex dressing change after his daughter was told that she would not be able to take him home with her, and a physician on the staff just found out his daughter was admitted to the psych ward for bulimia. In the busyness of completing the checklist, how aware are nurses of the complexities of their patients' or coworkers' lives? Or for that matter, their own stomachs or bladders? How well does ensuring the completion of a series of important tasks contribute to person-centeredness or enhance the patient experience?

Prior to COVID-19, a time and motion study was completed on a medical unit in Switzerland where two researchers (both RNs) performed continuous caregiver observations of 21 healthcare workers over 46 complete work shifts. Findings showed that less than one third of registered nurses' work time was spent with patients. They allocated the most time to communication, care planning and coordination and the least amount of time to optimizing the quality and safety of care, integrating and supervising staff, and patient education (Michel et al., 2021). These results are similar to those in the U. S. (Baker et al., 2019; Butler et al., 2018). Patients and families desire information, reassurance, acceptance, support, commitment, acknowledgment, competence, mutual decision making, vigilance, comfort, security, family engagement, and their basic human needs met (Duffy, 2018). They want to be treated as if they were a close relative of the care provider; they want to matter. Don't we all? Nurses consistently say they want to relate more to their patients doing what they were educated to do. They also want to work in environments with other health professionals who perform the same way. In other words, professional nurses desire a more relationship-centric environment.

BOX 12.10: Designing care delivery models that are relationship-centered while integrating health information technology (HIT) requires careful, reflective analysis of the work of professional nursing, identification of key role components, and tough decisions about how the work will be accomplished. Included in this analysis must be the fundamental understanding that professional nursing incorporates *both being with* and *doing for* in an integrated fashion. Thus, the use of a theory-guided model and standards of nursing practice to redesign patient care delivery can help provide the foundation for workflow redesign.

One approach to assessing whether a relationship-centric patient care delivery system is adequately represented in nurse work is the use of a table or diagram that "crosswalks" the relationships between theoretical concepts and components of nursing work that are typically described in job descriptions (see Exhibit 12.1). Such an illustration depicts how nurses incorporate aspects of the theory into everyday practice and can also serve as an aid in developing clinical advancement programs.

Difficult decisions are needed *now, in the best interest of patients and families*, while considering *nursing workflow*. For example, what will be the major components of RN work? Who will support RN work? What human and environmental resources will be required, and how will they be scheduled and assigned to optimize person-centered care? What means of communication will enhance RN work?

EXHIBIT 12.1: Example of Quality-Caring Model Concepts Linked to Nursing Work Major Model Concepts

Components of Nursing Work ↓	Humans in Relationship ↔	Relationship-centered Professional Encounters	"Feeling Cared For" ↔	Self-Advancing Systems
Person-centered care	Appreciates the illness experience; maintains self-awareness; remains present to situations by integrating being and doing; appreciates the whole person	Uses the caring behaviors; completes a holistic assessment and plan of care; integrates bedside report; includes patient/family in decisions; makes decisions based on best patient needs; checks in with patients regularly	Solicits feedback regarding patients' experiences; levels of comfort; sense of safety; dignity; inclusion, etc.	Individualizes patient outcomes
Practice improvement (PI) using evidence and research	Reflects on practice	Participates in PI and research using the caring behaviors; evaluates strength of the evidence for use in practice; protects human subjects according to system policy	Periodically, measures "feeling cared for"	Uses data/information to revise practice
Population health	Understands and uses the health parameters of community served	Uses targeted interventions with patients; engages in community groups using the caring behaviors; partners with community groups; advocates for population health	Solicits feedback from community groups	Incorporates community or population-based health parameters into care

(continued)

EXHIBIT 12.1: Example of Quality-Caring Model Concepts Linked to Nursing Work Major Model Concepts (*continued*)

Components of Nursing Work ↓	Humans in Relationship ↔	Relationship-centered Professional Encounters	"Feeling Cared For" ↔	Self-Advancing Systems
Quality and safety	Appreciates nursing and health systems role in improving healthcare, quality, and safety	Uses the caring behaviors to create just and safe cultures; implements evidence-based improvements in care using the caring behaviors; ensures healing environments	Participates in evaluation of intermediate quality and safety outcomes	Evaluates patient, employee, and systems outcomes for progress
Teamwork and collaboration	Recognizes the human person in healthcare team members	Actively participattes in collaborative rounds; delegates and follows up with teams using caring behaviors	Solicits feedback from team members regarding experiences	Routinely evaluates team effectiveness and efficiency
Professionalism	Reflects on one's actions and their consequences; demonstrates accountability for safe and quality care; remains sensitive to others' values and preferences	Advocates for peoples' right to self-determination; safeguards privacy, confidentiality, and autonomy in all interactions; demonstrates professional and personal integrity; complies with state nurse practice act; uses the caring behaviors	Solicits feedback from individuals and leadership regarding professional behaviors	Participates in peer evaluation
Personal, professional and leadership development	Engages in self-care practices; differentiates between personal and professional responsibilities	Participates in continuous learning; uses the caring behaviors with educators and mentors to support professional growth.	Solicits feedback on leadership performance	Modifies one's own leadership behaviors based on feedback and reflection

As caring relationships are tied to intermediate and terminal health outcomes for both patients and health professionals (see Chapter 7), nursing administrators are faced with balancing the competing needs of patients for human caring with the economic complexities of the current health system that is trying to recover from a pandemic. The value of nursing lies in its caring core. Leaders who can demonstrate a return on investment for the caring behaviors of professional nurses are needed. Evidence such as increased safety (for both patients and the healthcare workforce); enhanced experiences of care; faster and better attainment of clinical outcomes; improved long-term health outcomes such as reduced 30-day readmissions, increased functional status and return to work; improved nurse retention; and increases in the well-being of the workforce are needed to demonstrate how nurses use the caring behaviors to influence the performance of a healthcare system (self-advancing systems). Leaders who are able to rally an expert nursing workforce that incorporates the caring behaviors in their work will create health experiences that are safe, comfortable, optimistic, and preserve the wholeness of persons. In other words, inspiring the restructuring of professional nurse work that is delivered in a person-centered context will be increasingly tied to effective leader behaviors.

Engaging clinical staff through relational approaches, including joint decision-making, visiting frequently with patients and families (customers), cultivating meaningful caring relationships with healthcare colleagues, and continuously learning how to improve nursing practice builds a lasting legacy for the next generation of nurses; and in so doing, perhaps some of the productivity, staffing, and retention issues associated with the nursing workforce may improve.

BOX 12.11: In fact, creating a legacy of quality-caring so that others will sustain the provision of person-centered care is invigorating. Periodically asking, "Am I doing what enhances self-advancement? Am I preserving the essence of nursing? Am I operating from a relationship-centered base? Am I self-caring? Am I really practicing nursing?" provides consistent reinforcement and inner confidence.

In this developing *never before seen* system of healthcare delivery, rethinking the role of professional nursing as it has been previously expressed in health systems is vital. At the same time, upholding longstanding disciplinary values in the context of current evidence and social inclusivity may in fact lead to some confrontation. For example, in a resource constrained system that has just been through major disruption from an unexpected pandemic, CEOs and payors want action regarding reimbursement and throughput. Such discrepancies may lead to conflict and resistance. Upholding professionalism in this climate requires systematic, thoughtful, and courageous nursing leaders who seek to understand both future healthcare demands *and* clinical workforce needs. After all, connecting professional values to nursing work provides meaning and renewal.

In fact, *professionalism* and *professional identity* are learning domains in AACN's *Essentials: Core competencies for Professional Nursing Education* (AACN, 2021) that demand renewed focus on accountability, collaboration, and personal conduct in the promotion of ethical behavior, demonstration of social justice, and moral courage. The pandemic has tested nurses' and other health professionals' professionalism and for the most part, they have risen to the challenge. However, ongoing attention to issues such as the use of social media, including specific applications and internet sites, accountability for how human persons are treated, incivility, and cultural humility are needed. Actually, nurses' continued motivation "to care" is one of its greatest assets that appreciative leaders can exploit during the progression towards a newer health system.

Lastly, maintaining *a team of first-line managers* who value and focus primarily on high-quality nursing care, including caring relationships with patients and families and other health professionals is central to person-centered care. Today's first-line nurse leaders are responsible for large, diverse workforces and deal with complex, life-threatening patient situations every day. Additionally, they are responsible for legal, regulatory, budgetary, human and other resources, and safety standards in their units. So, on the one hand, they are responsible for quality patient care; and on the other, they are asked to prepare reports, attend numerous meetings, attain advanced education, attend to facilities, and reconcile the budget. However, this first-line nurse leader position is pivotal and linked to patient outcomes, staff nurses' satisfaction, turnover, nurse-reported adverse events, and the quality of patient care delivered (Kostich et al., 2021; Labrague, 2021; Saleh et al., 2018). Nurse managers themselves often perceive their role as inadequate, exhausting, and unsuccessful (Omery et al., 2019). In fact, first-line nurse managers often have many employees, large spans of control, limited real authority, and high levels of stress (Omery et al., 2019).

BOX 12.12: The connection between the work of nurse managers and the mission of health systems (quality patient care) is integral. Valuing and reinforcing this association daily is necessary to self-advancing systems.

Creating safe, transparent microsystems (nursing units) that successfully safeguard patients and families and guarantee quality outcomes, preserve the integrity of professional nursing, and contain organizational costs are often recorded on the written job descriptions of first-line nurse managers—a tall order indeed! This important work requires global awareness; analytical and sophisticated research and evaluation capacity; expert interpersonal relationship skills; self-caring ability; advanced knowledge of nursing, including nursing theory and professional practice models; the ability to collaborate, share successes, and acknowledge failures; and most importantly, the ability to express caring. Frequent contact by nurse executives (and others in the C-suite) in the actual practice setting helps top leadership appreciate the realities of the clinical practice environment, including first-line leader needs. Creating a safe space for frank dialogue and open, flexible communication; fostering self-caring practices in first-line leaders; expressing caring often through internal and external recognition; and most importantly, taking a hard look at the role to ensure that attention to quality patient care is the number one priority are essential. To build teams of first-line nurse managers capable of leading in a quality-caring practice environment, some nurse executives are using a coaching approach. Others have created dedicated self-caring meetings, participate in book clubs, attend off-campus gatherings once a month to work on mutual goals and support each other, attend to healthy eating, partner with universities to provide "internal" consulting or assistance with leadership evidence-based practice, and participate in annual nursing renewal ceremonies. Expecting and ensuring that future front-line nurse managers have the knowledge, skills, and values necessary to keep the focus on caring relationships means making hard decisions about what the preparation is for the role, whether who is hired is a good fit for the organization, how persons will be on-boarded, evaluated and rewarded, and how they can be retained.

BOX 12.13: Value-based health systems demand high-quality relationships, true person-centeredness, inclusivity, and ongoing optimism. This suggests attention to what enables others to "feel cared for," establishing partnerships and collaboration, empowering and engaging patients, families, and employees, and extending hope—for progress, new possibilities, and discovery. Each of these principles hinges on relationships.

In a recent cross-sectional web-based survey, results indicated that relationship-based competencies were prominent in the perceived importance of competencies among nurse managers at different levels (Liou et al., 2022). Often solving immediate problems feels more satisfying; however, this customary and rather easy substitute for attending to the real, underlying problems/concerns of a health system or profession drives out the more foundational, limiting leaders' effectiveness. Accordingly, leaders who make the hard decisions required for radical and lasting value know that today's urgency is relational. Patients, families, employees, and systems are acknowledging their needs "to matter, to be involved, to be heard, to feel valued, to belong" (Bourgault, 2022). Failure to act on these significant needs may undermine any lasting changes and/or further fragment the existing system.

Sustaining frontline nurse managers' relational leadership competencies while addressing the dynamically altered health system requires expecting caring relationships at all levels with skills in facilitating a safe space for learning, adaptation, engagement, acceptance of constructive criticism, and inspiring a workforce focused on human persons. The humanistic qualities inherent in caring relationships may offer the grounding needed by frontline nurse managers to promote excellence, ensure accountability, maintain integrity and safeguard workplace civility, and all components of professionalism. Applying coaching, learning labs, certification, comprehensive onboarding, mentoring programs, networking, and other continuing education programs may enhance nurse manager ongoing competencies.

Quality-Caring Education

Building a workforce of professional nurses who are competent; accountable; engaged; competently practice the caring factors; continuously monitor and perfect relationships with self, patients and families, other health professionals, and the community served; and who engage in opportunities to improve clinical practice requires educational programs that adequately prepare them for this role. Although many nursing faculty members are busy evaluating and revising their curricula in order to meet the new *Essentials* competencies (AACN, 2021), concerns exist in health systems that graduates' readiness for the realities of modern-day practice may not be realized (Grubaugh et al., 2021; Huston et al., 2018; Shatto et al, 2022).

BOX 12.14: Immediate needs for more experiential and reflective learning, including increased time in practice, attention to meaningful pre- and post-clinical conferences, the use of real situations in interprofessional classrooms or simulation laboratories, and increased use of evidence as the basis for practice is needed. Such learning requires the expertise of senior faculty members, comfort with open dialogue, student-led learning, multidisciplinary classrooms, closeness to the practice environment, ongoing and rigorous faculty development, and awareness of the characteristics of today's health professional students.

In a typical health professions' course today, the composition of the class might include an occasional baby boomer and a large number of generation X, generation Y, and generation Z students who are of varying ages, diverse in terms of gender, race, and ethnicity, and who, for the most part, are tech savvy. Many students are working, commuting, and raising families. Each of the represented generations of students has its own unique set of characteristics that have been shaped by the values, trends, behaviors, and events in place in society at that time. These generational characteristics create vast opportunities to learn, but the differences can also create challenges for faculty members who themselves may be of a different generation.

Using a caring pedagogy of embracing whole, unique persons, creating a safe space for learning, inclusive learning environments, and meaningful, shared (or co-learning) experiences, nursing educators will need to value caring relationships as essential to learning and health and be committed to the development of caring knowledge in themselves and their students. To promote a growing awareness of self and emerging professional identity, students need to be exposed to nursing early in their academic programs and build on the life experiences and characteristics they bring to the program. A focus on personal knowing or balancing inner and external knowledge is paramount. The days of planned content delivered in lecture format with a set course scheduling may not always be the best way to learn and be caring! Relational experiences with patients and families during clinical courses help students appreciate their value to healthcare outcomes and their own growth as a caring person. Designing such experiences is a role of the faculty. Crucial to such experiences is asking probing questions while in practice that stimulate students to think about their experiences with patients and families. Questions such as "What relationships are emerging?" "What is the quality of the relationships?" "What seems important to the relationship?" and "What are the potential consequences of the observed relationships?" provide opportunities for much more introspection.

Helping students to value and learn the caring behaviors through study, simulations, and role modeling creates situations in which students can test their interactions in a safe place under the guidance of experts. Grounding nursing simulations in caring relationships allows faculty to create environments in which the uniqueness of the human person and the fullness of nursing practice can be understood (Eggenberger & Keller, 2008). Likewise, in the online course environment, faculty members must ensure the wholeness of students is preserved. Integrating knowledge from multiple sources is a skill necessary for quality care; and therefore, less emphasis on textbooks and more emphasis on professional literature early and repeatedly is wise. Finally, ensuring caring competency through formative and summative evaluation helps prepare professional nurses "to be" as well as "to do" nursing.

Clinical faculty members are instrumental in facilitating students' capacity for caring as well as overall readiness for practice. Some argue that the caring behaviors of faculty members enable students to grow as caring professionals (Allari et al., 2020; Wei et al., 2021). Many learning strategies exist to facilitate such learning. For example, simulations, role playing, online learning modules, and use of expert patients have been studied (Ferri et al., 2019; Hofmeyer et al., 2018; Koch et al., 2021). Although there were some limitations, most of these studied approaches showed positive learning outcomes. It is evident that more research is needed on learning approaches; however, real-life situations in the clinical setting may have the richest influence on learning how "to care." Embedding caring processes—the essence of nursing (Watson, 1979, 1985)—in clinical situations more fully engages students in the everyday experiences that patients, families, and health professionals endure, linking them to students' evolving emotions about the profession. Forming caring relationships and enacting caring presence in real clinical situations requires reciprocity between faculty and students, where caring and technical skills are equally valued, modeled, and evaluated for competency.

BOX 12.15: Savvy nursing educators are needed who can effectively integrate new learning strategies with real clinical experiences in order to meet the demands of health systems for value. The pedagogical challenge for faculty is to help students find meaning in their nursing, connecting it with values that affirm caring relationships as central to clinical practice. Consistent dialogue with relevant affirmations, clinical practice, and reflection is crucial.

To effectively build caring relationships, students and teachers must learn how "to be" in relationship with each other and, in a sense, to co-learn. Through the relationship, the two become aligned in the learning process, and new information is tossed about, questioned, and grasped as pertinent or not pertinent to clinical practice. In this manner, caring nurse educators transform the learning environment from a passive acquisition of facts to an active relational investigation of new ideas and partnership, much like clinical practice.

Educators will also be tasked with evaluating caring competence, showing progression throughout academic programs, to effectively assure readiness for work.

Finally, facilitating the development of new knowledge about caring relationships through advanced inquiry is also a faculty responsibility that requires research mentors who understand its nature and who are involved with the science themselves. Research mentoring is crucial to building a future group of nurse scholars who can translate caring relationships into practice and demonstrate their impact. See AACN's latest white paper on the research-focused doctorate (American Association of Colleges of Nursing, 2022b).

ADVANCING THE SCIENCE OF CARING RELATIONSHIPS

Evaluating how caring relationships impact patient outcomes (safety and quality in particular), how to improve and widely disseminate them as the basis for care, and sustaining longer term caring relationships is demanding; however, as a central construct of professional nursing practice, knowledge of this core process is necessary to improve and accelerate its adequate translation into practice. Moreover, it provides needed feedback to health professionals about their practice, which is so often lacking in specialized departments. To extend the understanding and strengthen the evidence pertaining to caring relationships (specifically nurse caring) as a significant variable in the healthcare process, much more evaluation is necessary. However, there is a relative lack of data on the quality of nurse caring, its relationship to outcomes, and caring-based interventions. Inconsistencies exist among the many evaluation tools used to measure caring and little robust research has been conducted regarding variability of caring nursing practice. Furthermore, patient characteristics (such as acuity) and nurse characteristics (such as educational preparation, work experience, etc.) are not routinely used to adjust for differences in nursing performance. Linking nurse caring behaviors to important reimbursable outcomes is crucial to demonstrate nursings' vital, contribution to healthcare. In fact, "quantification of nursing's value across the healthcare delivery system" is a finding in the revised research agenda for nursing administration and leadership science (Chipps et al., 2021).

Nursing-sensitive outcome measures do showcase the value of nursing; however, many of these are reported as negative or adverse results of nursing care. Although the NDNQI indicators have been instrumental in generating awareness of and improving important nursing-sensitive indicators (Press-Ganey, 2022), there are numerous metrics that may more positively reflect the performance of nursing.

For example, hospitalized older adults frequently leave the hospital with poorer mental and physical function than when admitted (Chen et al., 2022). This is a national problem with significant cost and clinical burden, not to mention the personal burden it places on patients and families. Measuring and reporting differences in functional status from admission to discharge for older adults would showcase how nursing's attention to mobility during hospitalization saves both clinical burden and actual dollars (and might enhance the patient's experience). Those with chronic illnesses, such as heart failure, cancer, and chronic obstructive pulmonary disease (COPD), often are readmitted within 30 days of discharge, financially draining the U.S. health system. This burden may be lessened if nurses worked, through caring relationships, to activate patients in their care prior to discharge. Patient activation is a positive outcomes indicator that is measurable (Hibbard et al., 2005) during and at hospital discharge, and has been associated with decreased utilization and improved outcomes in certain patients (Dumitra et al., 2021; Shnaigat et al., 2022). It reflects the relational aspect of nursing care and could potentially raise positive regard for nursing-specific contributions to healthcare.

Other, more positive indicators such as comfort (versus pain), knowledge (versus knowledge-deficit), dignity, health-related quality of life (HRQOL), optimistic mood (versus depression), feeling "cared for," recovery time, adherence (versus nonadherence), contentment (versus anxiety), continence (versus incontinence), self-caring, cognition (versus cognitive impairment), empowerment, health-seeking behaviors, mobility (versus functional decline), symptom control, and skin integrity (versus pressure ulcers) are examples of affirming outcomes measures that could be used to report the outcomes of nursing care. Many of these indicators have well-documented instruments that would easily translate to the clinical environment, rendering measurement and reporting feasible; and the findings might provide some much-needed encouragement to nurses.

To extend the understanding and strengthen the evidence of caring (specifically nurse caring) as a significant variable influencing health outcomes, further research must be conducted and disseminated. Although studies of nurse caring over the last 3 years are few, studies of the benefits of person-centered care are emerging as are those related to health professionals' self-caring (relationship with self). For example, in a comparison study of 47 people with dementia, the person-centered care group showed statistically significant improvements in behavioral/neuropsychiatric symptoms and care quality (Chenoweth et al., 2022). In an observational study of 76 faith-community and hospital nurses, RNs did not report practicing self-caring at the highest levels, but did report the highest levels of self-caring when helping and giving love to others (Davis et al., 2022). Similar results were found in a descriptive qualitative study using semistructured interviews ($N = 19$). Researchers reported that although nurses think that self-compassion is important, they do not regularly practice it. Personal and organizational barriers limited oncology nurses practice of self-caring (Serçe et al., 2022).

Continuing to build on the foundation of existing caring knowledge using multiple methods will provide the evidence needed to demonstrate nursings' unique contribution to healthcare. Refining existing measures of caring using appropriate conceptual definitions and adequate psychometric properties, with particular emphasis on the patient's view, will allow for correlational studies and multisite comparisons. In-depth studies of outliers (those organizations and health professionals who successfully embrace quality caring principles), examination of how to improve relational competencies in organizations, the influence of work environments on caring relationships, how caring relationships with self can be fostered amid the current realities of health systems, and leveraging information technology to enhance caring relationships and person-centered care are all important questions for further study.

Continuing to study the link between caring relationships and specific nursing-sensitive patient outcomes will strengthen the evidence base regarding the importance of caring relationships in clinical practice; and linking caring relationships to reimbursable outcomes, such as patient experiences, readmission rates, and adverse outcomes may significantly impact hospitals' bottom line. Educational studies that examine the acquisition of deeper levels of caring and/or professionalism over the course of a program are necessary. Nursing administration studies that identify the contribution of health professionals' characteristics to the delivery of person-centered care and how well relationship-centered leadership adds to organizational relational capacity will also be valuable to the scientific base.

Developing caring-based interventions for testing is necessary to provide high levels of evidence for caring-based professional practice and to validate caring theory. Caring-based interventions are complicated to design, and practical limitations for testing can be challenging. Nevertheless, caring-based interventions must be studied through research investigations to better understand how they contribute to healthcare outcomes. Using empirical data and a caring-based conceptual framework to support the intervention, a detailed description organized to meet the needs of the population under study is paramount. Developing a protocol describing the content, strength, and frequency of the intervention allows for replication. Using probability sampling and longitudinal designs, questions such as, "What is the effect of the intervention on specific outcomes of care over time?" can be answered. Integrating cost-effectiveness components will add to the understanding of the intervention's worth.

BOX 12.16: Using strategies such as interprofessional teams, applying tools where data are pooled from multiple sites, and integrating biological, behavioral, and cost-effectiveness methods will eventually enable us to make predictions about how health professionals with certain characteristics perform the caring behaviors, the proper "dose" of caring for particular patient populations, the most effective ways to learn caring, and the relative worth of caring practices.

Relevant manuscripts and doctoral dissertations published in high-quality journals will continue to expose others to caring research. Likewise, presentations at meetings of professional organizations and use of the results of caring studies to create or revise existing policy add to the science. Through the daily application of evidence-based practice, nurses at all levels who critically appraise caring research to judge the trustworthiness of study findings and to translate credible results to the bedside will strengthen the work of nursing.

Applying new knowledge in the appropriate setting may help transform the work environment for nurses such that they find meaning in the important work they do.

Finally, drawing conclusions from research about caring theory helps to validate and refine it. Explicitly stating the caring theory that undergirds research studies adds valuable knowledge for the profession and provides the basis for future nursing care (Fawcett, 2007), supplies rationale for practice improvements, exposes the significant role of professional nurses in healing, and helps validate or reject existing theory. Professional nurses have a social responsibility to study, mentor, and facilitate scientific inquiry related to caring relationships, the cornerstone of their clinical practice.

THE PROMISE OF A VALUABLE HEALTH SYSTEM

Now what?

Postpandemic models of healthcare are unfolding, while healthcare payment options continue to evolve. Accelerated use of technology, evidence-based practice, person-centered care, and evaluation of the clinical workforce are going to continue dominating the national discourse. Although enrollment in BSN programs has increased since the pandemic started, it is not sufficient to meet the projected demand for nursing services (Seegert, 2022). In fact, the AACN's latest enrollment data showed a decline in RN-BSN, Masters, and PhD programs. More concerning is the fact that 91,938 applications were turned away, 76,140 from baccalaureate students alone! Most of the identified barriers included lack of faculty, preceptors, clinical sites, and other budgetary reasons (AACN, 2022a). Well-qualified, curious, and competent nurses are needed now more than ever; however, obstacles remain in terms of how to facilitate new graduates' transition to practice and to help practicing nurses feel valued and supported in the workplace.

It is obvious that a remodeled and different healthcare system is emerging—and it is not going to look or feel like the one that existed prior to COVID-19. It is an atypical and awkward time that continues to introduce disorder and instability. However, now is not the time to give up or give in. Nurses can seize this rare opportunity to remodel their work in a way that increases personal well-being and meaning, while positively impacting human persons—by using their ongoing trustworthy status to create more person-centered, relational workplaces that lend credibility to their importance in the health system. There is no time for delays as the world is rapidly moving all around us. Robust leadership is needed to facilitate top of practice nurse work, support wages aligned with the work and the health risks involved, and to really invest in nurses' well-being and career development. The sort of leadership needed is the human-to-human, caring, and uplifting type that reminds us of our similarities, common ground, and shared experiences as nurses.

Reviving our collective purpose "to care" by focusing attention on serving communities whose voices are easily diminished in these politically charged times and working together to achieve population health is a simple yet powerful concept that enables adaptive behaviors. Working *together*—community groups and health systems, universities and health systems, patients and providers, health providers and law enforcement, schools and primary care centers—in caring partnerships may generate strong, coherent groups of individuals who better respond to health problems in communities. Characteristics such as flexibility, resilience, reliability, durability, self-monitoring, and self-caring are necessary. There is no room on this list of adjectives for self-doubt, mistrust, disregard, roughness, violence, inattention, incivility, or despair. Rather the former characteristics are born of confidence, feeling safe and connected, included, and optimistic—all consequences of "feeling cared for."

Health professionals and health systems now have a real opportunity to reduce low-value healthcare by accelerating and extending new ways of doing clinical work, advancing their professions, themselves, and communities in the process. Thinking differently, flexibly, and collaboratively while simultaneously learning about the present allows novel ideas to become a reality. And *productive* dreaming (brainstorming) in caring environments enables emerging new ideas and strategies for achieving them to come to the forefront.

Acknowledging that the past may not always provide the right lessons, reshuffling roles, or adding new activities to existing ones is not adapting to complexity. For example, healthcare modification with a focus on technology, new care delivery models, employee well-being programs, or accepting increased numbers of health professional students by itself is not enough to influence a *different* healthcare system. Fundamentally shifting the focus from the system to the human person, arranging clinical work around person and community needs, ensuring safety and teamwork, reminding each other often how we are connected, demonstrating (though data) disciplinary contributions, and limiting excessive authority structures will embolden an engaged workforce capable of innovative practice.

Taken together, these principles have guided the evolution of the QCM such that it incorporates a holistic, sustainable, integrated set of assumptions, propositions, concepts, and empirical indicators from which to guide professional practice and innovation. Although originally intended to blend the human caring aspect of patient care with the evidence base needed for quality outcomes, more recently, the model has focused on enhancing the *quality of caring relationships* in an effort to meet the demand for high value (and self-advancing) health systems amid the confusion of a post-pandemic world. It is within this dynamic paradigm that attending to the *quality* of caring relationships is a global health priority.

BOX 12.17: As significant as caring is to the profession of nursing, it is now being extended to the larger health system. Enabling caring relationships to flourish by acknowledging the good work health professionals do, deriving meaning in that work, expertly performing the caring behaviors, and continuously improving clinical practice offers health professionals and health systems a way to demonstrate their significance to society. Displacing the disease-based, negative outcomes paradigm with one that focuses on well-being, wholeness, and positive outcomes transforms the future outlook to one of possibility, hope, and advancement.

Although health professionals themselves have stretched to meet the demands for health services in the past 3 years, the anchoring foundation of caring must also be stretched, providing energy (and renewal) for high-value outcomes. The one enduring principle of healthcare practice that can support this work remains the same: Effectively and efficiently advancing health and well-being in the context of caring relationships. This fundamental principle takes hard work—showing up day after day, searching for "what matters," authentic collaboration, multiple smaller innovations at the point of care, discipline, genuine concern, inclusion, openness, and acceptance. Today's workforce has the tools—but must be supported while taking responsibility for living these principles.

BOX 12.18: Genuine, adaptive teams of health professionals developed and led for the purpose of providing expert caring to persons that acknowledge the need to do better, where learning from the work is the norm, and real-time patient data prevail are beginning to transform health systems to ones "centered on persons." Health systems and health professionals must decide whether to sit on the sidelines and watch this unfold or risk organizing around the caring needs of human persons.

Turmoil and instability sometimes prevent consideration of what really matters; in this case, professional nursing's primary function, caring relationships. However, it is precisely at this time that the caring essence of professional nursing (Watson, 1979, 1985) may provide the strength necessary to carry out dramatic change. Refocusing skill acquisition and tasks/procedures to caring competencies and teamwork, building relational capacity, and measuring "feeling cared for" and other patient-defined positive outcomes demonstrate and extend nursing's relational core to other health professionals and health systems. Taking advantage of this unique time in history to prioritize all human persons and adapt in new ways that leverage nursing's often hidden power will facilitate self-advancement, adding value to those who need it most!

SUMMARY

Reflections about the future were presented. Particular attention was paid to healthcare value and the challenges of person-centered health systems. Nurses, who practice from a caring stance are already learning and adapting for tomorrow. Several outliers are mentioned with current examples, and clinical practice, leadership, and educational challenges are presented. In particular, reducing adverse outcomes attributed to nursing, redesigning clinical workflow to be person-centered, sustaining professionalism, and creating teams of first-rate front-line managers are reviewed. Principles of appreciative leadership are reiterated with emphasis on responding positively to complexity. In education, using caring relationships as the basis for learning and evaluation, experiential learning with additional and meaningful clinical time, and partnering with service are advocated. Evaluating and researching how caring relationships impact selected outcomes and widely disseminating findings are significant. Using patient-derived feedback and more positive nursing-sensitive indicators might shed new light on nursing contributions to patient outcomes.

The revised QCM provides a framework for modern clinical practice that offers hope for future generations. Rethinking how clinical work is organized to add value is paramount. Finally, nurses who are experts in caring relationships can facilitate adaptation, driving self-advancing systems that will make a profound impact on human persons.

CALL TO ACTION

Relationships, specifically caring relationships, as the basis for actions and decision making are necessary to revive valuable health systems. Highly developed, inclusive, and interdependent professional nurses who understand the significance of the whole and whose practice is based on caring relationships are the critical mass that can lead the health system toward a sustainable future. **Choose** to believe (caring intention) in the power of caring relationships—they drive actions. **Assume** that others care—look for the positive—it changes the dynamic of relationships. **Walk the talk**—it establishes your credibility. **Identify** the caring leaders you can turn to for guidance. **Discover and imitate** the caring experts in your health system. **Create** transparency, **clarify** expectations, and **keep** commitments. **Embody** your nursing values.

A mindful, engaged, and relational professional workforce that remains true to its caring roots will help shift the disease-based, task-oriented, shift-focused approach of today to a relational, health-based, holistic, theory-based practice that invigorates the healthcare system. Regularly **participate** in self-awareness practices and research. **Internalize** the significance of caring relationships to health. Rethinking the task-focused work of clinical practice is a national priority. The nonlinear and multiple relationships so common to healthcare work require a completely different focus of attention—one that is driven by persons and that embraces little structure and form, but allows for relationships to generate ideas and conditions for innovation. The goal of the leader is to enable the healthcare system to emerge and self-advance by increasing the number and quality of interactions, developing caring–healing–protective environments, and being mindful of the unfolding world in which they function. **Generate** new ways of thinking about nursing work. Demonstrating a return on investment for the caring behaviors of professional nurses will be a leadership responsibility. **Offer** some practical evidence of nursing's value to your organization. Nursing educators who value and use caring relationships as the basis for learning and design meaningful clinical experiences that emphasize caring relationships as essential to health will ensure the clinical competency needed for tomorrow's practice.

Reflective analysis on the future work of professional nursing, including the identification of role dimensions, effective and efficient clinical workflow, the ongoing challenges in the nursing workforce, particularly related to the value of any new models that arise, meeting the needs of health professionals for healthy work environments that include a focus on well-being, and meeting local populations' health needs. All this will require difficult decisions about how the work of nursing and healthcare will be accomplished while also guarding available financial resources. **Think about** the meaning of person encounters, including the skills and attitudes required. Expecting caring relationships in all interactions minimally demands civil discourse. No tolerance for verbal or other abuse in the workplace starts with relationship-centered leadership that continuously focuses on what is best for patients and families. **Role model** caring relationships. How front-line nurse managers are prepared, hired, evaluated, rewarded, and retained for a work environment focused on caring relationships requires in-depth analysis and crucial decision making. **Challenge** front-line nurse managers to **embrace** caring professional practice models. Weaving the caring core of nursing with positive, patient-derived feedback about the process strengthens and forms new connections that influence the future. **Engender** hope and possibility.

REFLECTIVE QUESTIONS/APPLICATIONS

For Professional Nurses in Clinical Practice:

- How can professional nurses extend caring to health team members? Be specific.
- Explain how you have learned life lessons from authentically relating to patients and families.
- Create a future scenario (50 years from now) of a patient situation from your area of expertise. What is different about professional nursing then, and what remains the same?
- Remember a time when you chose caring over some other response to a patient's needs. How did it feel?
- Can you identify leaders in your health system who regularly use caring relationships as the basis for their practice? How are they different from others? Does their behavior impact others? How?

For Professional Nurses in Educational Practice:

- Describe how a sophomore nursing clinical course could be enhanced through caring relationships with patients. What would be required of faculty and of students? How would the course be evaluated?
- What are the necessary thinking patterns that will have to occur in graduate students in order to meet the challenges of relationship-centered caring?
- Create a future clinical nursing scenario emphasizing relationships either for the simulation lab or for use as a case study. Evaluate it with real students and revise as necessary.
- Design a leadership course introducing the QCM. Include course competencies and link it to AACN's new *Essentials*. How would you know if

the students could apply the model to their practice? What would be the basis of your evaluation of student learning?

■ Choose a proposition from the QCM. Using a population of interest, present a research question that could test this proposition. Include relevant variables and hypotheses. What instruments might be used to test your hypotheses?

■ Evaluate the necessity of more meaningful clinical time for undergraduate nursing students. What would need to happen?

■ Discuss with fellow faculty members the redesign and testing of one undergraduate and one graduate course using the domain of person-centered care from AACN's New Essentials (2021). What would the course competencies look like? Who would teach it? How would the students and faculty be evaluated?

For Professional Nurses in Leadership Practice:

■ Record the methodology you would use to justify a team-based patient care delivery system with a RN leading others in nursing care for an inpatient acute care medical unit. How would you evaluate its impact?

■ Create a plan for dramatically altering RN work at your organization to enable *real* person-centeredness. Who would be involved? What methodology would be used? How long would it take? What implications for RN staffing and scheduling would occur? How would you ensure that all opinions and ideas were heard? How would you evaluate it?

■ What critical knowledge and skills concerning caring relationships has the nursing leadership team in your organization acquired? What caring knowledge and skills do they lack? Create a plan for attaining the requisite knowledge and skills for relationship-centered caring.

■ How do *you* help nurses stay focused on caring relationships in their day-to-day practice?

■ What nursing-sensitive indicators do you track? How could they be more person-centered? What suggestions do you have to focus more on "positive" outcomes indicators?

■ How would you go about working with first-line nurse managers to enable healthy work environments focused on learning and well-being?

■ What will your legacy be? What will you leave the next generation of nurses and patients?

REFERENCES

Agbo, C. C., & Mahmoud, Q. H. (2020). Blockchain in healthcare: Opportunities, challenges, and possible solutions. *International Journal of Healthcare Information Systems and Informatics (IJHISI)*, 15(3), 82–97.

Allari, R. S., Atout, M., & Hasan, A. A. H. (2020). The value of caring behavior and its impact on students' selfte and Graduate Programs tundergraduate nursing students. *Nursing Forum*, 55(2), 259–266.

American Association of Colleges of Nursing. (2021). The essentials: Core competencies for professional nursing education. https://www.aacnnursing.org/Portals/42/AcademicNursing/pdf/Essentials-2021.pdf

American Association of Colleges of Nursing. (2022a). 2020–2021 Enrollment and graduations in baccalaureate and graduate programs in nursing. Author.

American Association of Colleges of Nursing. (2022b). The research-focused doctoral program in nursing: Pathways to excellence. https://www.aacnnursing.org/Portals/42/News/Position-Statements/Pathways-Excellence-Position-Statement.pdf

American Hospital Association. (2022). Hospital-at-home. https://www.aha.org/hospitalathome

Baker, K. M., Magee, M. F., & Smith, K. M. (2019). Understanding nursing workflow for inpatient education delivery: Time and motion study. *JMIR Nursing, 2*(1), e15658.

Barbour, C. M., & Volkert, D. (2021). Nursing students' perspective of faculty caring using Duffy;s quality caring model: A Q-methodology study. *International Journal of Caring Sciences, 14*(1), 18–28.

Bartosiak, M., Bonelli, G., Maffioli, L. S., Palaoro, U., Dentali, F., Poggialini, G., Pagliarin, F., Denicolai, S., & Previtali, P. (2022). Advanced robotics as a support in healthcare organizational response: A COVID-19 pandemic case study. *Healthcare Management Forum, 35*(1), 11–16.

Bourgault, A. M. (2022). Difficult times without easy solutions: Nurses want to be heard! *Critical Care Nurse, 42*(1), e1–e3. https://doi.org/10.4037/ccn2022577

Butler, R., Monsalve, M., Thomas, G. W., Herman, T., Segre, A. M., Polgreen, P. M., & Suneja, M. (2018). Estimating time physicians and other health care workers spend with patients in an intensive care unit using a sensor network. *The American Journal of Medicine, 131*(8), 972-e9.

Centers for Medicare and Medcaid Services. (2020). National health expenditure projections 2019–28. https://www.cms.gov/files/document/national-health-expenditure-projections-2019-28.pdf

Chen, Y., Almirall-Sánchez, A., Mockler, D., Adrion, E., Domínguez-Vivero, C., & Romero-Ortuño, R. (2022). Hospital-associated deconditioning: Not only physical, but also cognitive. *International Journal of Geriatric Psychiatry, 37*(3), 5687. https://doi.org/10.1002/gps.5687

Chenoweth, L., Williams, A., Fry, M., Endean, E., & Liu, Z. (2022). Outcomes of person-centered care for persons with dementia in the acute care setting: A pilot study. *Clinical Gerontologist, 45*(4), 983–997. https://doi.org/10.1080/07317115.2021.1946233

Chipps, E. M., Joseph, M. L., Alexander, C., Lyman, B., McGinty, L., Nelson-Brantley, H., Parchment, J., Rivera, R. R., Schultz, M. A., Ward, D. M., & Weaver, S. (2021). Setting the Research Agenda for Nursing Administration and Leadership Science: A Delphi Study. *Journal of Nursing Administration, 51*(9), 430–438. https://doi.org/10.1097/NNA.0000000000001042

Clipper, B. (2022). Going boldly … into digitally enabled care models. *Nurse Leader, 20*(2), 141–144. https://doi.org/10.1016/j.mnl.2021.12.015

Cowie, M. R., & O'Connor, C. M. (2022). The digital future is now. *Heart Failure, 10*(1), 67–69.

Davis, K. C., Duffy, J. R., Marchessault, P., & Miles, D. (2022). Self-caring practices among nurses: Findings from an online survey. *Holistic Nursing Practice, 36*(1), 7–14.

Duffy, J. (2018). *Quality caring in nursing and health systems: Applying theory to clinical practice, education, and leadership.* Springer Publishing Company.

Dumitra, T., Ganescu, O., Hu, R., Fiore, J. F., Kaneva, P., Mayo, N., Lee, L., Liberman, A. S., Chaudhury, P., Ferri, L., & Feldman, L. S. (2021). Association between patient activation and health care utilization after thoracic and abdominal surgery. *JAMA Surgery, 156*(1), e205002–e205002.

Eggenberger, T., & Keller, K. (2008). Grounding nursing simulations in caring: An innovative approach. *International Journal for Human Caring, 12*(2), 42–46.

Fawcett, J. (2007). Nursing qua nursing: The connection between nursing knowledge and nursing shortages. *Journal of Advanced Nursing, 59*(1), 97–99. https://doi.org/10.1111/j.1365-2648.2007.04325.x

Ferri, P., Rovesti, S., Padula, M. S., D'Amico, R., & Di Lorenzo, R. (2019). Effect of expert-patient teaching on empathy in nursing students: A randomized controlled trial. *Psychology Research and Behavior Management, 12*, 457–467. https://doi.org/10.2147/PRBM.S208427

Fotis, T. (2022). Digital nursing and health care innovation. *Journal of PeriAnesthesia Nursing, 37*(1), 3–4.

Grubaugh, M., Africa, L., & Mallory, C. (2021). Where do we go from here? The impact of COVID-19 on practice readiness and considerations for nurse leaders. *Nurse Leader, 20*(2), 134–140. https://doi.org/10.1016/j.mnl.2021.12.016

Grundy, Q., & Malone, R. E. (2017). The "as-if" world of nursing practice. *Advances in Nursing Science, 40*(2), E28–E43.

Harrison, J. M., Aiken, L. H., Sloane, D. M., Brooks Carthon, J. M., Merchant, R. M., Berg, R. A., McHugh, M. D., & American Heart Association's Get With the Guidelines–Resuscitation Investigators. (2019). In hospitals with more nurses who have baccalaureate degrees, better outcomes for patients after cardiac arrest. *Health Affairs, 38*(7), 1087–1094.

Hartman, M., Martin, A. B., Washington, B., & Catlin, A. (2022). National health care spending in 2020: Growth driven by federal spending in response to the COVID-19 pandemic. *Health Affairs (Project Hope), 41*(1), 13–25.

Hibbard, J. H., Mahoney, E. R., Stockard, J., & Tusler, M. (2005). Development and testing of a short form of the patient activation measure. *Health Services Research, 40*(6 pt 1), 1918–1930.

Hofmeyer, A., Toffoli, L., Vernon, R., Taylor, R., Klopper, H. C., Coetzee, S. K., & Fontaine, D. (2018). Teaching compassionate care to nursing students in a digital learning and teaching environment. *Collegian, 25*(3), 307–312.

Huston, C. L., Phillips, B., Jeffries, P., Todero, C., Rich, J., Knecht, P., Sommer, S., & Lewis, M. P. (2018). The academic-practice gap: Strategies for an enduring problem. *Nursing Forum, 53*(1), 27–34.

Kakemam, E., Hajizadeh, A., Azarmi, M., Zahedi, H., Gholizadeh, M., & Roh, Y. S. (2021). Nurses' perception of teamwork and its relationship with the occurrence and reporting of adverse events: A questionnaire survey in teaching hospitals. *Journal of Nursing Management, 29*(5), 1189–1198.

Kerfoot, K. M. (2022). Leadership and the great reset: Rethinking possibilities for the future of nursing. *Nursing Economics, 40*(1), 38–41.

Koch, A., Ritz, M., Morrow, A., Grier, K., & McMillian-Bohler, J. M. (2021). Role-play simulation to teach nursing students how to provide culturally sensitive care to transgender patients. *Nurse Education in Practice, 54*, 103123.

Kostich, K., Lasiter, S., Duffy, J., & George, V. (2021). The relationship between staff nurses' perceptions of nurse manager caring behaviors and patient experience. *JONA: The Journal of Nursing Administration, 51*(9), 468–473. https://doi.org/10.1097/NNA.0000000000001047

Labrague, L. J. (2021). Influence of nurse managers' toxic leadership behaviours on nurse-reported adverse events and quality of care. *Journal of Nursing Management, 29*(4), 855–863.

Lakeland Regional Health. (2022). Our vision, mission and promises. https://www.mylrh.org/vision-mission-promises/

Liou, Y. F., Lin, P. F., Chang, Y. C., & Liaw, J. J. (2022). Perceived importance of competencies by nurse managers at all levels: A cross-sectional study. *Journal of Nursing Management, 30*(3), 633–642. https://doi.org/10.1111/jonm.13545

Lowell General Hospital. (2022). 2021 Cupola award recipients. https://www.lowell-general.org/careers/employee-appreciation-and-recognition/cupola-awards/2021-cupola-award-recipients

Malloch, K., Porter-O'Grady, T. (2022). *Appreciative leadership: Building sustainable partnerships for health.* Jones & Bartlett.

Massachusetts Department of Health and Human Services. (2017). National telenursing center. https://www.mass.gov/info-details/about-the-national-telenursing-center#ntc-education-and-training-model-

McCauley, L., Kirwan, M., & Matthews, A. (2021). The factors contributing to missed care and non-compliance in infection prevention and control practices of nurses: A scoping review. *International Journal of Nursing Studies Advances, 3*, 100039.

Michel, O., Garcia Manjon, A. J., Pasquier, J., & Ortoleva Bucher, C. (2021). How do nurses spend their time? A time and motion analysis of nursing activities in an internal medicine unit. *Journal of Advanced Nursing, 77*(11), 4459–4470.

O'Brien, D., Knowlton, M., & Whichello, R. (2018). Attention health care leaders: Literature review deems baccalaureate nurses improve patient outcomes. *Nursing Education Perspectives, 39*(4), E2–E6.

Omery, A., Crawford, C. L., Dechairo-Marino, A., Quaye, B. S., & Finkelstein, J. (2019). Reexamining nurse manager span of control with a 21st-century lens. *Nursing Administration Quarterly, 43*(3), 230–245.

Pinilla, L., Barbé, F., Guerra, J. M., Llorente-Cortés, V., & de Gonzalo-Calvo, D. (2022). Epigenetics in precision medicine of cardiovascular disease. In J. L. Garcia-Giminez (Ed.), *Epigenetics in precision medicine* (pp. 347–368). Academic Press.

Press-Ganey. (2022). Clinical excellence. https://www.pressganey.com/products/clinical-excellence

Rainbow, J. G., Gilbreath, B., & Steege, L. M. (2021). Risky business: A mediated model of antecedents and consequences of presenteeism in nursing. *Nursing Research, 70*(2), 85–94.

Rochefort, C. M., Labelle, J. B., & Farand, P. (2022). Nurse staffing practices and postoperative atrial fibrillation among cardiac surgery patients: A multisite cohort study. *CJC Open, 4*(1), 37–46.

Rosenfeld, P., DeMarco, K., & Rodenhausen, N. (2022). Forever changed: RNs speak of their COVID-19 experiences through a system-wide nursing web site. *JONA: The Journal of Nursing Administration, 52*(1), 12–18. https://doi.org/10.1097/NNA.0000000000001097

Saleh, U., O'Connor, T., Al-Subhi, H., Alkattan, R., Al-Harbi, S., & Patton, D. (2018). The impact of nurse managers' leadership styles on ward staff. *British Journal of Nursing, 27*(4), 197–203.

Seegert, L. (2022). The current state of nursing. *AJN: The American Journal of Nursing, 122*(2), 18–20.

Serçe, Y. Ö., Partlak, G., Çelik, I., & Zeybekçi, S. (2022) Experiences of oncology nurses regarding self-compassion and compassionate care: A qualitative study. *International Nursing Review,* 1–10. https://doi.org/10.1111/inr.12747

Shatto, B., Meyer, G., Krieger, M., Kreienkamp, M. J., Kendall, A., & Breitbach, N. (2022). Educational interventions to improve graduating nursing students' practice readiness: A systematic review. *Nurse Educator, 47*(2), E24. https://doi.org/10.1097/nne.0000000000001145

Shnaigat, M., Downie, S., & Hosseinzadeh, H. (2022). Effectiveness of patient activation interventions on chronic obstructive pulmonary disease self-management outcomes: A systematic review. *Australian Journal of Rural Health, 30*(1), 8–21. https://doi.org/10.1111/ajr.12828

Shorey, S., Chan, V., Rajendran, P., & Ang, E. (2021). Learning styles, preferences and needs of generation Z healthcare students: Scoping review. *Nurse Education in Practice, 57*, 103247.

Swanson, K. (2008). *Living caring*. Presentation Delivered at the International Association for Human Caring Conference, Chapel Hill, NC.

Taylor-Clark, T. M., Swiger, P. A., Anusiewicz, C. V., Loan, L. A., Olds, D. M., Breckenridge-Sproat, S. T., Raju, D., & Patrician, P. A. (2022). Identifying potentially preventable reasons nurses intend to leave a job. *JONA: The Journal of Nursing Administration, 52*(2), 73–80.

Triberti, S., Durosini, I., La Torre, D., Sebri, V., Savioni, L., & Pravettoni, G. (2022). Artificial intelligence in healthcare practice: How to tackle the "Human" challenge. In C. Chee-Peng Lim, A. Vaidya, K. Jain, V. U. Mahorkar, & L. C. Jain (Eds.), *Handbook of artificial intelligence in healthcare* (pp. 43–60). Springer.

University of West Georgia. (2022). Tanner health system school of nursing. https://www.westga.edu/academics/nursing/index.php

Watson, J. (1979). *Nursing: The philosophy and science of caring*. Little, Brown and Company.

Watson, J. (1985). *Nursing: Human science and human care*. Appleton-Century-Crofts.

Wei, H., Henderson, D., Peery, A., & Andrews, A. (2021). Nursing students' perceptions of faculty caring as a predictor of students' caring behaviors. *International Journal for Human Caring, 25*(2), 123–130.

Weston, M. J. (2022). Strategic planning for a very different nursing workforce. *Nurse Leader, 20*(2), 152–160. https://doi.org/10.1016/j.mnl.2021.12.021

Williams, G. A., Fahy, N., Aissat, D., Lenormand, M. C., Stüwe, L., Zablit-Schmidt, I., Delafuys, S., Le Douarin, Y.-M., & Muscat, N. A. (2022). Covid-19 and the use of digital health tools: Opportunity amid crisis that could transform health care delivery. *Eurohealth, 28*(1), 1.

APPENDICES

APPENDICES

APPENDIX A

Quality and Caring Resources on the Internet

Affordable Care Act (www.healthcare.gov/law/full/index.html)

Agency for Healthcare Research and Quality (www.ahrq.gov)

American Association of Colleges of Nursing (www.aacnnursing.org)

American Council on Education (www.acenet.edu/pages/default.aspx)

American Health Care Act of 2017 (www.govtrack.us/congress/bills/115/hr1628)

American Organization for Nursing Leadership (www.aonl.org)

Association of American Medical Colleges (www.aamc.org)

The Berkana Institute (www.berkana.org)

Bureau of Health Workforce—Health Resources and Services Administration (bhpr.hrsa.gov)

Centers for Disease Control and Prevention (www.cdc.gov)

Centers for Medicare & Medicaid Services (www.cms.gov)

The Commonwealth Fund (www.commonwealthfund.org)

The Daisy Foundation (www.daisyfoundation.org)

Institute for Healthcare Improvement (www.ihi.org/Pages/default.aspx)

Health Equity: Prioritization, Perception, and Progress IHI 2021 Pulse Report (https://www.ihi.org/Topics/Health-Equity/Pages/Pulse-Report-Health-Equity.aspx)

Institute of Medicine (www.ihi.org/resources/Pages/OtherWebsites/The InstituteofMedicine.aspx)

International Association for Human Caring (www.humancaring.org)

The Joint Commission (www.jointcommission.org)

National Association for Healthcare Quality (www.nahq.org)

National Council of State Boards of Nursing (NCSBN) (https://www.ncsbn.org/index.htm)

National Database of Nursing Quality Indicators® (NDNQI®) (https://www
.pressganey.com/products/clinical-excellence/national-database-nursing
-quality-indicators)

National Institute for Nursing Research (www.ninr.nih.gov)

National League for Nursing (www.nln.org)

Nursing Theory (https://www.clayton.edu/health/nursing/nursing-theory/
index)

Patient-Centered Outcomes Research Institute (www.pcori.org)

Picker (picker.org)

Plexus Institute (www.plexusinstitute.org)

Quality and Safety Education for Nurses (www.qsen.org)

Relational Coordination Collaborative (https://heller.brandeis.edu/relational
-coordination/about-rc/index.html)

Relationship Centered Health Care (www.rchcweb.com)

Example Health Systems Translating Quality-Caring Theory to Professional Nursing Practice

Association of Women's Health, Obstetric and Neonatal Nurses, Washington, DC

Banner Gateway Medical Center, Gilbert Arizona

Children's Mercy Hospital and Clinics, Kansas City, Missouri

Department of Health and Human Services, National TeleNursing Center, Boston, Massachusetts

International Association of Forensic Nurses, Elkridge, Maryland

Jefferson Health System, all 18 hospitals

Lakeland Regional Medical Center, Lakeland, Florida

Loma Linda University Health, Loma Linda, California

Lowell General Hospital, Lowell, Massachusetts

MD Anderson Medical Center, Houston, Texas

Methodist Hospital, Henderson, Kentucky

Miriam Hospital, Providence, Rhode Island

Moffitt Cancer Center, Tampa, Florida

Montefiore Health, New York City, New York

Novant Health Forsyth Medical Center, Winston-Salem, North Carolina

Novant Health Presbyterian Medical Center, Charlotte, North Carolina

St. Barnabas Health System, Livingston, New Jersey

St. Joseph's Medical Center, Towson, Maryland

South Florida State College, Avon Park, Florida

SwedishAmerican Hospital, Rockford, Illinois

Texas Health Resources, Arlington, Texas (multiple hospitals)

Torrance Memorial Hospital, Torrance, California

UMC Health System, Lubbock, Texas

University of California at San Diego Medical Center, San Diego, California

University of Colorado Anschutz Medical Campus, Aurora, Colorado

University of West Georgia, Carrollton, Georgia

West Virginia University Hospitals, Morgantown, West Virginia

Winchester Medical Center, Winchester, Virginia

Nursing Implications Based on the Quality-Caring Model©

NURSES IN CLINICAL PRACTICE

- Know the state of nursing quality in your organization.
- Accept responsibility for your own professionalism.
- Use nursing theory to guide your practice.
- Develop competency in the caring behaviors.
- Focus on caring relationships as the foundation of nursing work.
- Use the caring behaviors to effectively collaborate with health team members.
- Remind yourself often of the important work you do.
- Listen to patients and their families—they are the best source of information and life lessons.
- Practice caring for yourself.
- Balance "being" and "doing."
- Understand and value your role on the health team.
- Evaluate your caring intention.
- Use communication strategies that convey caring.
- Engage in ongoing practice improvement.

NURSES IN EDUCATIONAL PRACTICE

- Set the tone for student success.
- Increase clinical learning experiences.
- Familiarize yourself with PCORI.
- Test the Quality-Caring Model
- Center learning around patients and families versus disease and geographic areas.

- Teach enduring nursing concepts in depth.
- Sustain caring relationships with students.
- Use caring as a pedagogy.
- Mentor emerging relational scientists.
- Evaluate the caring capacity of students.
- Care for yourself, patients and their families, health team members, and the community served.

NURSES IN LEADERSHIP PRACTICE

- Evaluate and redesign nursing work; organize it for effective person-centered relationships.
- Build professional practice models and design patient care delivery systems that embrace caring relationships as the foundation for nursing practice.
- Revise roles and responsibilities of first-line nurse leaders to focus on caring relationships.
- Understand how the context influences caring relationships.
- Appreciate and preserve the important work nurses do.
- Partner with those in academia.
- Recognize, reward, and incentivize nurses for their caring practice.
- Make tough decisions in the best interests of patients and families.
- Practice caring for yourself, your staff, your patients, health team members, and the community served.
- Focus on the fundamental work of the health system—high-value patient care.
- Lead from within.
- Use principles of appreciative leadership.

APPENDIX D

Using the Caring Behaviors to Keep Patients Safe

- Help patients and families understand threats to their safety.
- Listen to patients' concerns.
- Clarify questions.
- Routinely check in, offering assistance with basic human needs.
- Anticipate patient and family needs.
- Ensure availability.
- Call patients and families by their preferred name.
- Allow patients to choose when and where they receive care.
- Remove noxious stimuli—lights, noise, and smells.
- Position and reposition often.
- Know what is important to patients.
- Relieve muscle tension through range of motion massage, exercises, and relaxation techniques.
- Provide fast and effective pain relief and then evaluate its effectiveness.
- Assist patients with food, sleeping arrangements, and elimination.
- Maintain privacy and confidentiality.
- Protect patient information.
- Be alert for environmental variables that represent risks to safety.
- Provide gentle, sensitive, physical care.
- Use anticipatory guidance.
- Engage family members in patient care and decision making.
- Communicate (including shift report and other handoffs) at the bedside, including the patient in the discussion.
- Use consistent and caring verbal and nonverbal behaviors.
- Show patients that they can depend on you by walking the talk.
- Help patients understand their illnesses.

- Accept feedback from patients and their families.
- Look for and praise safe behaviors.
- Allow family members to stay and engage them in safe practices.

APPENDIX E

Using the Caring Behaviors to Advance Quality Health Outcomes

- Listen attentively to patients' health and illness stories.
- Provide information about specific illnesses and lifestyle modifications to patients and their families.
- Use multiple formats to present information.
- Allow patients and their families to ask questions about living with their illnesses.
- Ask patients to teach *you* about living with their illnesses.
- Encourage forward thinking.
- Recognize patients' rights.
- Praise attainment of intermediate goals.
- Allow expression of both positive and negative feelings.
- Follow up often.
- Set up transitional activities.
- Know what is important to patients and their families.
- Avoid assumptions.
- Routinely assess patients' perceptions of "feeling cared for."
- Understand the patient's frame of reference.

Assessment of Professional Work Environments for Evidence of Quality-Caring Practice

Directions: To answer the question, "Where are caring relationships evidenced at your institution?" evaluate the following activities for the presence and/or links to the caring behaviors. List the specific caring behaviors. Next, evaluate how well they are integrated into the professional practice environment on a scale from 1 (poor) to 5 (extremely well). (Note: Higher scores reflect better representation of caring professional practice).

ADMISSION

The admission process 1 2 3 4 5
Admission database—Is it holistic? 1 2 3 4 5
Care plans—Are they nurse, system, or patient-driven? 1 2 3 4 5
Documentation system—How are caring behaviors recorded and monitored? 1 2 3 4 5

DAILY PROCESSES

Shift report/handoffs 1 2 3 4 5
Delegation of responsibilities to patient care assistants 1 2 3 4 5
Hygiene and mobility care 1 2 3 4 5
Transfers and "road trips" 1 2 3 4 5
Preventative management 1 2 3 4 5
Patient education materials 1 2 3 4 5
Discharge planning processes 1 2 3 4 5
Decision making at unit level 1 2 3 4 5
Family visitation 1 2 3 4 5

PHYSICAL ENVIRONMENT

Family waiting areas 1 2 3 4 5
Bulletin boards 1 2 3 4 5

Meeting areas and learning resources for staff 1 2 3 4 5
Staff meetings 1 2 3 4 5
Scheduling/staffing 1 2 3 4 5
Assignments 1 2 3 4 5

TEAM CARING

Interprofessional rounds/physician visits 1 2 3 4 5
Engagement in practice improvement 1 2 3 4 5
Team meetings 1 2 3 4 5

PATIENT OUTCOMES

Routine measurements of nursing-sensitive outcomes 1 2 3 4 5
Routine measurements of shared outcomes 1 2 3 4 5
Routine measurements of "feeling cared for" 1 2 3 4 5
Feedback mechanism for outcomes reporting 1 2 3 4 5

POLICIES

Policy and procedure manuals 1 2 3 4 5
Protocols 1 2 3 4 5
Practice guidelines 1 2 3 4 5

Potential Research Questions

- How do caring relationships contribute to specific nursing-sensitive outcomes?
- What are the characteristics of environments and communities that are perceived by patients to be caring?
- How does nurse caring influence patient outcomes in specific settings or patient populations (e.g., long-term care, schools, home healthcare)?
- What contextual factors influence nurse-caring capacity?
- How effective are caring-based interventions on health promotion, quality of life, self-caring, patient experiences of care, decreased adverse outcomes, illness knowledge, and hospital readmission rates?
- What is the relationship between nurse-caring capacity and collective relationship capacity?
- Does patient feedback in real time influence the delivery of person-centered care?
- What is the relationship between nursing leadership and nurse-caring capacity?
- What are the psychometric properties of caring tools for specialized patient populations?
- How do professional nurses differ in terms of nurse caring capacity?
- What improvements in nursing-sensitive patient outcomes are linked to nurse caring?
- What is the nature of the student–teacher relationship? Explain with reference to undergraduate and graduate students.
- What is the relationship between faculty caring and student learning?
- How does caring practice affect reimbursable outcomes (e.g., length of stay, readmission rates, experience of care)?
- What is the best approach to mentor nursing students in relationship-centered research?
- How are caring relationships with healthcare professionals best sustained over time?

- How do outcomes of care differ between those sites that use caring-based professional practice models and those that do not?
- Does appreciative leadership improve organizational relational capacity?
- What hiring and orientation practices influence relational capacity?

APPENDIX H

Reflections on Practice

- Think about someone you have experienced as a caring leader. Identify their key attributes. Do these attributes correspond to the caring behaviors? If yes, how?

- Reflect on an experience in your professional career in which a patient or a family member taught you something about life. Did you use these lessons in your own life? If yes, how?

- Reflect on a time your practice was truly "professional." What were you doing? What did it feel like?

- Think about the last time you worked. How did you connect with the health team? What did you do? What did you learn?

- In your last patient interaction, what nonverbal behaviors did you convey? How do you know?

- Remember the last time you cared for yourself. What did you do? How did it feel? When will you do it again?

- What reminders in the practice environment would help you stay focused on relationships? List them.

- Do your patients/employees "feel cared for"? How do you know?

- Are you creating value in your health system? Describe how. What indicators do you use to evaluate it?

APPENDIX I

Quality-Caring Organizational Self-Assessment Tool

Directions: Please check the box associated with how often you think the statement is occurring in your setting.

Domain	Item	Low = 1	2	3	4	High = 5	Comments
Leadership	Clear statements of commitment to QCM exist.						
	Explicit expectations, accountabilities, and measurements related to QCM exist.						
	QCM included in nursing philosophy, policies, procedures, and guideline development.						
	Nurse leaders set clear expectations for professional practice (consistent with the QCM).						
	Nurse leaders understand and can inform others about all components of the QCM.						
	Nurse leaders assume accountability for ongoing support and development of the QCM.						
	Clinical nurse leaders champion the QCM.						
	Nurse leaders facilitate research and evidence-based practice.						

Domain	Item	Low = 1	2	3	4	High = 5	Comments
	There is an established succession plan to ensure sustained professional practice.						
Performance Improvement	QCM informs nursing strategic plan, QI plans, performance metrics.						
	QCM evaluation data are used in future planning.						
Personnel	QCM informs hires, RN job descriptions, and clinical advancement.						
	Overall employee norms of behavior reflect the QCM.						
	Nurses and other employees can articulate elements of the QCM.						
	RNs provide care that best utilizes their full scope of practice.						
Environment	RNs assume accountability for exemplary professional practice.						
	The QCM is perceived by RNs as compatible with RN work.						
	Employees are comfortable expressing their opinions and report "feeling heard."						
Professional Development	Web portals provide specific resources for the QCM.						
	Orientation contains information and expectations related to QCM.						
	Multiple sources of continuing education are available for the QCM.						

Domain	Item	Low = 1	2	3	4	High = 5	Comments
	Educators understand and embrace the QCM.						
Documentation	There is evidence of QCM language in the medical records.						
Care Processes	Families participate in discussions, rounds, and change of shift reports.						
	Family presence assured 24/7.						
	Patients engage in collaborative goal setting with the care team.						
	Patients express feeling listened to, respected, and treated as partners in their care.						
	Patients are actively involved in planning and care transitions.						
	Patient discomfort is respectively managed in partnership with patients and families.						
	Patients report feeling safe.						
	Patient information is held confidentially.						
	Patients' basic human needs are attended to consistently and in a timely fashion.						
	Patients' understanding about their illness is achieved through tailored educational approaches.						
	Patients are routinely monitored for changes in their condition.						

QCM, Quality-Caring Model; QI, quality improvment.

IMPROVEMENT PLAN

_____

_____

_____

_____

_____

_____

_____

Index

Printed in the United States
by Baker & Taylor Publisher Services

Printed in the United States
by Baker & Taylor Publisher Services